THE DEVELOPMENT OF SCIENTIFIC MARKETING IN THE TWENTIETH CENTURY: RESEARCH FOR SALES IN THE PHARMACEUTICAL INDUSTRY

STUDIES FOR THE SOCIETY FOR THE SOCIAL HISTORY OF MEDICINE

Series Editors: David Cantor
Keir Waddington

TITLES IN THIS SERIES

THE DEVELOPMENT OF SCIENTIFIC MARKETING IN THE TWENTIETH CENTURY: RESEARCH FOR SALES IN THE PHARMACEUTICAL INDUSTRY

EDITED BY
Jean-Paul Gaudillière and Ulrike Thoms

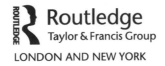

Routledge
Taylor & Francis Group

LONDON AND NEW YORK

First published 2015 by Pickering & Chatto (Publishers) Limited

2 Park Square, Milton Park, Abingdon, Oxon OX14 4RN
711 Third Avenue, New York, NY 10017, USA

Routledge is an imprint of the Taylor & Francis Group, an informa business

First issued in paperback 2017

BRITISH LIBRARY CATALOGUING IN PUBLICATION DATA

The development of scientific marketing in the twentieth century: research for
sales in the pharmaceutical industry. – (Studies for the Society for the Social
History of Medicine)
1. Drugs – Marketing – History – 20th century. 2. Pharmaceutical industry –
History – 20th century. I. Series II. Gaudilliere, Jean-Paul, 1957–, editor. III.
Thoms, Ulrike, 1962–, editor.
338.4'76151'0904-dc23

ISBN-13: 978-1-8489-3559-4 (hbk)
ISBN-13: 978-1-138-63011-6 (pbk)

Typeset by Pickering & Chatto (Publishers) Limited

CONTENTS

LIST OF CONTRIBUTORS

Christian Bonah is a professor of the history of medical and health sciences at the University of Strasbourg and a member of the Institut Universitaire de France. He has worked on the comparative history of medical education, the history of medicaments and the history of human experimentation, and was one of the initiators of the ESF drug network and the GEPHAMA project. His recent work includes research on risk perception and management in drug scandals as well as studies on medical film. Selected publications include: *L'expérimentation humaine. Discours et pratiques en France, 1900–1940* (Paris: Les Belles Lettres, 2007) and *Harmonizing Drugs: Standards in 20th Century Pharmaceutical History* (Paris: Glyphe, 2009).

Tricia Close-Koenig has been part of the GEPHAMA project as a post-doctoral researcher. She completed her PhD at the University of Strasbourg in 2011, with a thesis that analysed the emergence of medical lab analyses as medical and economic entities within a theoretical framework of knowledge-based economies. In 2011 and 2012, she worked on the DFG-ANR GEPHAMA project, before she became the project manager for the INTERREG project, Projections du Rhin Supérieur, Rhinfilm (SAGE UMR7363, University of Strasbourg), and a collaborator in the ERC project Ways of Writing (Institute for the History of Medicine at the Charité-Berlin). Her main interests are the history of management and administration in medicine, through collecting and cataloguing, notably in French cancer institutes, and the pathological anatomy practices of diagnosis. Her on-going work further considers the history of medical film.

Stephan Felder studied contemporary history, religious studies and philosophy at the Freie Universität Berlin and the Technische Universität Berlin until 2008, when he moved on to study medicine at the Charité Universitätsmedizin Berlin. He participated as a scientific assistant in the GEPHAMA project of the Institute for the History of Medicine at the Charité Berlin (2009–12). His interests focus on the history of medicine, knowledge and belief systems. He works as a physician.

Jean-Paul Gaudillière is a senior researcher at the French Institute for Health and Medical Research (INSERM), Paris, and the director of the Center of Medicine, Sciences, Health, Mental Health and Health Policy (CERMES3). He was one of the initiators of the ESF drug network and the GEPHAMA project. His works cover the fields of the history of biomedicine and biomedical innovations, the relations between science, industry and medical practice, the transformation of medical research in the twentieth century and the history of globalization. Among his many publications are the special edition *Standardizing and Marketing Drugs in the 20th Century, History and Technology*, 26 (2013), which he edited together with Ulrike Thoms, 'Une marchandise scientifique? Savoirs, industrie et régulation du médicament dans l'Allemagne des années trente', *Annales – Histoire, sciences sociales*, 65 (2010), pp. 89–120, and *Ways of Regulating Drugs in the 19th and 20th Centuries* (Basingstoke: Palgrave Macmillan, 2013), which he edited together with Volker Hess.

Lucie Gerber is a PhD candidate in the history of science at the Ecole des Hautes Études en Sciences Sociales in Paris. Her dissertation focuses on the history of animal experimentation in the fields of Alzheimer's disease and depression since the 1960s and analyses sources from scientific, industrial and institutional archives, interviews and field observations. It is funded by the French National Foundation on Alzheimer's disease and related disorders, and supported by the Centre National de la Recherche Scientifique (CNRS) and the Institut National de la Santé et de la Recherche Médicale (INSERM).

Nils Kessel has studied modern and contemporary history, medical history and French in Freiburg, Germany, Bordeaux and Basle. He has been a research fellow in several research projects funded by the German Science Foundation, among them the GEPHAMA project on the history of marketing in the twentieth century, and has taught at the Universities of Freiburg, Germany and Strasbourg, France. He is currently completing his PhD on 'Pills, Magic Bullets, Scandals: Medical Drug Consumption in Germany, 1950–1990' at the University of Strasbourg. Among his publications are '"Doriden von Ciba": Sleeping Pills, Pharmaceutical Marketing, and Thalidomide, 1955–1963', *History and Technology*, 29:2 (2013), 153–68 and 'La médecine, l'opinion publique et le scandale', in C. Bonah et al. (eds), *Sciences humaines, médecine et santé. Manuel du Collège desenseignants de SHS en médecine et santé* (Paris: Les Belles Lettres, 2011), 340–9.

Quentin Ravelli is researcher in sociology at the Centre National de la Recherche Scientifique, Ecole Normale Supérieure, in Paris. He received a PhD in sociology from the University Paris-Ouest and held fellowships at Berkeley, as Fulbright visiting researcher, and Casa de Velázquez in Madrid. His work focuses on the sociology of dangerous commodities such as antibiotics and subprime mortgage credit as a means to understand recent transformations of the capitalist economy. Among other publications, he has published a book, *The Strategy of the Bacteria* (Paris: Le Seuil, 2015), and an article on pharmaceutical marketing, 'Medico-Marketing between Use Value and Exchange Value: How Political Economy Sheds Light on the Biography of Medicines', *Medische Antropologie*, 23:2 (2011), pp. 243–4.

Lisa Malich is a PhD candidate in history at the Institute for the History of Medicine and Ethics in Medicine at the Charité Berlin. Her work focuses on the history of reproduction and contraception, concepts of gender, cultural aspects of emotions, studies of endocrinology and representations of pregnancy. Recent publications include 'Die hormonelle Natur und ihre Technologien: Zur Hormonisierung der Schwangerschaft im 20. Jahrhundert.' *L'HOMME*, 26:2 (2014), pp. 71–86, and 'Vom Mittel der Familienplanung zum differenzierenden Lifestyle-Präparat: Bilder der Pille und ihrer Konsumentin in gynäkologischen Werbeanzeigen seit den 1960er Jahren in der BRD und Frankreich', *N.T.M.*, 20:1 (2012), pp. 1–30.

Anne-Sophie Mazas was supervised on her PhD by Professor Jean-Paul Gaudillière at the Cermes3. Her work focused on the history of scientific marketing practices in the pharmaceutical field during the post-war period in France.

Ulrike Thoms is a researcher with a focus on the history of medicine, science and technology, the role of the public and the expert, the history of consumption and the body. In her work she has combined approaches from economic, cultural and medical history, thereby integrating perspectives from the history of knowledge and innovation as well as from business history. She works at the Max Planck Institute for the History of Science in the research program on the history of the Max Planck Society, 1945–2002. Among her recent publications are the special issue *Standardizing and Marketing Drugs in the 20th Century*, *History and Technology*, 26 (2013), which she edited together with Jean-Paul Gaudillière, and 'The Contraceptive Pill, the Pharmaceutical Industry and Changes in the Patient–Doctor Relationship in Germany,' in Teresa Ortiz Gómez, María Jesús Santesmases, Agata Ignaciuk, Nicolas Tschudy (eds.), *Gendered Drug Standards from Historical and Socio-anthropological Perspectives* (Farnham: Ashgate, 2014), pp. 153–77.

LIST OF FIGURES AND TABLES

ACKNOWLEDGEMENTS

This book originates in the French-German research project on the history of pharmaceutical marketing, 'From Advertisement to Marketing: Pharmaceutical Enterprises, Patients, Physicians and the Construction of Drug Markets' (GEPHAMA). The French Agence Nationale de Recherche and the German Research Association / Deutsche Forschungsgemeinschaft generously supported this venture. We would like to thank all the participants in the GEPHAMA project: Christian Bonah, Tricia Close-Koenig, Stefan Felder, Volker Hess, Nils Kessel, Fabien Moll-François and Anne Rasmussen; as well as the contributors and organizers of the workshops linked to the project, such as Sergio Sismondo, Elizabeth Watkins, Alexandre Marchant and Jeremy Greene, for their time, ideas and commitment.

Likewise we would like to thank the European Science Foundation for the support it provided to the European DRUGS Network. The conferences the network funded and organized have offered a unique and stimulating atmosphere in which we could discuss our findings in the long run with highly knowledgable researchers participating in the renewal of the historiography of pharmacy.

We thank the Society for the Social History of Medicine for their offer to publish this volume in its Studies for the Society for the Social History of Medicine series and especially David Cantor as the editor of this series. He has given invaluable advice on the first versions of the papers in this book, while Marina Urquidi has been a tremendous help in improving the linguistic form of the papers. Both helped to carve out the ideas in this volume. Of course, all remaining mistakes are our responsibility.

Finally, a special thanks goes to our families, who had to carry the burden of our absence while we were researching, writing and revising the outcomes of the GEPHAMA project.

INTRODUCTION

Jean-Paul Gaudillière and Ulrike Thoms

'Who will pay for this?' was the headline of a short article published in May 1974 in the critical German journal *Arznei-Telegramm* (Drug Telegram), an independent, advertising-free bulletin that had been published since 1969. The article was supplemented with a table containing data from market surveys conducted by the renowned Institute for Medical Statistics.[1] The table showed that the twenty-five leading German pharmaceutical companies spent nearly DM 250 million each year to cover the cost of advertising in journals, mass mailing and pharmaceutical representatives' visits to physicians' offices.[2] One firm in particular came under special criticism: Nattermann, a pharmaceutical company which accounted for nearly 20 per cent of this expenditure.

This did not come as a surprise to the authors given that Nattermann's drug portfolio depended mainly on the much-discussed Lipostabil, an 'essential phospholipid' used to lower blood cholesterol levels. As the authors of the article stated in their short notice, however, Lipostabil was obviously ineffective.[3] They also suggested that only ineffective drugs needed to be advertised at all. This was therefore a case of double waste since a lot of money was spent on advertising rather than on more useful actions and, on top on that, the drug would not even cure patients.

Unsurprisingly, Nattermann did not take kindly to this criticism and filed a lawsuit against the *Arznei-Telegramm*. The firm complained of unbalanced reporting and demanded that the journal stop publishing negative results without including positive outcomes too. Instead, the *Arznei-Telegramm* justified its article with citations from the recent American and German medical literature. Above all, it pointed to the fact that the drug had not been licensed in the USA, where the Food and Drug Administration (FDA) allegedly only allowed the marketing of efficient drugs. Ultimately, the court ruled that the journal was free to choose which articles it would publish. This would not be the end of the story for the *Arznei-Telegramm*. It continued to request that Nattermann explain why its advertising material insistently claimed that the drug was effective even though positive effects were at best unproven, if not purely imaginary. The *Arznei-Telegramm* ironically mocked the firm's use of imprecise terms and formulations, for instance in adverts stating that Lipostabil 'support[ed] expansion of the collateral' and took over its 'protection'.[4] This statement in the advertisement seems to be intended as an expert claim but is obviously meaningless. The editorial board finally explained complacently that Nattermann's owners had refused to answer their questions on efficacy, while a specialist in internal medicine filed another lawsuit in which he accused the firm of misleading advertising.

These events are not as spectacular as the drug scandals that in the past twenty years have attracted the attention of many observers from the media, the political world or academic circles, including the social sciences. The *Arznei-Telegramm* was, and still is, a journal with a relatively small audience, read by physicians only. Lipostabil-type altercations are however routine in the contemporary world of industrial pharmacy. This was one example out of dozens every year of recurrent and everyday struggles between pharmaceutical firms and their critics, physicians as well as muck-raking journalists, who often play the card of 'evidence-based medicine' while the industry claims that its investments in 'research and development' (R&D) provide the basis of the quality of its products.

Claims and counterclaims are nonetheless not made on a level playing field. Although they are both competing for doctors' and patients' attention, the pharmaceutical industry and its critics are not playing the same game. Their respective resources and scale of operations are barely comparable. This becomes obvious when considering the ability to launch investigations and produce data, but it is also true of communication. At the time of the Lipostabil discussion, practising German doctors were confronted with a massive amount of information on new drugs, their effects and their uses. As EMNID (Erforschung der öffentlichen Meinung, Marktforschung und Meinungsforschung, Nachrichten, Informationen, Dienstleistungen), an institute for opinion and market research, had already stated in a 1958 survey, doctors were getting increasingly irritated with the massive amount of leaflets, brochures, adverts and mailings they were receiving.[5] Given the asymmetric power between pharmaceutical firms and single physicians, doctors had indeed many reasons to feel overwhelmed by marketing campaigns and incapable of deciding whether the claims on safety and efficacy they spread were reliable or not.

This is the visible face of the scientific marketing of drugs as it has existed since the 1960s: a problematic by-product of the transformation of pharmacy into a fully fledged capitalistic industry; an industry that finances its massive research activities with high income from drugs that are protected by patents and are marketed aggressively. Beyond this visible face, scientific marketing is more than just a problem of conflict of interests and boundaries between science and marketing. It is rather a work of articulation and association through which science facilitates the construction of drug markets while the latter inform the making of relevant knowledge. Scientific marketing is based on complex arrangements for making market-relevant knowledge and to establish it between many different actors beyond drug representatives and their physician targets, including professional associations, administrative bodies, government scientists, lawyers and academic researchers. These arrangements touch upon questions of professional expertise, administrative regulations, public health policies and market-based mass consumption of therapeutic agents.

These linkages as well as the conflicts between science of drugs and their marketing do not come out of the blue. There is a vast amount of literature on the practices of pharmaceutical marketing provided by investigative journalists, former executives of marketing departments or health economists.[6] Business historians have examined the development of the pharmaceutical industry and pharmaceutical companies as a typical example of modern corporations investing in R&D.[7]

Historians of science and historians of medicine for their part have reminded us that drug marketing must be understood against the background of the larger process of industrialization, standardization and the increasing reliance of pharmacy on laboratory sciences. What the work of S. Chauveau, V. Quirke, D. Tobbell, D. Carpenter, W. Wimmer and many others in the past fifteen years teaches us is that post-war reorganization of the Western world of drug making can be characterized by five main features: (1) the changing scale of a market increasingly supported by the extension of benefits provided by health insurance; (2) the mergers and disappearance of vast numbers of small family-run firms that had originated in pharmacies established by graduate professionals; (3) the introduction of whole new classes of drugs, opening the door to chemotherapy in areas that had either not at all been working with therapeutic substances (cancer) or not doing very successfully with them (tuberculosis); (4) the rising importance of administrative rather than professional or industrial regulation; which led to (5) the generalization of chemical-biological-clinical screening as the dominant path to drug invention, which in the eyes of most firms gave them the possibility of finding radically new active substances rather than copying, modifying and combining those included in the pharmacopoeia, therefore legitimizing massive investments in internal research infrastructures.[8]

The advent of scientific marketing must be placed against this background. Until the late nineteenth century, drugs in their majority were prepared in pharmacies and apothecaries, where a learned craftsman – whose expertise was guaranteed by the possession of an academic diploma – was obliged to provide the population with the drugs described in the national pharmacopoeia and in turn received some legal protection of his rights by the state. Nevertheless, from the mid-nineteenth century onward, drug production was increasingly taken over by industrial companies, some of which had developed out of traditional pharmacies, such as Dausse, Roussel, Merck, Schering or Boehringer, while others like Bayer or Rhône-Poulenc were chemical companies entering the drug business.[9] Industrialization did not only mean changing the scale of production, it also implied the making of new products and practices. This is well illustrated with the changing status of the pharmacopoeia.[10] These regulatory tools participated in the standardization of drugs but their aim was to establish references for the preparative work of pharmacists; they contributed less to the regulation of industrial activities than to the regulation of professions, i.e., of the duties and rights of the pharmacists and of the division of labour between them and physicians.[11] When the industrial production of pharmaceutical substances took off in the late nineteenth and early twentieth centuries, it went together with the development of different kind of specialities, i.e., mass-produced, standardized and possibly purified. Parallel to this process the long-discussed balance of power between doctors and pharmacists was replaced by new arrangements, new 'ways of regulating', which furnished the industry with ever greater impact on the structure of the drug business.[12]

The escalating role of the industry has therefore not gone unnoticed in the history of American and European medicine and pharmacy. Investigations have however often focused on the production of knowledge and on the role of industrial research.[13] What is often forgotten is that the industrialization of pharmacy was part of more general developments in business and corporate capitalism. As a consequence, and although an interest in the general history of marketing has emerged in the past years, especially in the US context, the history of pharmaceutical marketing has been neglected.[14] Only recently Jeremy Greene and Elizabeth Watkins in their path-grounding work on the history and changing patterns of medical prescription in post-war United States have carved out the dense web of relations linking practitioners and industry in a world increasingly associated with clinical trials, quantitative risk of diseases, and new modes of scientific promotion.[15]

One may wonder about the reasons for a neglect that is especially striking when it comes to the European history of pharmacy. One explanation may be that the drug business is often seen by the actors involved but also by historians and social scientists as something special because what is at stake are not only drugs but people's lives. This special dimension is used to argue about the inevitable conflicts between public health and the logic of the market. Ironically, it is also mobilized to advance the opposite argument, i.e., that pharmaceutical companies are atypical corporations because their unique goal is not just profit making – given that they are dealing with health, they have as a consequence adopted ethical practices by investing in proper drug evaluation and refraining from aggressive marketing and false claims. These two positions are utterly incompatible unless the role of the market is seriously considered, which is to create both use value and financial value. In this respect, there is nothing atypical about the drug sector.

As clearly revealed by the history of drug patents and their problematic normalization during the twentieth century, the specificity of the drug sector is less a question of ethics than a problem of balance of powers and of the relationship between the industry (which replaced producer pharmacists) and practising physicians.[16] The professional medical organization and the existence of state regulations that mandated prescription for the most powerful (eventually dangerous) drugs prevented firms from advertising or marketing many of their drugs directly to patients and final consumers, who were seen as lacking the necessary knowledge to evaluate the usefulness of a treatment and its alternatives.

Just as pharmacists had opposed patents, in the early twentieth century most doctors refused advertising for drugs and pointed to the 'secret-remedy trade' as a reprehensible business making false promises and exaggerating the effects of drugs.[17] The growing role of the industry changed this perception. In order to distance themselves from these dishonourable practices, the so-called 'ethical' firms developed a business model that focused on the central role of the physician as prescriber, addressed them rather than the end buyers, and underscored the scientificity of both their production and clinical claims. This first mode of scientific promotion was not based on in-house research but rather on informal, quite personal collaborations with selected university scientists and hospital physicians.[18] This was by no means a one-way relationship as physicians and clinicians benefited from a connection that allowed them to access new substances or technical knowledge while opening new opportunities for them to carry out trials, publish articles and establish themselves as renowned scientists. Firms would then feel free to use this research for promotion.[19] They produced abstracts or offprints, which were then sent out to doctors or brought to them by representatives, who would then use the content as an entry point for conducting a conservation 'between scientists', thus paying tribute to the physician's claim to being a man of knowledge and expertise.

Initially, this model was rather successful. After all, it acknowledged the prestige of physicians and scientists by giving them access to technologies and production sites while making the knowledge of the latter available to the companies. What made it obsolete during the second half of the twentieth century was the changing scale and nature of the operations performed by pharmaceutical firms. With the transition from advertising to marketing, the focus moved from mere selling to building markets by mobilizing science. This move embraced three different developments, which will be analysed in the contributions to this volume.

First, advertising was professionalized: new publicity agencies specializing in pharmaceuticals sprang up. In the same line, special textbooks on marketing were written, often based on the practice of existing firms, which had developed their own curricula for their apprentices, trainees and young employees. Second, and at the same time, marketing developed as a research activity going far beyond the observation of sales figures and their analysis and focusing on techniques for planning and building an organization centred on therapeutic classes and product divisions.[20] Third, this was linked to massive changes in the nature of the research conducted by drug companies. These changes included the growth of in-house R&D capabilities, the generalization of large-scale screening procedures, an increasing emphasis placed on chemistry, purity and molecular structures, and the organization, by the companies themselves, of controlled clinical trials.

All three developments began before the beginning of World War II, partly as responses to the economic crisis of the 1920s and early 1930s, but they achieved their full potential after 1945 in the context of the 'therapeutic revolution'. Marketing then became scientific in two different ways: (1) it evolved into a research activity, which was observed, analysed and steered according to the newest findings of social and communication sciences; and (2) it increasingly mobilized biomedical research to build drug markets.

Instead of presenting innovations to be advertised and accepted or rejected, the firms now tried to understand competition and the structure of the market, how physicians prescribed, the needs of patients and the epidemiological landscape. Research not only provided knowledge about market niches and putative new drug use, but helped to integrate promotional activities into uniformly and purposefully designed marketing campaigns. This process was not so much connected to the use of new advertising channels – given that the arsenal of advertising means already covered the whole range of communication channels in the 1920s (print advertising in the professional and lay press, flyers, shop window advertising, posters, films and drug representatives) – as it was related to the integration and scaling-up of all these tools.

Second, during the same years, marketing developed into a series of practices that not only *used* scientific facts as advertising *arguments*, but merged pharmacological and clinical research with promotional activities. Firms did not only spread scientific knowledge; they began to shape research and scientific discourse on the basis of perceived market potentialities. The internalization of clinical research was in this respect a decisive development. It not only meant that toxicity and efficacy trials were increasingly financed and coordinated by company managers and salaried physicians, it also produced a new integrative space. In the 1960s and 1970s, 'marketing' and 'medical research' departments of large drug companies increasingly worked together and finally joined to form departments that organized all activities related to single drugs from research to advertising. This implied that new substances were tested with an eye not only on the regulatory exigencies but also on the future marketing campaigns, while new screening targets and procedures were intentionally defined according to market surveys and feedback from the promotional apparatus. With their own clinical research departments, firms would from the 1960s and 1970s onwards actively participate in the definition of medical practices, categories and needs. This in turn implied a new hierarchy of marketing tools such as: (a) the growing role of printed material resembling academic journals and reference manuals; (b) encounters such as conferences where company scientists and physicians could meet and 'key opinion leaders' be identified, addressed and used as multiplicators; and (c) sponsorship of medical societies and cultural events.

The analysis of the rise of scientific marketing presented in this volume evolved from a French-German research project entitled 'From Advertisement to Marketing: Pharmaceutical Enterprises, Patients, Physicians and the Construction of Medical Markets'. The aim of the project was not only to explore the validity of the two regimes' hypothesis outlined above but also to gather information on the specific trajectory of drug marketing in Europe to foster comparison with the less badly known developments in the United States. Such comparison was badly needed given the stronger role played by the professional organization of pharmacy in Europe, the longer history of many firms with a background in apothecaries, the early socialization of drug costs or the (relatively) late generalization of marketing permits, administrative regulation and clinical trials. The project was jointly financed by the Deutsche Forschungsgemeinschaft and the Agence Nationale de Recherche from 2009 to 2012.

It ended with a conference called 'The Birth of Scientific Marketing' organized in Berlin in June 2012 at which drafts of most of the chapters in this volume were first presented and discussed. In contrast to a previous series of papers published in *History and Technology* and focusing on the two regimes of drug promotion, this collection addresses the post-war changes and the dynamics of scientific marketing in Europe. This allows for a more specific understanding of the two meanings 'science' has taken in the set of practices, which became standards of drug market construction during the therapeutic revolution, i.e., the mobilization of biomedical, first of all clinical, research and increasing reliance on market research while planning firms' operations. Moreover, the focus of these papers on development in France and Germany helps understand how, within the context of an increasingly global market, the practices of US companies as well as the regulatory requirements of the FDA became pervading references in spite of the longer history of scientific marketing in large European firms, especially German ones. In other words, the new *glocal* nature of drug markets proved critical in generalizing the system of professionalized and knowledge-based marketing. The volume is accordingly organized into three parts.

The first three papers are centred on marketing research and the problem of innovation, which is considered to be one of the pharmaceutical industry's major driving forces. Pharmaceutical companies' marketing strategies strongly insist on the revolutionary, ground-breaking or simply innovative character of newly introduced products. Even critics who question the innovative character of many pharmaceutical products by asking whether they are 'true' innovations share the idea that the main goal of pharmaceutical companies should be innovation.

As Nils Kessel's paper agues, innovation as an essential condition for both medical and entrepreneurial progress has so far dominated the history of drugs. A closer look reveals, however, that 'new' substances, or the 'improved efficacy' or the 'increased safety' of a product, do not necessarily reflect the structure of consumption, which may be seen as the result of the consumer's expectations with regard to drugs. In fact, the story of post-war drug consumption and marketing is less about innovation and more about tradition than the 'blockbuster' stories nourished by media attention and launch narratives would like us to believe. Nils Kessel thus points to the market relevance of therapeutic groups such as cough and cold medicines, laxatives and anorectic drugs, which are often neglected and regarded as non-scientific, empirical and traditional, if not old-fashioned, and should not have been able to compete with the iconic products of the therapeutic revolution seen in the glossy advertisements of today. Using sales figures, the paper is a counter-narrative to the story of a seemingly almighty pharmaceutical industry, which uses marketing successfully to place drugs on saturated markets in order to sell the 'new', where in fact both physicians and consumers prefer 'old', well-proven products. The paper underscores the fallacies of following the narrative of permanent innovation that drug companies have used time and again in their marketing campaigns and is still used today by associations of pharmaceutical producers in their public relations campaigns.

Ulrike Thoms in her paper questions innovation from another angle, referring to the pivotal role it plays in the self-promotion of pharmaceutical companies as 'scientific' and 'ethical'. The novelty of certain products has been used as a major, if not the central sales argument in almost every branch of industry from the very beginning of advertising, but nowhere has it played a greater role than in the pharmaceutical sector. Here it has not only been a sales argument, it has also proved a crucial element in competition and thus a precondition of economic success, as only new drugs are granted the patents that will protect the producers and help them achieve high profits. These mechanisms are rather old, but in the post–World War II era they became central to the success of new drugs for two reasons. First, while the number of really new and innovative drugs decreased, research expenses increased enormously. The planning of research and costly promotion thus played an ever-growing role. Second, only new and improved drugs were allowed to enter the market and were protected against imitation.

The paper then explores how the life-cycle concept, which until today is an indispensable part of the theoretical toolbox of business studies, came into being as a tool to estimate the most probable success of a drug. It shows that the concept was influenced by the then-emerging field of cybernetics, the organization of science and business studies, which aimed to analyse and grasp the different factors influencing the trajectory of an industrial product in order to help to estimate its life span and economic potential. The promise here was to be able to steer these factors for the sake of increasing sales and profits. A growing awareness of the new systemic thinking led company marketing departments to be granted a much more prominent place during the 1960s and 1970s, especially as a new generation of managers entered the firms, who were familiar with the use of these theoretical models to forecast future developments. As the paper shows, however, the pharmaceutical industry did not only *use* this model for its marketing, which many believe to have been implemented later than in other industrial branches. The opposite is true. As with the theoretical model of the 'opinion leader', which originates in the context of industry-sponsored social research in medical innovation, the pharmaceutical industry was at the very forefront of investigating and implementing research planning and its economic exploitation. In parallel, the life-cycle model as well as the theory of innovation became cornerstones of entrepreneurial thinking in the drug business and the very foundation of modern marketing theory. This development was strongly related to the emergence of systems research, which was used to analyse the relations between different actors in the market and formed part of the development of social science and communication science, which were to become indispensable parts of basic marketing knowledge and of standard marketing routines. These then helped to minimize the risks associated with the launch of new innovative drugs.

The final paper of this part, by Quentin Ravelli, broadens the perspective to the global scale and to the problems and possibly massive consequences of scientific marketing. 'Marketing Epidemics' discusses the role of scientific data, which has always been essential in drug marketing: it is a way of convincing doctors to prescribe a firm's drugs and to obtain market authorization from public administrations. This same type of information, often generated by clinical trials, is also used by regulatory agencies to restrain pharmaceutical markets. Here again, science plays an ambivalent role: as a tool for and as an obstacle to market forces. Are regulatory agencies really *limiting* markets by controlling scientific data? Would it not be more accurate to describe their activity as *adapting* medical needs to market realities?

The case study of antibiotics highlights this ambiguous role of scientific regulation between states and corporations, medical needs and corporate profit. Over the last decade, multi-resistant bacteria, known since the 1940s, has emerged as a global health issue: doctors are now facing clinical 'dead end' situations that are not confined to emergency care units only but are threatening larger outpatient communities. For public health promoters, the solution is to find new drugs and to limit the prescriptions of older ones, those responsible for the growth of resistances. Pharmaceutical corporations, however, consider antibiotics as one of the less profitable classes in terms of research investment and try instead to increase the market shares of their old antibiotics. Trying to fill this gap, but dependent upon pharmaceutical corporations, regulators do not only try to restrain marketing activities but also seek to include them in their agenda.

Ravelli's paper concentrates on the case of pristinamycin, which was launched in 1973 for skin infections, but soon shifted its indication to bronchopulmonary infections in 1988. Through genetic and chemical engineering the active principle was improved and used to create a new product called Synercid, which obtained FDA approval in 1998. At that time resistant strains had been identified as a major health concern in the United States: a healthcare deal was then cut between the firm and the agency to authorize a drug both for 'compassionate use' and for more traditional markets.[21] This case shows how scientific regulation can oscillate between market and public health concerns and how hard it is for government agencies to counter the enormous financial potential of firms and their marketing activities.

The second part discusses the changing tools and practices of marketing with a special interest in the ways in which the professionalization of promotion was linked to visualization as an essential dimension of scientific marketing. The first contribution in this part by Stephan Felder, Jean-Paul Gaudillière and Ulrike Thoms displays the major findings of an extensive analysis of advertisements in two major medical journals, one in France and one in Germany, during the period from the 1920s to the late 1970s. The chapter discusses the methodology, then the choice of an approach that combines quantitative and qualitative analyses. Based on the evaluation of several thousand drug advertisements, the paper demonstrates that the period under discussion was not only marked by a vast growth in the number of advertisements, but also by a change in their appearance, structure and informational content. The increasing use of elements such as brand signs, logos, colours or pictures not only illustrates the professionalization of marketing and the changing fashions in design, but also borrows from the practice of scientific publishing and brings in more technical information, which is typical of scientific marketing. Moreover, as the paper shows, there are major national differences that cannot merely be explained by different regulatory frameworks and practices; these are also related to the two countries' different therapeutic cultures as well as to different consumption patterns in France and in Germany.

Christian Bonah's paper presents medical films as a marketing tool by using the case of Sandoz. The paper is not centred on what could be understood as advertising films, which had for instance been used since the 1930s in the form of animated cartoons to underscore the beneficial effects of certain drugs in countries with a low literacy rate. Instead it discusses the ambitious artistic and educational films made by renowned film directors and artists with the support of pharmaceutical companies who wanted to acquire social and cultural benefits from their sponsorship. The marketing value of these films was twofold. First, as they often dealt with general biological and medical topics, they were used as a vehicle to visualize the effects of specific drugs for the sake of doctors. Second, these films addressed physicians as part of an intellectual elite habitus in a prestigious way that created a common ground between physicians and pharmaceutical companies in that it referred to education and culture as a social and cultural capital that they shared. These films were very often artistically innovative and crafted with sophistication by well-known film artists. What was then at stake was less the shaping of prescription patterns than the establishment of a shared social and cultural world in which it was suggested that both physicians and companies were striving for the same goals.

Anne-Sophie Mazas's analysis of print advertisements highlights that in France, post-war advertisements referred to science in a very different mode than ads from the pre-war period. Advertisements increasingly cited research results and used graphics or charts, but this was only the tip of the iceberg. Blending information and promotion involved less direct, more complex visualization strategies. The systems of signification – which integrated research, information and promotion – thus connected meanings and products to selected sets of images, icons, slogans and specific symbols, building new medical narratives. In France, the development of 'scientific' advertising was immensely influenced by American practices that were brought to France by French marketers returning from trips to America and by the translation of American books, and speeded up by the growth of a massive European market. An additional specificity of developments in France was the regulation of publicity. From the 1950s onwards, a visa system was set up, intended to reinforce the informative value of advertising to physicians by stating that if a producer wanted to be allowed to advertise his product without getting a special advertising permit from the health administration, it had to include a certain number of elements regarding composition, dose, price, etc. In this framework, visualization was a particular matter of concern. The paper then presents a typology of visualization techniques, such as tropes, emblems and colour codes by analysing advertisements identified from a corpus of advertisements combining the GEPHAMA database and the archives of companies such as Geigy, which sold psychotropic drugs in France.

In contrast to this general approach to visualization strategies, Lisa Malich in her paper on the French and Western German marketing of oral contraceptives uses a set of ads from the period between 1961 and 2006 to analyse how ideas of standardization were represented. Two different uses of standardization can be found. On the one hand, the pill was presented as a standard drug that promised safety building on the notion of the woman as a patient in need of medical advice. On the other hand, in a second phase, during the 1980s and 1990s, the women taking the pill were, in the promotion material, increasingly diversified. The advertisements identified bodily differences as well as diverse female gender roles and consumer types with distinct wishes. In both cases, however, representations of standardization reduced random variability and produced controlled variation in drugs and women. This way, they emphasized both the safeness and the uniqueness of the advertised product. Malich identifies strong national differences. In Germany, preparations of synthetic oestrogens and progesterone were quickly marketed as contraceptive, whereas in France the 'pill' was advertised as a multi-purpose drug. In a second step her paper analyses how pill advertisements referred to standardization and how standards were employed.

The other paper of this part, authored by Tricia Close-Koenig and Ulrike Thoms, demonstrates how insulin was used as an inroad to create an entire market of products for diabetics. Insulin holds a special place in the history of biological medical products. The role played by patients in the successful treatment of diabetes was recognized very early on as these had to control their diet, monitor injections and later survey their blood sugar concentration. Diabetics would therefore not only need insulin, they would also need devices such as syringes, measuring devices and diagnostic tests. Patient organizations such as the Deutscher Diabetiker Bund and the Association Française des Diabétiques, founded in 1931 and 1938, respectively, helped to convey the necessary knowledge on treatment and devices to the patients and pleaded for greater autonomy. As such, they became marketing targets. The paper analyses the ads in the journals of the mentioned diabetics' associations and documents strong relations between these organizations and the producers of specialized goods for diabetics. It suggests that diabetics were regarded somewhat differently from other patients. The state did not prosecute the firms that advertised prescription drugs such as insulin to laypeople in these journals, although this was prohibited by law in both countries. The ads are deciphered in regard to the definition or conception of the diabetic as a consumer of special, remarkably profit-making goods, showing, for instance, how the ads for insulin and later on for oral anti-diabetics were by far outnumbered by ads for special diet products and medical devices, often produced by the very same firms that sold the prescription drugs. In this respect, the paper sheds some light on today's pharmaceutical companies' much discussed strategies to use self-help and patient groups, the position of patients as well as diabetes specialists, and their relations to the industry, to serve their own economic interests.

The third part of the book pursues the question of the relationship between science and marketing by focusing more precisely on the first meaning of the term, namely the mobilization of biomedical research to build markets and the looping effects of the markets on the development of in-house industrial research. The paper by Jean-Paul Gaudillière approaches the advent of scientific marketing by using the case of Ludiomil, an antidepressant developed and marketed by the Swiss firm Ciba-Geigy. It argues that this shift took place towards the end of the 1960s in the context of the merger between Geigy and Ciba. On the organizational side it was linked to major changes inside Geigy both in terms of how clinical research was conducted and how marketing was organized. Until 1970 this work had been structured into two departments: publicity and sales, and medicine. The new organization occasioned a major growth in in-house and collaborative research with the development of pharmacological screening and clinical trials, while the institution of a marketing department led to new modes of research on prescription and sales. Based on the Ciba-Geigy archives, the paper analyses how the advent of scientific marketing, i.e., the massive use of clinical research in promotion and the rise of marketing research for the purpose of strategic planning, contributed to shifting the boundaries of depression.

In the early 1970s, Ciba-Geigy organized a whole series of initiatives (workshops, publications and training of its sales representatives, as well as the enrolment of physicians, general practitioners or specialists in clinical trials). They concerned the changing status of the disease, what seemed to be its generalization worldwide, how this generalization was related to the changing roles of psychiatry, the use of antidepressants outside the hospital, and the proper ways of handling an emerging mass of depressive patients. Special attention is paid to the ways in which the relationship between the company, a core set of psychiatrists engaged in long-term collaboration with Geigy and general practitioners, made the problem of depression visible in general practice and stabilized a new category, 'masked depression', the diagnosis and treatment of which were widely advocated through the multi-layered organization of scientific marketing.

Lucie Gerber investigates similar 'marketing loops' by analysing the links between Geigy's marketing and the development of psychopharmacological screening. As she argues, a whole range of new psychotropic drugs gradually entered clinical practice in the late 1950s and early 1960s. When in 1952 chlorpromazine became the first chemotherapeutic treatment of psychoses it opened up a market for such drugs that promised a high sales potential. Nevertheless, knowledge on aetiological and pathophysiological mechanisms underlying psychiatric afflictions was still very limited, and this posed a severe problem for developing new drugs quickly and at low cost. The paper examines how animal models were developed for this purpose and as tools for psychopharmacological screening. Based on printed sources as well as on sources from the Geigy archives, it analyses in detail how the local understanding of the market structure and of its prospects nurtured the establishment of a screening system aiming to discover 'big antidepressants' that could compete with tranquilizers. Putting aside the psychological and mental dimensions of depression, industrial pharmacologists focused on a limited and selected set of secondary manifestations, such as loss of vitality and psychomotor retardation. Once this model was developed it was exploited for matching clinical targets and commercial goals by grouping different psychiatric disorders alongside their symptoms. As the paper demonstrates, with the development of psychopharmacological screening, a complex feedback system between the market, the clinic and the laboratory was established, and this led to shifting the focus from diagnosis-based therapy to drug-induced behaviour change.

Altogether these chapters show that it is possible to develop a history of science and medicine that acknowledges the centrality of pharmaceutical markets and their complex construction. Drugs are and are not goods like any other. They are like any other because they are industrial products, massively promoted and massively used. They are not like any other because the fact that they are appropriated and commercialized by large capitalistic firms remains a matter of open controversy as it is perceived as detrimental to health. A history of drug marketing thus goes far beyond the history of consumption, which emphasizes discourse and culture and ignores the uneven balance of powers, the hierarchies and their relations to the making of knowledge and expertise.[22] Power is distributed unequally and according to hierarchies; moreover it is linked to knowledge and expertise, and access to these resources differs enormously depending on the different groups of people, organizations and professions. As shown in the papers in this volume, these imbalances have been built not only into the marketing practices but also and even more radically into the structures of drug companies, including their research apparatus. Viewed from this perspective, the question of 'capture', of the influence of marketing on drug prescription, consumption and regulation, appears in need of reformulation that will give firms a central but not isolated and all-powerful role. Marketing can be understood as a technique aimed at influencing the multiple actors in the pharmaceutical system in order to increase sales. This works mainly through the collection and production of a vast body of information as the precondition for taking any action. In this system agency remains unequal not only because of unequal access to financial or technical resources, but also because of the strong power gradient associated with unequal roles in the production, control and circulation of biological, clinical, social and economic knowledge. Taking stock of these differences and hierarchies is a precondition for any reflection on change.

1 BEYOND INNOVATION: PHARMACEUTICAL MARKETING, MARKET STRUCTURE AND THE IMPORTANCE OF THE 'OLD' IN WEST GERMANY, 1950–70

Nils Kessel

Innovation is everywhere. In the world of goods (technology) certainly, but also in the realm of words: innovation is discussed in the scientific and technical literature, in social sciences like history, sociology, management and economics, and in the humanities and arts. Innovation is also a central idea in the popular imaginary, in the media, in public policy and is part of everybody's vocabulary. Briefly stated, innovation has become the emblem of the modern society, a panacea for resolving many problems, and a phenomenon to be studied.[1]

Most historians specialized in the pharmaceutical industry will probably agree that innovation actually is 'the emblem of the modern society ... and a phenomenon to be studied'. Both the pharmaceutical industry and many of their critics share the common belief that innovation is the most important, if not the only legitimate cause for bringing new drugs into the market. Not surprisingly, many historical studies on pharmaceuticals and drug marketing deal more or less explicitly with 'innovations' when describing the discovery, development and production of new drugs.[2]

I would however like to argue that this focus on innovations occults another very rich history of 'old' drugs and their marketing. It could even be said that the history of innovation is the top of the history iceberg in the field of drugs. By concentrating on selected research-intensive drugs, it does not have much to say about the drug market as a whole.

In contrast, this paper looks at post-war West Germany's markets, which were dominated by old products rather than the latest innovations, particularly by the markets for analgesics, hypnotics and tonics. It focuses on three aspects: first, market shares of older products and substances in the field of analgesics;

second, advertising of prescription-free analgesics and tonics as modern panaceas; and third, prescription figures, which shall illustrate how older concepts
of disorders such as vegetative dystonia (*vegetative Dystonie*) continuously made
older, panacea-like medicines relevant. The paper thus contributes to a historiography of technology, which is sensitive to the fact that 'innovations do not
necessarily substitute one technology by another'.[3] As argued by the historian
of technology David Edgerton, old products are more present in our daily lives
than the latest innovations.[4] They often get little attention, however, be it from
observers of their time or, later, from historians. As a consequence, innovation-
centred historiography supports progress narratives that are a poor reflection of
the existence and uses of technology in everyday life.

Innovation, or the Goose's Golden Therapeutic Eggs

> Nearly all the valuable new drugs of the last 30 years – penicillin and streptomycin
> are notable exceptions – have been discovered in the manufacturers' laboratories.[5]

When discussing the capacity of pharmaceutical companies to find 'valuable
new drugs', the head of the British Drug Safety Committee, Derrick Dunlop,
did not call for 'innovation'. He wished to have 'valuable new drugs' instead. For
Dunlop, a trained physician, pharmaceutical companies contributed to medical
progress through the development of drugs that were 'valuable' for the medical
community thanks to their therapeutic properties. At the climax of the Cold
War, Dunlop even felt obliged to protect the industry against tightened regulations: 'We must therefore be careful not to kill the goose which has laid so
many golden therapeutic eggs by excessive bureaucratic restrictions – still less
by nationalization'.[6] Dunlop's defence of the pharmaceutical industry is of interest to us here because of its explicit promise that the industry, which had 'laid
so many golden therapeutic eggs', would continue to do so. What the British
physician had in mind was research-intensive development of drugs that were to
bring up new molecules to heal incurable diseases or at least add substantial benefits to existing drugs. With this understanding of pharmaceutical companies'
social 'task', company-friendly Dunlop's position was not that distant from that
of critics of the pharmaceutical industry: 'While all innovations are commercially important for manufacturers, it is those which offer significant therapeutic
advance that are most valuable to patients' health'.[7] Both imagine a 'valuable new
drug' or an 'innovative' drug as a 'New Chemical Entity' (NCE) or 'New Molecular Entity' (NME).[8] Yet NMEs as technological (or radical) innovations are
not what drug markets are mainly made of.[9] Combinations of well-known molecules outnumber products with new therapeutic agents by far. Furthermore,
a restrictive definition of innovation such as that of an NME fails to take into

account the potential advantages of drugs for which the galenic composition has been slightly modified, for example to improve their metabolism or their taste.[10] In addition to such a restrictive – therapeutic – understanding of innovation, the economic literature usually applies its wider and general definition inspired by David Ricardo and Joseph Schumpeter. In this view new products placed on the market can be considered as innovative just on the basis of their new characteristics, even if their therapeutic benefit is minor. Not surprisingly, the introduction of new pharmaceutical products is often then accompanied by diverging judgement of the 'value' of the new product for therapy. Nevertheless, beyond their profound differences in judgement, manufacturers and critics alike share the idea that the main objective of pharmaceutical companies should be innovation.[11] This discourse on innovation as an essential condition for both medical and entrepreneurial progress also dominates much of the work in drug historiography:

> The aim [of the European Science Foundation (ESF) Research Networking Programme, Standard drugs and drug standards (DRUGS)] is to evaluate the contribution of industrial, administrative and clinical standardization to the 'therapeutic revolution' (1920–1990) in which a series of 'miracle' drugs changed the face of Western medicine.[12]

These 'miracle' drugs are, for example, sex hormones, insulin, oral anti-diabetics, new antidepressants, many cardiovascular drugs and some cancer medications, but also cyclosporine in transplantation medicine and others.[13] The life cycle of the few 'old' blockbusters such as aspirin has been mostly put forward to highlight the shortening life cycles of new drugs. Nevertheless, the historiography of drugs still focuses on important therapeutic 'advances'.

Notwithstanding, although the term 'innovation' is historically specific and its meaning somehow contingent, so are the controversies on the potentially innovative character of a drug. From a historian's point of view it then becomes essential to reflect on and clarify the use of the concept. I therefore suggest moving beyond identifying 'advances' or 'innovations' by considering 'innovativeness' as being a contingent judgement that tells us more about medical beliefs of the day than about a molecule or a product itself. Historical analyses interested in drug markets and the use of drugs should then turn away from a concept so normative and blurred, and privilege a symmetric view on 'old' and 'new' drugs. This is the intention of this article. It first requires combining two perspectives on drug markets. The first is interested in markets for different product groups classified according to their chemical identity or to their therapeutic group. The markets for hypnotics or analgesics can be looked at, for example, or the markets for benzodiazepines or amphetamines. Such perspectives, however, are incomplete unless users' perspectives are integrated in terms of symptoms and disease categories. Users, who can be either physicians or patients, choose drugs to treat pathological states or to (re-)establish wellbeing.[14] My account thus looks at drugs and drug groups 'in the shadow' of most progress and innovation histories.

The Pill-o-Maniac's Headache

Post-war West Germany had a high number of drugs on the different pharmaceutical markets. The number of available products on the West German market between the 1950s and 1970s ranges from 18,000 to some 70,000.[15] Medical experts have often criticized the size of the market and an assumed 'irrational' drug use by patients. Overprescription and prescription errors have been mentioned, but far less frequently than patients' excessive demand for drugs. Particularly, pharmacologists, psychiatrists and specialists in internal medicine in university hospitals and research have criticized 'irrational' drug use harshly.[16] According to post-war psychiatrists, starting in the 1950s pharmaceutical consumption seemed to have risen faster than ever before.[17] The less these experts recognized the 'therapeutic value' of a drug group, the more their criticism of companies manufacturing those drugs was harsh. Drugs for 'minor' problems were particularly criticized: products against digestion problems, laxatives that could be used to lose weight, anti-cold drugs, anorectic drugs, tonics, liver products, liver protection drugs and many more. No therapeutic group, however, has raised as many concerns in the 1950s as the many 'headache pills' with their commercial success. These painkillers usually contain salicylic acid, paracetamol or phenacetin as an analgesic agent. Often manufacturers have added stimulants such as caffeine, and sometimes calming agents have been added, too. In Hoffmann-La Roche's Swiss version of Saridon, for example, chemists had added the company's own sedative agent Persedon intended to calm nervousness. In the language of marketing, caffeine was to provide a feeling of 'refreshment' while the analgesic agent attenuated the pain.[18] Analgesic preparations with caffeine and Vitamin C were sold as anti-cold drugs.

The diversity of pain as both a symptom and a syndrome allowed marketing to continue advertising with panacea-like dimensions. When in 1961 the pharmaceutical manufacturer Much AG began selling a new, stronger version of its bestselling analgesic Spalt, the company's advertising insisted on the variety of pain that could be treated. The range of indications shown in painkiller advertisements mentioned such diverse problems as headache, toothache, neuralgia, migraine, articular gout, sciatic pain syndrome, rheumatism or menstrual cramps.[19] A syndrome the advertisers called 'nerve pain' (*Nervenschmerzen*) was also listed. When translated into medically correct terms, it was perfectly synonymous to the above-mentioned neuralgia, but in advertisement language it opened up the field to a vast range of possible uses.

In this sense, analgesics too were advertised as modern panaceas. Despite the fact that pain by definition is a general phenomenon accompanying many diseases, advertisements for painkillers tried to extend the uses of analgesic pills as much as was possible. Many university physicians were particularly dissatisfied with this kind of advertising for prescription-free drugs. Nephrologists in particular protested against this advertising for pharmaceuticals and lobbied for stronger regulations as they had to treat patients suffering from severe nephrotoxic effects due to long-term use of certain analgesic compounds.[20]

None of these analgesics was particularly 'innovative' in the eyes of their contemporaries. They were all made of analgesic agents that dated back to the turn of the century. Big pharmaceutical companies knew of the negative image of drugs such as analgesic combinations of aspirin, caffeine and Vitamin C. In an industrial branch for which reputation was mainly built on the scientific nature of its production, it could be useful for both marketing purposes and economic rationalization to separate the research-based 'ethical' drug business from the production of prescription-free every-day drugs, so major companies sold their prescription-free headache drugs through their subsidiaries. The corporate group Bayer in Germany had set up a formally separate company, Drugofa, while Ciba in Switzerland sold these products via Zyma-Blaes. One of the most successful companies selling analgesics was Karl Thomae GmbH in Biberach, a subsidiary of the C. H. Boehringer Sohn AG in Ingelheim. While the latter produced highly sophisticated cardiovascular drugs and psychopharmaceuticals, the former was well-known for its analgesics Thomapyrin and Thomapyrin N. Sometimes these subsidiaries could make more profits with these prescription-free painkillers than the parent company with its 'serious' products.

Painkillers did clearly outweigh every psychiatric drug, even Valium, in numbers of consumed units.[21] They were best-selling drugs. Based on the 1974 sales figures from the pharmaceutical market research company IMS, out of all the analgesics on the West German pharmacy market, the best-selling drug in number of units sold was Spalt-Tablette, introduced as early as 1931.[22] Contrary to the assumption that the market is mainly dominated by new products, a comparison of introduction year and market shares shows the impact of older products, in this particular case of analgesics, including both prescription-free products and drugs under prescription. We examined a sample of fifty analgesic products to gain greater understanding of the novelty of products on the West German market in 1974. These drugs were used and advertised against headaches and similar nervous pain, but not exclusively. For a better perception of the market trajectories, we refer to the year of introduction of the therapeutic agent, rather than to the year of discovery, which is the more common reference. Out of the fifty products, only seven were introduced in 1970 or later. Fourteen were put on the market during the 1960s and six during the 1950s.[23] The remaining twenty-three products, almost half of all the products, were older than twenty-five years, including nineteen older than forty years and eleven older than fifty. Nonetheless, the year of introduction is still a fairly imprecise way of identifying the relative novelty of drugs historically, as it does not allow consideration of simple modifications of existing therapeutic agents and their combinations. Looking at product families, out of the twenty-one analgesics introduced after 1960, seven, or one-third of them, were only new combinations or new galenic forms of older products, such as Aspirin plus C added to the existing Aspirin, or Brausende Spalt, which is simply the effervescent version of Spalt. The dominance of older products is particularly highlighted when looking at the number of units sold.[24]

Ironically, the commercial success of analgesics undermined their reputation, given that they were ultimately depicted as one of the 'seven sins of humanity' and as the drugs of a presumably pill-addicted society.[25] Mass media were all too willing to level harsh criticism at users, calling them 'pill-o-maniacs' (*Tablettomanen*), no matter that the magnitude of consumption on a nationwide scale was unknown.[26]

Grandpa's Pills

Another psychotropic therapeutic subclass, hypnotics and sedatives, strengthens the assumption that in several therapeutic classes older products remained very important. Hypnotics and sedatives are a particularly interesting group because they include many new chemical groups such as piperidinedione derivatives (e.g., products containing thalidomide (Distaval/Softenon) and gluthethimide (Doriden)) or benzodiazepines (e.g., Librium or Valium).[27] They also include barbiturates and their derivatives.[28] While the first two groups were considered to be innovative in psychiatry and in general practice when discovered in the early and mid-1950s, respectively, barbiturates had been well known since the beginning of the twentieth century.

Hypnotics and sedatives in the IMS classification are differentiated as barbiturates or barbiturate-free drugs, and as pure products or combinations. This chemical differentiation also provides information about the relative novelty of a product, because pure products usually appear before combinations of several therapeutic agents.[29] West German 1974 sales figures for hypnotics and sedatives indicate that in the mid-1970s barbiturates and their combinations still accounted for significant market shares despite the fact that they had several disadvantages including the risk of over-dosage and of 'hangover'. Of course, all these listings only include the drugs that were still on the market, not all the products. For example, products containing thalidomide are no longer listed. Nevertheless, as withdrawals are quite rare and mainly due to commercial, not regulatory, reasons, these figures can be used for a better identification of innovation clusters and of the novelty of many of these products. The term 'innovation cluster' refers to the fact that the invention of a new therapeutic agent of a new chemical group is often the beginning of a whole series of research activities exploring the potential of related substances. For example, a first wave of pure barbiturate-free products arrived on the market in the 1950s, including drugs such as Doriden or Contergan. Regarding our initial question of product novelty – analysed here with 1974 IMS data – it can be shown that an older chemical group, barbiturates, and more particularly their combinations, accounted for high pharmacy purchases. Forty per cent of all purchased hypnotics and sedatives contained barbiturates.[30] At first glance it may be surprising that many of the barbiturate combination drugs that produced high sales figures were in fact introduced as late as the 1960s. This might be a potential consequence of the thalidomide disaster and the disappearance of Contergan and Contergan forte, the two bestselling products containing the noxious agent thalidomide. Both products had concentrated about 40 to 60 per cent of the hypnotics and sedatives market at the beginning of the 1960s.[31]

Another finding heightens this still rather blurred impression of the innovative character of products. When looking at the year of introduction of the therapeutic agents used in products and not at the year of introduction of the product itself, the dominance of 'older' drugs is confirmed. Out of the seventy-two hypnotics and sedatives on the West German market in 1974, the therapeutic agent used in fifty-nine of them had been introduced before or in 1950 while only thirteen had been discovered after that. This observation questions assumptions made on a very general level about the importance of innovation. Using the German company Bayer's sales in 1960, which depended up to 60 per cent on products put on the market since 1945, the economic historian Werner Abelshauser argued, for example, that technological knowledge would rapidly become obsolescent in the chemical industry. Abelshauser's argument is however quite general and only true for a few 'innovative' therapeutic groups such as oral antidiabetics, cardiovascular drugs and some psychotropic drugs.[32] It is less convincing for the profitable analgesics and hypnotics markets, which were strongly dominated by 'old' drugs. The introduction year of anti-diabetic drugs that were on the market in 1974 can serve here as an example for comparison. Anti-diabetic drugs have been an important field of research since the beginning of the century (insulin) and again since the 1940s (oral antidiabetics). It can then be assumed that technological innovation in the many new barbiturate-containing products put on the market in the 1960s had been rare. We instead see a recombination of therapeutic agents that dated back to the first half of the twentieth century but were introduced as commercial innovations in the second half of the century.[33] Consumption of these 'old' substances for which the risks were well known raised serious fears in the medical community as their sales increased sharply in the late 1960s. The German political magazine *Der Spiegel* ultimately criticized this revival of older substances in one of its articles, ironically calling them 'pills from Grandpa['s days]'.[34]

Keep Calm: Take Carmelite Balm Water

There is therefore a strong orientation towards innovation in both expert and public/lay discourses, but many products in daily use do not reflect the ideal of innovative, research-intensive drugs. In fact traditional tonics such as the famous German Klosterfrau Melissengeist (Carmelite balm water) are found amongst the drugs most sold. Essentially containing alcohol, this tonic has been used by many people as a sort of panacea. Not surprisingly, it has not had good press amongst protagonists of scientific medicine. The commercial group of tonics confirms the observation made about hypnotics-based combination products: that the most successful products were already quite old in the mid-1970s. Lecithin products were commonly sold as tonics, including the very famous Buerlecithin. Well-known and commercially successful products such as Doppelherz, Klosterfrau Melissengeist or Buerlecithin dated back to the 1920s. Throughout the 1960s, however, the manufacturing companies diversified their product range considerably. They did so either by adding new galenic forms such as capsules, said to be more modern, or by bringing new combinations into the market that were only slightly different from the original products.[35] Products of this kind were less contested for their therapeutic value because tonics were of great use in cancer and postoperative therapies, but they were also welcome for older patients. Almost completely ignored by modern drug historiography, the marketing of tonics such as Klosterfrau is an excellent example of successful product branding of traditional medicine. Developments in advertising and branding of Klosterfrau Melissengeist, for example, were no more than just nuances, with continuity of the nun's image maintaining the traditional character of the tonic, which even became a sort of 'cultural icon'.[36] The advertising continued to insist on traditional knowledge and used the image of the nun to remind the users of the pre-modern origins of religious healing knowledge and the natural base of the product.[37] Its 'cure-all' character was particularly visible in advertisements before the restrictions issued in the 1965 law on drug advertising. For example, one Klosterfrau Melissengeist advertisement recommended the drug, which contained essentially alcohol, as a treatment against 'pill addiction', suggesting that drug dependence could be treated by using a prescription-free alcoholic tonic.[38]

An explicitly 'calming' drug, Klosterfrau covered an important range of indications as shown in the advertising copy published in the mainstream magazine *Bunte* in 1955:

> Our Nerves! Yes, our nerves. They are so often the source of daily troubles in our restless times. Keep calm: the true Klosterfrau Melissengeist has rendered much service against nervous troubles, against the 'disturbed harmony of the nerves ['Spannungsmissverhältnisse'].
>
> Those who are seriously nervous should turn to a doctor. But those who only occasionally need help to calm down can trust in the use of our established traditional household remedy: the true Klosterfrau Melissengeist. As an all-around household remedy it should be readily on hand everywhere. For example*, use it when you are suffering from a common cold: stir 1–2 teaspoons of [KM] into a cup of hot sugar water or tea. Drink it – as hot as possible – before going to bed. Experience shows that it provides good help.
>
> *Read further examples in the package instructions.[39]

This advertising copy provides particular insight as it illustrates both the marketing strategies of these panacea-like drugs and the regulatory framework partly shaping the advertising copy.[40] In 1950s West Germany, an imperial edict dating back to 1901 allowed advertising for drugs outside pharmacies as long as they were 'prophylactic' (*Vorbeugungsmittel*).[41] Since 1941, however, advertising for sleeping pills and 'calming' drugs has been restricted to the medical community even though the drugs were still available prescription-free in pharmacies.[42] The advertising strategy for Klosterfrau is reflected in the added second paragraph: while in the first paragraph the company was clearly advertising a 'calming' drug for daily use, the second paragraph served to avoid problems with the legislation. After having advertised the product more generally for nervous problems, the advertisement differentiated between 'nervous problems' and 'serious nervous problems'.

Vegetative Dystonia: A Syndrome to Catch All Disorders

Before the 1965 West German law on drug advertising (*Heilmittelwerbegesetz*) put an end to many advertising practices – including panacea-like promises for drugs – many manufacturers had sold and advertised tonic preparations and fortifiers for the heart and nerves. Drugs were sold by mail order for treatment against 'circulation problems' (*Kreislaufstörungen*), vegetative dystonia, rheumatism and 'nervous disorders' (*Nervenleiden*).[43] In the 1950s and early 1960s, many of these products were being advertised as drugs against vegetative dystonia. Advertisements published in the German tabloid magazine *Bunte* in the 1950s show a large spectrum of possible symptoms ranging from fatigue, non-chronic depressive moods, 'nervous heart irritation', nervousness, sleeping disorders, loss of appetite and testiness to somatic symptoms such as digestion disorders or palpitations.[44]

From a prescriber's point of view, vegetative dystonia could cover the same field of disorders that neurasthenia and hysteria had done previously.[45] Vegetative dystonia was a strongly gendered disorder primarily addressing women. Statistics confirm the over-representation of women in all psychiatric medication prescriptions that I have analysed. Even neurasthenia, culturally gendered as a male disorder complementary to female hysteria, saw a fairly stable distribution between the genders within the range of 25 to 35 per cent for men and 65 to 75 per cent for women.[46] Advertisements were jointly responsible for producing the gendered image of the disorder by showing exclusively women as affected by vegetative dystonia. Ironically these advertisements argued that this condition was a consequence of modern life and women's multiple particular and stressful 'obligations'. Women in these advertisements had to use drugs to fit into a clearly drawn role model as pleasant partner to men. They were expected to maintain their 'beauty' – understood as physical youth – while complying with the needs of modern household management and work. The advertisements argued that 'hurry and stress' (*Hast und Hetze*) had to be compensated pharmaceutically in order to allow women to work and have fun without showing signs of fatigue.[47] Advertisements such as those for the tonic Frauengold (women's gold) addressed women directly, claiming that Frauengold would help them find good recovery sleep so they could be 'beautiful', have 'youthful freshness' and be able to 'manage daily life'.[48] Turning away from sales figures towards prescription habits, we must acknowledge the 'national' specificity of several factors influencing prescription habits, such as medical traditions, regulatory frameworks submitting certain products to prescription while allowing prescription-free sales of others, and the relevance of product names and indication ranges, which may vary from country to country. We have chosen the example of vegetative dystonia, which is a perfect illustration of these national specificities that were of such great relevance for marketing strategists. As described above, vegetative dystonia was a rather fuzzy concept summing up symptoms at the margins of both clinical psychiatry and normal living conditions. In psychiatric diagnostics it was mainly related to mild forms of neurosis, but it rapidly became a fill-in concept for all forms of mild mental problems that did not meet the psychiatric criteria of mental disease but where a frequent disorder was felt by patients. Interestingly, 'vegetative dystonia' was used synonymously to terms such as 'stress disorders' or 'psychophysical fatigue'. A majority of general practitioners (82 per cent) identified the symptom much more frequently than internal medicine specialists (15 per cent) and neurologists and psychiatrists (1 per cent).[49] In the current state of research there can only be speculation to explain the over-representation of general practitioners in prescriptions for vegetative dystonia. First, this preference might be due to the fact that general practitioners had to face patients suffering from minor mental problems more often than psychiatrists did. Second, general practitioners were not specially trained in psychiatry and might have preferred broader definitions of disorder and disease when writing prescriptions.[50] Also, in the 1970s the reputation of psychiatrists as 'insanity doctors' (*Irrenärzte*) might have motivated patients to begin by seeing their general practitioner, who generally remained the first health professional to get in touch with.[51]

The rise of the concept of depression did not lead to the disappearance of vegetative dystonia, although its symptomatic description was strikingly similar to the early definitions of depression. While diagnostic manuals such as the *Diagnostic and Statistical Manual of Mental Disorders* (*DSM*) had already switched to modern concepts of depression, vegetative dystonia continued to be indicated as a syndrome on general practitioners' prescription sheets.[52] Meanwhile, pharmaceutical marketing integrated those older disorder schemes as an indication for the new antidepressants.[53] Vegetative dystonia remained popular amongst physicians even during the 1970s, a period generally associated with the rise and spread of the concept of depression. Almost unknown in Anglo-Saxon countries, it was a well-known syndrome amongst both medical and lay people in German-speaking as well as in Latin countries. The vegetative dystonia syndrome says a lot about the relationship between the uses of old and new drugs and the shaping of drug markets through marketing practices.

Conclusion, or Why Write a History of the 'Old' in Drug Marketing?

This article has shown the importance of older products that were no longer considered innovative or therapeutically relevant. Instead, very often, they were considered as dangerous leftovers of a less advanced past by pharmacologists and clinicians.[54] Notwithstanding, these products are in fact important both in terms of sales and of packages sold. Besides, the focus on therapeutic innovation does not sufficiently take into account that neither physicians nor patients necessarily share the therapeutic enthusiasm that motivates scientific experts or pharmaceutical manufacturers when it comes to the introduction of new drugs.

In consequence, future scholarship on the history of drugs, and the historiography of twentieth-century history of medicine and health in general, should take into account older technologies in our apparently innovation-driven world.[55] Such a change in perspective would probably question interpretations put forward by historians of drugs during the last years. Focusing on drug development and essentially based on industry archives and media sources, studies on the history of vitamins or modern psychopharmacology have contributed to strengthen the idea that science-based pharmaceutical industry in the mid-twentieth century has revolutionized drug therapy.[56] For example, Beat Bächi's valuable history of Vitamin C gives the impression that drug markets can be created through coalitions of scientific, political and economic actors.[57] Finally, such a vision of pharmaceutical markets comforts the interpretation of 'pharmaceuticalization' processes.[58] The latter concept, suggested by sociologist John Abraham, insinuates that, first, drug therapy does expand to more and more fields and that, second, this expansion is mainly controlled by health professionals and the industry. Yet, one can doubt whether things are as simple as that. Criticizing the concept of medicalization as empirically weak, Nicolas Rose has argued in 2007 that consumers do understand themselves as autonomous actors, too. Marketing then rather tries to identify their desires in order to orient them towards specific consumptions than to invent them as such.[59] Once again, a view on older drugs can contribute to a better understanding of if and how those desires could be satisfied *before* the 'innovative' drug has been introduced.

As for the field of marketing, the persistence of old, well-known products in a sector in which the main marketing argument is medical progress makes it necessary to compare standard branding strategies with the argument of therapeutic innovation. Today, in the history of drug marketing, it is far from clear whose marketing strategies proved successful in which situations. Not only have innovators had to face their competitors' marketing strategies, they have also had to deal with peoples' habits. Marketing has not – as both 'success stories' and polemics might argue – change prescription or consumption habits easily. In addition, the pharmaceutical sector has specificities in the realm of marketing and advertising. Attempts to influence prescription or consumption directly have been complicated by regulatory barriers. Scientific companies depending on physicians', and especially clinicians' good will for their reputation have had to avoid being categorized as 'quacks', not only those accused of fraud but also those who have not taken into account modern scientific knowledge and continued to rely on 'old-fashioned' concepts of disease. Pharmaceutical companies seem to have dealt with this problem in their usual discrete way: it is in the physician files that the companies kept for their medical representatives that remarks can be found regarding each doctor's prescription habits and his or her openness to modern therapy.[60]

Although schematic and reductionist, the distinction between the 'new' and the 'old' makes it possible to take into account the diversity of users and uses. If on the one hand we look at innovation, scientists, public health experts and large-scale research come into focus. If on the other hand we look at old-fashioned, somehow dubious, sometimes scientifically obsolete drugs, then users and general practitioners who *continue* to use these products – very often against scientific advice and reasoning – enter the scene as independent actors who sometimes even oppose the conceptual hegemony of university medicine. In the field of marketing, we can observe the existence of very traditional forms of marketing, such as mainstream-product marketing in tabloid magazines, which have been given up by companies trying to appear as serious, innovative (because research-based) companies. This perspective influences which historical actors historians look at and to whom historians grant or refuse credit.

Finally the desire of both practitioners as prescribers and consumers to keep 'their' products should not be underestimated. On the contrary, this preference for well-known products could at least partly explain the need for manufacturers to multiply the number of medical representatives as a response to the greater difficulties they meet when placing products in growing markets. Marketing in this sense needs to be considered not only as a progressive tool of modern industry but also as a reaction to an increasingly difficult situation in which to sell new products.

2 INNOVATION, LIFE CYCLES AND CYBERNETICS IN MARKETING: THEORETICAL CONCEPTS IN THE SCIENTIFIC MARKETING OF DRUGS AND THEIR CONSEQUENCES

Ulrike Thoms

In June 1973 a meeting of the Special Market Research Committee was held at the pharmaceutical company Bayer. The foundation of this committee had been part of a large restructuring process of the firm, during which a department for pharmaceutical market research had been established. In June it was still busy implementing the new organization and taking stock of the firm's situation, which a member of the new committee summed up with the statement:

> At the moment 18,000 pharmaceutical products are on the market. The main target group of marketing activities is doctors as prescribers of the preparations. Problem: on average the German doctor is 53 years old, he knows 200 products, receives 29 written information notices per day and about 66 samples per week.[1]

The statement documents an enormous discrepancy between the roughly 18,000 products on the market and those prescribed on a more or less regular basis. Moreover it points at the high input of information on supposedly new drugs. Introducing new drugs was indeed a risky venture, and even more so as expenses for research and development as well as for marketing had skyrocketed in the second half of the twentieth century while the number of newly found substances had decreased. Of the many newly introduced drugs, only a few would become blockbusters and refinance research investment. The German pharmaceutical industry, which had formerly dominated the world market in pharmaceuticals, was now facing a 'technological gap' between Germany and the United States and a general feeling of lagging behind in technological and organizational development. Although the business executives of German companies realized their need for new, successful drugs, they feared failure; to overcome the crisis, they were therefore open to new methods of innovation management and new organization models.[2]

This paper asks for the role that cybernetics and the life cycle model played in this context. It will show that neither of them surfaced suddenly out of the blue but rather in the context of long and complicated processes that began in the late 1940s and the 1950s and lasted until the 1980s. The pharmaceutical industry did not simply take over these concepts and theories from economics. Instead it was actively and prominently involved in the development of strategic thinking and long-range planning from the very start. Activities were very much centred around the life cycle concept of pharmaceuticals. Surprisingly, this concept has rarely been evaluated in recent work on pharmaceutical marketing, although the existence of a product life cycle is widely accepted as a matter of course.[3]

The paper will show that the concept of the product life cycle was perceived first as key to the management of data in the pharmaceutical market and second as a tool to assess and fully exploit the commercial potential of drugs. The first section of this paper will thus pay particular attention to the role of innovation in the pharmaceutical business, and the second will turn to the concept of the role of cybernetics and systems research. A third chapter will then examine the implementation of these new approaches, while a fourth will examine the impact of the discussed processes on the codification of marketing knowledge and techniques. The conclusion will question the long-term effects of the previously discussed developments.

Innovation and its Associated Risk

Innovation and the novelty of products have always been a central argument for advertising in competitive markets. As innovation incorporates the idea of progress, it is also strongly associated with progress which, since the Enlightenment, has been imagined as being inherent to science and specifically to medicine.[4] In this perspective, science is expected to introduce new drugs and improve existing ones.[5] Based on this idea physicians and even critical consumer organizations have accepted the idea that advertising helps to spread important novelties.[6]

For pharmaceutical companies innovations have always been extremely important to demonstrate their research orientation, which distinguishes them from charlatans.[7] The only problem was that only a minority of newly introduced drugs became successful innovations that paid back the investments made in them, or, in the words of an employee at Bayer: 'every month a new product surfaces and either soon disappears or stagnates. The approximately one million marks that have been spent in massive propaganda are lost – as we can surely assume'.[8] How, then, could doctors be made to take notice of new products when they complained of the quantities of printed ads they received and threw them away unread?[9] In terms of new products, addressing doctors as researchers or scientists seemed to work best to make them hope for and expect new products. As put by a pharmacist at Bayer in November 1901, it would be excellent for the firm if a clinician, when meeting a firm representative in the street, would eagerly ask him: 'Do you have anything new for me?'[10]

From the 1920s on, the strong position of innovation was supported by economic theory. According to Joseph A. Schumpeter's very influential book of 1939, *Business Cycles*, economic development was driven only by innovation and the innovative entrepreneur.[11] He argued that innovation constituted the basis for an entrepreneur's monopoly in a specific field and allowed him to get outstanding income as he could charge higher prices, but, just as life was ruled by the cycle of birth and death, business relied on the cycle of production and destruction of products, making room for other, new, products.[12] Practically speaking, this idea had been present in drug marketing ever since, but, starting in the 1930s, it permeated the theoretical works on pharmaceutical marketing and branding.[13] Like Schumpeter, who believed in the creative power of the 'entrepreneur', proponents of the brand article believed that goods could simply be 'made' and made successful by advertising.

Nevertheless, the failure of innovations and products was a common experience in business. Risks were especially manifold in the drug business, and the cases of Contergan, Phentermin, Stalinon or Mediator are good illustrations of the possible consequences of risk taking. According to estimates, 70 to 90 per cent of all innovative products will fail, and only one out of three marketed products will pay back its investments.[14] Most new products are withdrawn from the market within their very first year of existence. Although a general historical awareness of the history of failure is growing, drug histories have neither taken notice of these 'failed' drugs, nor have they fully acknowledged that until the end of the 1960s most drug company sales were not of new but of old drugs.[15] Consequently, the history of the successful construction of pharmaceutical markets has almost exclusively concentrated on the trajectories of commercially successful drugs and especially of psychochemical drugs.[16]

Failure is nevertheless an important element in drug history, and firms have tried to learn from it. As long as the discovery of new therapeutic principles depended mainly on chance or on the research activity of external university professors, the flop of a newly introduced product was no big deal because investments in research and development were still low. This changed after World War II under the influence of the fierce competition of American and Swiss companies with new types of products such as antibiotics and psychotropics. When German firms finally returned to the market, they relied on licensed production of these new classes of drugs. They were all too aware that they needed new and innovative products to be able to compete. The only problem was to find them.

They therefore decided in the 1960s to invest massively in research. Schering built its own toxicological research centre in Bergkamen in 1961, and Bayer opened its rebuilt research centre in Wuppertal in 1967.[17] As a consequence there was an increase in the number of employees in Schering's research department. Their number had already stood at 619 in 1960, but it was multiplied by four by 1984, while their share of the total number of employees climbed from 12 to 23 per cent.[18] In parallel, the average expense per employee was multiplied by more than eight. According to a member survey of the German Pharmaceutical Industry Association firms spent 10 per cent of their expenses on research in 1973, and this figure rose to 14.5 in 1984.[19] In other words, firms were under increasing pressure to decide where to invest their money, whether in research or marketing. The developments brought structural changes that reduced the financial flexibility of the firms, even more so as 'expenses for advertising can be reduced at any time, while the steadily growing costs for research and sales and counselling mean trouble, because they very quickly become permanent in almost 100% of the cases'.[20] This made it even more important to make reasoned decisions.

Cybernetics, Systems and Communication Research

The answer to the problem of investments was forecasting and systems research, both of which made a remarkable career during the 1950s and 1960s against the background of future research. First applied in business economics, they soon made their way into research planning.[21]

These new concepts benefitted from cybernetics models. Theorized by Norbert Wiener in the 1940s, cybernetics was first applied to military research by the U.S. RAND Corporation during World War II, where it demonstrated its enormous potential to speed up research processes by analysing and planning the necessary measures carefully. Communication was the central feature in Wiener's concept, and it was not by accident that social scientists like Margaret Mead and important communication researchers like Paul Lazarsfeld and Claude Shannon took part in the Macy conferences, which furthered the spread of cybernetics as an interdisciplinary concept.[22] Different from earlier stimulus response models, which attributed colossal influence to mass media and advertising, cybernetics told a more complicated story and introduced quite a number of variables into communication research. The model made it possible to isolate, describe and analyse the many relations, circuits and loops between the different actors in the communication process. In fact, cybernetics and systems research made a remarkable career in post-war Germany and other European countries, especially in research planning, opinion and market research, and business administration and marketing, where they stimulated the mathematization of economic processes.[23]

It has gone almost unnoticed that although they reacted differently, pharmaceutical companies played a very important role in this process. Ciba, which for some of its activities worked indirectly through the Ciba Foundation, was one of the very active firms in this field. The foundation had been instituted in 1949 to 'promote international co-operation in medical and chemical research among scientists from all parts of the world'.[24] Starting in 1949, the foundation organized six to ten three-day symposia, three or four one-day study groups per year and several informal meetings at its house in London.[25] Over the years, the foundation organized about one hundred symposia on different topics, including the famous 1963 symposium, 'Man and his Future', which assembled some of the most distinguished scholars of the time, including Julian Huxley, Gregory Pincus, John B. S. Haldane, Joshua Lederberg and Albert Szent-Györgyi, who presented projections on the future of their research fields.[26] Starting in 1953, reports on these symposia were issued periodically while all the contributions to every symposium were published in edited volumes.[27] Covering almost every area of medical research, particularly pharmacological, most of the symposia charted scientific progress and the state of the art in one specific field of modern bioscientific research, such as toxaemias in pregnancy in 1950, the chemical structures of proteins, mammalian germ cells, drug resistance or the neurological basis of behaviour, to name just a few. On the occasion of its tenth anniversary Ciba published *Significant Trends in Medical Research*, a book intended to take stock containing representative work on modern biosciences and on methods of quantitative research.[28] Interest in research planning continued, as shown by publications from the symposia such as *Decision Making in National Science Policy* (Amsterdam: Elsevier, 1968), *Medical Research Systems in Europe* (Amsterdam: Elsevier, 1973) and *The Future as an Academic Discipline* (Amsterdam: Elsevier, 1975). As chairman of the latter symposium, the geneticist Conrad H. Waddington from the Institute of Animal Genetics in Edinburgh argued in his introduction: 'we can't escape from a whole lot of feedback circuits, interactions and non-linear effects. Thinking in terms purely of cause and effect in the old-fashioned way is totally inadequate in our present situation'.[29]

In fact, systems research helped to organize and systematize the existing massive bulk of information in such a way as to provide an overview of the relations between the actors and the different streams of information. Its promise was to improve assessment and coordination given the means and the aims, or, in other words, to provide the grounds to make reasoned decisions in an environment characterized by insecurity and an increasing risk of unwise investment and failure. It was by no means accidental that communication and opinion research gained momentum in exactly this situation.[30] What had dominated thus far had been the theory of mass society. Called the 'Hypodermic Needle Theory', it was rooted in a simple model of stimulus and response, arguing that stimuli necessarily caused effects, and the stronger the stimulus, the stronger the reaction to it.[31] For advertisers this meant the more advertising, the more the goods were sold. Companies who had run their advertising on the basis of such models, however, had had their own, less favourable experience as enormous advertising spending did not necessarily lead to high sales figures.[32] In this experience there was no direct link between the strength of the stimulus of advertising and the response, i.e., the sales or prescriptions. Firms had realized that advertising was a rather complicated and multi-staged communication process.[33] These experiences were confirmed by the results of the new discipline of mass communication research, which was driven from different fronts such as psychology, communication science and market research. Market research was extremely important as it contributed massively to the revenues of the many new research institutes.[34]

One of these, the Bureau of Applied Social Research, was run by the sociologist Paul Lazarsfeld. His studies of the presidential elections in the USA had not been able to confirm the otherwise assumed strong influence of propaganda on opinion.[35] This finding was ground breaking as it challenged the belief in the power of propaganda and advertising and their ability to manipulate people.[36] What Lazarsfeld and his research team found was that the media were only able to strengthen opinions and that communication did not only work directly but also through communication agents called 'opinion leaders', who were marked by their tendency to use the media massively and by a strong position in the community. These findings were probed in a series of four subsequent empirical studies, one of which examined the diffusion of a new antibiotic amongst doctors.[37]

The study was rooted in the institute's broader interest in the impact of personal relations on information behaviour, which also targeted doctors, especially as the pharmaceutical industry was a potent financier of studies. Members of the institute had published many studies in this field. Herbert Menzel, for example, had published a study on the flow of scientific information in the medical profession in 1954 and in 1959 his dissertation, 'Social Determinants of Physicians' Reactions to Innovations in Medical Practices'; a year later he published, together with Elihu Katz, a first summary of the institute's work in the paper 'Social Relations and Innovation in the Medical Profession: The Epidemiology of a New Drug'.[38] Unnoticed by the working group around Lazarsfeld – and by many historians – the economist and marketer Theodore Caplow had already published a very similar study in 1952 in the *Harvard Business Review*.[39] The latter was widely acknowledged by business economists, who were increasingly interested in the effectiveness of promotion.[40] A third player in the game was Raymond A. Bauer, a professor of business studies and Caplow's colleague at Harvard University, who was generally interested in forecasting questions and particularly interested in marketing.[41] Bauer used the results as an entry point to the question of how information was used to reduce risk.[42] These studies were in fact not so much used by companies to assess the cost-and-effect relationship in their pharmaceutical promotion as for the development of a theoretical communication model.[43] The specific merits of these studies were to point to the 'entire web of potentially relevant relationships within which the doctor is embedded', to know about the information sources and their impact on doctors' willingness to accept the associated risks of using newly introduced drugs.[44] This knowledge was extremely useful to marketing experts for optimizing the choice of communication channels and speeding up innovation processes. General interest in these themes was testified to in Roger Everett's seminal study *Diffusion of Innovations*, published in 1962.[45] Everett's book summarized the state of the art and helped to popularize the above-mentioned studies on doctors.

German firms began to look out for planning methods in the 1960s and showed particular interest in the somewhat bizarre ideas of futurology and prognosis. Bayer's house journal *Bayer-Berichte,* for example, published an article on the 'art of prognosis' ('Die Kunst der Prognose') in 1969. This essay was written by one of the most distinguished German scientists, Carl Friedrich von Weizsäcker, a member of highly ranked state commissions on research policy and planning.[46] Three years later, the systems researcher Karl Steinbuch published the article 'Futurologie auf dem Weg zur Systemtheorie' (futurology on the way to systems theory) in the same journal, and six years after that another relevant article was published there written by Heinz Maier-Leibnitz, the chairman of the German Research Association (Deutsche Forschungsgemeinschaft, DFG).[47] In other words, cybernetics made its way into the German pharmaceutical industry and was used in it to reorganize the firms and to work out promotion plans.[48] Underscoring the usefulness of feedback loops, the firms organized existing information and exploited it with the statistical methods of econometrics, thus analysing the past and extrapolating it to the future in order to assess coming developments and to decide on the possible need for action.[49]

The Life Cycle Concept

It was precisely in this context that the 'life cycle concept' was developed and applied to drugs.[50] The concept incorporated the idea of the business cycle and resonated with physicians' prescientific impressions of the permanent replacement of older drugs by newer, improved drugs that were expected to work better and have fewer side effects.[51]

The basic idea of the concept was rather simple. Theodore Levitt, a professor of business economics at Harvard, defined the life cycle of products as the 'history of their passing through certain recognizable stages'.[52] A citation analysis from the Web of Science shows that this model is still popular today as the number of publications that use the concept is still on the rise.[53] Levitt, however, aimed at broadening the perspective of business executives to the many factors influencing their sales figures and to their task to 'create and capitalize on growth opportunities'.[54] Publications visualized these stages in idealized curves that usually showed the phases of introduction, growth, maturity and decline. It was fully acknowledged that different marketing methods were needed for the different phases of the life cycle. A proper assessment of life cycles was seen as a means to plan the marketing process and to choose the appropriate promotional means.[55] In 1963, William Cox published an extensive study that examined the usability of this model for the pharmaceutical industry. Based on an analysis of the life cycle of 754 drugs that had been introduced in the United States between 1955 and 1960 he classified the drugs according to the shape of their life curve and found six different types.[56] There were: the standard bell-shaped curve with its phases of introduction, growth and decline; a curve showing steadily increasing revenues; a curve that showed a fast take-off followed by a quick and steady decline; a curve that was, in fact, a line showing steady sales figures; and the standard curve that, close to its end, moved downwards before taking a new upswing, marking the 'second life' of the drug. The last, sixth type showed a similar development, but with decline starting already at half of the life span.[57] These curves were clearly idealized, but they were based on accumulated experiences, and they helped to forecast the further developments of a drug after its recent development had been analysed and compared with the ideal curves. Executives could then decide whether to withdraw a drug or invest some money to influence the curve, as, for example, to give the drug a second life. In any case the curves helped to visualize the recent developments of a drug and to estimate its future development. Ending marketing expenses for products that were already dead helped to save money.

The model was also used by European firms, most remarkably the Swiss firm, Ciba, which commissioned a study on the life cycles of its drugs from its employee, René Abt, who had written his dissertation on the subject.[58] Abt's study was clearly inspired by futurology and cybernetics, as well as studies on American opinion research, and he obviously saw these as a means to plan and steer products to success.[59] Remarkably enough, this publication provided some insight on Ciba's performance as well as on its marketing practices, though the figures he gave were somewhat vague as a way of paying tribute to business secrets. While the first part of his book presented the state of the art, the second part discussed his empirical findings for forty of Ciba's products, which were analysed with regard to turnover, advertising expenses and profit margins. What he found was that new drugs reached their maximum sales figures during the first eighteen to thirty months of their life, while the decisive phase was between the sixth and twelfth months. Only a very small number of drugs were economically successful in the sense that sales actually covered the investment costs within the first three years of their existence. This underscored the importance of choosing the right marketing strategy and of promoting the drug just enough through the right channels.

To measure the effect of promotion on the monthly sales of products, Abt used a complicated quantitative marketing model that had been developed at Ciba to examine the fate of eleven different drugs more closely.[60] The work resulted in a hierarchy of promotional tools: in the case of seven products (63 per cent of them), he proved that samples had the highest impact on sales figures and increased them by a factor of five to fifteen. In contrast, he found a statistical effect of journal advertising for only five of the examined products. The result for mailings was similar, though a bit lower. In his studies of communication research, his findings on the effect of sales representatives came as the biggest surprise: in only three cases was he able to prove any influence at all, while in most cases the returns did not even cover the expenses of this category of personnel. This contradicted the long-established promotional practices of the pharmaceutical industry, which spent about two-thirds of its promotional budgets on its salesmen.[61] Nevertheless, the findings of communication research were so well established that Abt did not dare to challenge their core position. Instead he pointed to former findings of Coleman, Katz and others and underscored that representatives made the drug known in a first phase of promotion, while the decision to use it was made later, after the doctors had studied scientific publications. As the representative's visit thus only prepared the physician's decision, there might not have been any quantitative relationship between the representative's activities and the turnover at all. On the other hand, given the high cost of the sales force, a suboptimal use of the representative would have worse results than the wrong use of other promotional tools. Abt argued that success depended on four main factors: first, addressing the right physicians; second, promoting the drugs wanted by doctors; third, doing so with arguments relevant to them; and fourth, doing this at the right point in time and in a psychologically appropriate manner.[62]

Abt nonetheless remained concerned and irritated by the weak impact of representatives. He concluded that it obviously made no sense to use them as simple advertising tools. He thus proposed to switch their field of activities to information, to visit only those doctors for which the visit would bear some influence, and to integrate their needs, for example by visiting a physician as often as the doctor needed them to solve his problems instead of just presenting product information. To do so, the reps would need thorough and profound education, but, as Abt hoped, this would free them from the odium of advertising and might help to create goodwill toward them amongst the doctors.

The Codification of Marketing Techniques in the Drug Business

Abt's book formed part of the development of pharmaceutical marketing as an applied science with its own specific methods and tools. When his book appeared on the market, major changes were underway. As it was put by an employee at Bayer in the 1970s:

> In the past the best administration of the existing was at stake. Situations changed relatively slowly and seldom, so that one could always manage the reactions that were caused by the changes. We could manage because our capacities were sufficiently free ... thanks to on-going innovation. But this policy has been basically withdrawn, and the situation in the field of production is typical of this.[63]

He went on to explain that it was henceforth necessary to commercialize new products in an ever-decreasing time span, so that all the information processes were to be sped up. Above all, it was necessary not to act passively, but to plan all activities actively. This was exactly what Abt aimed for. In the following years, marketing practices were codified in handbooks, and systematic planning became part of the entrepreneurs' toolbox. The first German handbook of pharmaceutical marketing was co-authored by Abt and Harald Friesewinkel, a well-established Swiss marketer.[64] It started with an extensive discussion of the life cycle concept, from which it developed a model for the marketing of pharmaceuticals. Walter Gehrig's handbook of 1987 followed this same scheme of drawing on practical experiences in the field.[65] Like Abt, he had earned his PhD in this field with a study on the role of central product management in the pharmaceutical industry.[66] Publications were convinced that none of the theoretical efforts would have any effect if they did not result in organizational changes.[67] Significantly, the structures were presented by flow charts, as they had been established by cybernetics. Furthermore, firms now presented their new organization flow charts as examples for others.[68]

Executives of German firms had been massively unsatisfied with the compartmentalization of their different departments. It was not until the late 1950s that Bayer felt the need to change its somewhat messy organization in order to coordinate the many different tasks. Though a system of different conferences had tried to organize information exchange at the director's level since around 1900, there was no place for coordination and communication in the lower and middle levels of the company.[69] As a response to the disadvantages of such an arrangement, organization by product and by division was introduced. The establishment of a new information system and the development of an integrated planning system formed part of this process. By taking these measures, research operations were expected to help to increase the flexibility and speed of decisions, to set up manageable and forceful areas of accountability, to integrate sales, production, technology and research as operational units at different levels (lines, divisions, commissions and conferences), and to define the allocation of tasks, responsibilities and competences more clearly. In addition, the new organization aimed at increasing delegation of responsibilities at all levels in order to lighten the burden on top management.[70] Reorganization began with the establishment in 1958 of project management groups whose task was to coordinate work on specific products and, notably, their marketing.[71] From then on, scientists and administrative employees, who had been ranked differently thus far, had equal status. In 1966 research and development were reorganized to optimize the flow of information, coordination and the use of means.[72] In this context the research commissions were to monitor the market situation in certain fields, rank new projects according to their importance, develop plans for future activities and oversee their completion. Three years later, in 1969, product committees were introduced to coordinate all activities related to certain products. Netplans were set up for supervision, in which the different work steps were fixed for the introduction of new products. At the same time, new priorities were set that were oriented towards perceived consumer needs, now registered well beyond market surveys.[73] In 1969, the marketing department had already conducted an opinion poll amongst 10,000 physicians. The same year saw the establishment of a circle of medical advisers to discuss research needs and doctors' information needs.[74] At the same time, research efforts were increased and a new research centre was built. These changes were codified in an organizational handbook.[75] Contacts were made with university professors in order to learn more about the state's research planning activities and their impact on the collaboration between the industry and the university.[76]

All organizational and economic activities were summarized in the staff organization (*Stabsbereich*), while all scientific marketing activities were now under the responsibility of the newly introduced line organization.[77] The 'Scientific Marketing' department then included scientific market research, scientific information and product advice, and was organized along different product groups. This organization allowed close collaboration between marketing, the medical department, and research and development. All in all, experiences with this kind of organization were positive, though it turned out that the product group differentiation was too detailed and that product managers needed to be given more responsibilities.[78]

On 12 January 1970 a meeting of Bayer's 'chief ideologists' with representatives from other pharmaceutical firms was held during which the problems of advertising and rising criticism of advertising were discussed. The pharmaceutical industry had begun to monitor its public image regularly and launch systematic image campaigns.[79] Firms established departments that were to keep track of general developments in the economic and social system. The now central positioning of marketing in the firm's organization turned out to be by no means easy.

There was passive resistance and there were many conflicts between the different departments and divisions. As the board of directors had been very clear about the need to keep track of any of these developments as well as of general business trends, it established a special market research commission (*Fachkommission Marktforschung*) that was subordinated to the board of directors.[80] The commission met for the first time on 28 February 1973 and considered the state of market research and the consequences of a market-oriented organization of the firm, the specific activities of the central marketing department, as well as general questions about the strict market orientation of company management, such as the use of prognosis and its methods.[81] In its work it followed up on the general trends of the pharmaceutical market and particularly the health system, and its structures and changes.[82] To an ever-greater extent, the protocols of this commission underscored the importance of research for planning, developing and surveying research projects in order to oversee and evaluate their potential, and for making reasoned strategic decisions.[83] One of the tools and theories discussed was the life cycle. The presenter concluded that its value was not so much that it facilitated a reasoned decision on the strategies to be used, but that it had a particular ability to control the development of a specific product and its economic evaluation.[84] And so it was incorporated into the toolbox.

Conclusion

This paper has described and analysed the reception and implementation of cybernetics and systems research, and particularly the development and implementation of the concept of the life cycle of pharmaceuticals in the pharmaceutical industry. It has shown that these approaches matched the needs of the troublesome 1940s quite well and in a productive way, and helped to bring companies closer to the markets. The overall aim was to reduce the number of failed drug innovations and thus to balance the relationship between investments in the research and development of drugs in a way that achieved the highest profit possible.

Was this tool really of any use at all? Philipp Aumann in his book on the history of cybernetics in West Germany judged that cybernetics were no more than a fashion that at some point silently disappeared.[85] To his regret, no scientific discipline such as 'cybernetics' was established. Consequently, he rated cybernetics as a fad that had quickly lost impact and relevance after the 1970s. Economists who had evaluated the value of the life cycle concept criticized it as early as 1969 for having too little empirical evidence to support it: there was no such thing, they stated, as the ideal life cycle.[86] Some went so far as to advise: 'Forget the Product Life Cycle Concept!'[87] The ending of the theoretical discussion seems to point in the same direction as the fact that the *Journal of Historical Research in Marketing* did not value the product life cycle as a key concept in marketing. So is the concept obsolete?

I would argue that this is not the case. The life cycle concept has not passed away. In fact it is still almost everywhere in business, though practically invisible, and forms part of all introductions to marketing and business theory. Rather, I propose to look at its development according to the categories of Norbert Elias's studies on the civilization process. Elias has argued that the thematization of codes of behaviour did not wane over time because the rules were disregarded. As he explained, the opposite was true. Their wide acceptance made it unnecessary to discuss and disseminate them further through books and pamphlets.[88] The very same seems to be true for cybernetics and the life cycle concept, which are as active as ever, albeit behind the scenes and despite the flood of publications starting in the 1960s having somewhat dried up. The life cycle concept has nonetheless remained, as well as the ideas behind it: even though doubts have arisen, it was able to grasp relevant ongoing developments correctly. Abt was well aware that it was not its now hotly contested reliability of prognosis that constituted the value of the concept, but its contribution to the organization of firms and to the development of strategies. 'Since we have used the probability curve for active substance requirements', Abt stated more than ten years after he finished his dissertation:

> the most valuable result has not been that we now get any better single number, such as mean, mode or any other figure, but that we have the curve at all. No longer do production people and market forecasters accuse each other because a figure is 'wrong'. Both sides are aware of the uncertainties and therefore their dialogue has become more constructive. Decisions are made and the results are reviewed in light of the curve, which represents our best judgement when action is required. Thus our principal benefit has been an improvement in the quality and coordination of management efforts in production planning and resource allocation.[89]

In fact, similar organizational charts – with feedback loops and circuits – have moved from business practice to society. They are the theoretical foundation of health economics, which has developed to help NGOs and state bodies get a better understanding of the mechanisms behind the system in general and the pharmaceutical market in particular. It was worked out in the same context that made firms look out for new tools to assess the options of new drugs, a context that was determined by increasing competition and increasing financial pressure, if not the perceived beginning of a crisis in the German health system. This crisis made it all the more necessary to look out for methods and ways to steer and reduce health expenses. Tellingly, one of the most important proponents of the development of health economics in Germany, Philipp Herder-Dorneich, had published the book *Soziale Kybernetik* (social cybernetics) as early as 1965.[90] In 1973, the Institute for Health System Research in Kiel was founded by Fritz

Beske and the sickness funds set up their own scientific institute, which was administered by Ulrich Geissler. The federal ministry for research and technology, Bundesministerium für Forschung und Technologie, launched its first, systems-related research programme to enhance research and development in health in 1978, while Ulrich Eimeren established an institute for medical computer science and systems research (MEDIS) in 1980, to name only a few of the early institutes to show continued developments.[91]

In other words, cybernetics models have become a multipurpose tool for analysing and steering the health and drug market. While economists and pharmaceutical companies were at the very forefront of its theoretical development and used it to avoid unwise investment and to extend their profits, health policy took over the very same model as a tool to analyse the ongoing processes and to set limits to an ever-expanding health market. But it remains questionable if using this model is the right way to solve, or at least steer, the increasing problems of a profit-orientated drug and health market. The use of this model inhibits any new beginning and the development of alternatives. Instead it transforms the entrepreneurial logic with its emphasis on innovation and the market, business and company structures into an attempt to get hold of the devastating increase in spending and the constant extension of services, which is driven forward by industry and professionals for their own sake.

3 MARKETING EPIDEMICS: WHEN ANTIBIOTIC PROMOTION STIMULATES RESISTANT BACTERIA

Quentin Ravelli

Over the last decade, bacterial resistance emerged as a global health issue: the European Center for Disease Prevention and Control (ECDC) reported 25,000 deaths resulting from antibiotic-resistant bacteria in Europe in 2009.[1] In the United States alone, among 90,000 hospital-related deaths estimated by the Infectious Disease Society of America, 70 per cent are caused by drug-resistant bacteria,[2] and according to the Alliance for the Prudent Use of Antibiotics, doctors face 900,000 antibiotic-resistant infections every year.[3] What used to be an intimate controversy, born in the 1950s and confined to hospital communities and scientific networks until the 1980s, has become a worldwide political and social issue in the first decade of the twenty-first century. Following Polish epistemologist Ludwik Fleck, we may say that bacterial resistance, once an exclusively scientific fact enclosed within 'esoteric circles', has become a widely publicized 'exoteric' problem.[4] Among recent examples that made the newspapers headlines is the New Delhi super-resistant bacteria NDM-1, insensible to last-resort intravenous antibiotics, and the German *E. coli* outbreak,[5] which triggered diplomatic quarrels between Spain, Germany and Egypt over the origins of the mutant micro-organism. Apart from these fluctuating media coverage and political skirmishes, both focusing on isolated cases, many physicians from all over the world are now facing clinical 'dead end' situations that are not limited to emergency care units, prisons and locker rooms, but threaten larger outpatient communities.

Since the early 1950s, antibiotics overprescription has been criticized: Maxwell Finland, an American expert on infectious diseases, was already suspecting 'untherapeutic prescription' to arouse resistance to penicillin, terramycin and aureomycin among staphylococci, even if he considered it 'difficult, of course, to say whether these phenomena were a consequence of the widespread use of antibiotics or merely a temporary and transient increase'.[6] Sixty-two years later, the causal link between consumption and resistance is well established.[7] But what are the social and economic reasons for this persistent situation? What is the role of scientific marketing by pharmaceutical corporations? One of the main causes of this looming pandemic is a global antibiotic overuse, partly sustained by corporate advertising strategies. These strategies are driven by the two main engines of scientific marketing: biochemical and clinical research results used as promotion to build antibiotic markets; and economic, psychological and sociological methods used to increase patients' and doctors' consumption of antibiotics. These two sides of scientific marketing constantly intertwine, in such a way that marketing and science are part and parcel of the same activity. Here, we shall analyse how scientific marketing shapes the issue of resistant bacteria in favor of antibiotic prescribing: it does so first by *subordinating antibiotics use values to their exchange values*, and second by *emphasizing the notion of individual efficiency over the notion of global safety*. Each antibiotic can therefore appear more as the solution to resistance than the source of resistance, even if they all contribute, globally, to worsening the same problem.

After a brief introduction to the global social structure of this medical dead end in the first section, we will turn to France, where a particularly strong antibiotic market is linked to high resistance rates, and where I gathered first-hand sociological information during fieldwork at Sanofi, the largest European pharmaceutical corporation, in the second section. But public health policies, dealing with powerful marketing strategies and a lack of research and development, did not find a proper solution to resistant bacteria, as indicated in the third section.

From Darwin to Marketing: Social Structures of a 'Medical' Dead End

Biologically speaking, resistance consists of a Darwinian mechanism known by physicians at least since the seventeenth International Congress of Medicine in 1913, when Paul Ehrlich, four decades before the massive consumption of antibiotics, explained we had to 'hit hard and fast' against pathogenic micro-organisms, otherwise they would naturally develop resistances. Later on, in the years following the discovery of penicillin in 1928, Alexander Fleming noticed that bacteria developed resistances when the dose or the length of penicillin treatment were insufficient: under the selective pressure of antibiotics, any population of bacteria will be reduced to resistant individuals which will grow and spread their resistance traits. In 1942, scientists described the first resistance to penicillin G (marketed in 1941), in 1961 to methicillin (marketed in 1960), in 1983 to beta-lactam (marketed in 1981), in 1946 to streptomycin (marketed in 1946), and in 1987 to vancomycin (marketed in 1958).[8] After a few years or a few decades, every antibiotic launched to the market systematically plants the seeds of its own failure.

Since this golden age of antibiotic discovery, the phenomenon of resistance is more precisely understood. We know bacteria can exchange mobile genetic materials, such as plasmids, and therefore transform the statistical hazard of natural resistance into the global health threat of acquired resistance. If the 1970s, 1980s and 1990s had been the decades of 'complacency', 're-emergence' and the 'dawning realization' of bacterial multi-resistance threat, the 2000s were to be the years of 'reactivity'.[9] Many countries have then launched public health campaigns: 'search and destroy' in the Netherlands, 'antibiotics are not automatic' in France, and World Health Day 2011 dedicated to antibiotic resistance instigated by the World Health Organization, which acknowledged 'an inherent conflict of interest between the legitimate business goals of manufacturers and the social, medical and economic needs of providers and the public to select and use drugs in the most rational way'.[10]

Within these global and national public campaigns, three main lines of argument started to emerge: we need to control resistance mechanisms; we need to find new antibiotics; and we need to limit the use of old antibiotics. To control, to push and to pull – but on each front of the fight against multi-resistance, these public campaigns hit a solid wall. The first wall is the *exacerbation of a natural process in a context of hospital crisis*. With a global crisis affecting public budgets and healthcare systems, an efficient control and monitoring of resistance dissemination is not considered as a political priority, despite urgent medical needs, because the costs of detection, training in hygiene measures and patient confinement are too high for tight hospital economies.

This healthcare crisis wouldn't be so acute if new antibiotics, with novel mechanisms of action against resistant pathogens, were launched every year. The resistances created by older generations of antibiotics would be defeated by the newer generation. But the second wall precisely consists in the *increasing weakness of antibiotic research and development* (R&D): considering antibiotics as one of their less profitable products, pharmaceutical corporations have diminished their scientific activities aiming at designing new antibiotics. The result of this industrial choice is clear: from 1983 to 1987, sixteen new antibiotics were registered by the FDA, only seven from 1998 to 2002, and two from 2008 to 2011.[11] The consequence of this pipeline shrinkage is that doctors often have to deal with bacteria with resistance traits that cannot be fought by any new antibiotic. From a capitalist point of view, developing an antibiotic is not as economically profitable as developing drugs against chronic diseases such as cancer, diabetes, mental or musculoskeletal disorders.[12]

This dry pipeline wouldn't be so dramatic without the third wall of the dead end, *the wall of antibiotic misuse and overconsumption*. In many countries, antibiotics are massively used as growth factors in agriculture and prescribed *larga manu*, or inappropriately, by physicians: many of them prescribe antibiotics for self-solving infections or for viral infections, antibiotics known to be inefficient on the targeted pathogen, antibiotics with a too broad spectrum, or antibiotics that should be kept as a second line treatment to avoid new emerging resistances. All these medical behaviours increase a selective pressure accelerating the Darwinian process responsible for the dissemination of resistant genes.

Many factors can be evoked to explain this situation, including the pressure exerted by patients to get an antibiotic or the lack of independent continuous medical training in antibiotherapy. One factor, however, is more important than the others because it relies on powerful networks of trained employees paid according to physicians' levels of prescriptions: antibiotic promotion by a pharmaceutical sales representative, supported by advertising of clinical trials in scientific reviews, and designed by marketers. The marketing strategies for Zithromax, Augmentin and Biaxin illustrate this scientific marketing game. In 2000, Pfizer launched a wide advertising campaign for Zithromax – azithromycin – and by 2003 this antibiotic became the fifth most commonly prescribed medicine in the US, with 1.5 billion sales.[13] Pfizer's marketing strategy included direct-to-consumer ads, a controversial pre-school television show, a distribution of thousands of plush zebra toys to physicians – for 'letter Z as in Zithromax' – and even the donation of a real zebra, Max, to the San Francisco zoo. On the global market, this antibiotic was competing with Pfizer's 'Bix the bulldog' designed in 1996 for Biaxin – clarithromycin – by whimsical ad icons creator Abelson-Taylor, and with GlaxoSmithKline's 'Auggie Froggy' for Augmentin – amoxicillin-clavulanate. Prescribed for infections like bronchitis, tonsillitis and pneumonia, which don't required antibiotic treatment most of the time, these three antibiotics are produced, distributed and promoted on a worldwide scale, and contribute to the global development of resistant strains.

However, the scientific information disseminated by sales representatives doesn't mention this social and medical issue of antibiotic resistance. Far from being understood and depicted by marketers as the *source* of resistance, antibiotics may even be explicitly presented to physicians as a *solution* to it: in 2003 an Australian advertisement for Augmentin features a young professional-looking woman under the headline 'Sue wants to recover in time to see her project launched. For Sue's sake take a closer look at resistance. Augmentin delivers first time'.[14] Such a presentation of antibiotic resistance misleadingly suggests this product should be used as first-line therapy to avoid resistance, even though a smaller message details the 'restricted benefit' of the drug: 'Augmentin should be used in infections where resistance to amoxicillin is suspected or proven'. Here, promotional materials reflect the conflict between the use value and exchange value of antibiotics, but also the fact that the exchange value shapes the use value. It results in a confusing message in which the chemical properties of the drugs are not clearly said to be responsible for bacterial resistance, but instead appear to be an efficient tool against it. The individual efficiency of each drug overshadows the global harm to safety.

As we will see in the case of the antibiotic market in France, where antibiotic consumption is one of the highest in the world, this situation cannot be analysed from within doctors' offices only, as if individual practitioners should be personally held accountable. It is a collective socio-economic mechanism in which the role of market-driven scientific data is an essential cog. For this reason, we have to look at the manufacturer's side, to understand this situation from the point of view of pharmaceutical corporations that have an economic interest in maintaining some of the factors responsible for antibiotic overuse and misuse.

Market Forces and Antibiotic Over-Prescription in France

Pharmaceutical representatives, whose role consists in implementing marketing strategies conceived at commercial head offices, have to convince doctors they should prescribe more of their products. Sociologically speaking, we can consider this activity as a way to *influence medical habits*, or, more precisely doctors' 'dispositions', to use a term coined by French sociologist Bernard Lahire; a disposition is the 'result of an (explicit or implicit) passed socialization, it can only be constituted on the long run, i.e., through repetition of relatively similar experiences'.[15] In the case of pharmaceutical promotion, many medical habits are not only generated by physicians themselves, or from within scientific fields, but come from outside: they are the fruits of long-lasting commercial strategies designed by marketing departments, where marketers try to shape specific therapeutic use values that can favour the exchange value of pharmaceutical commodities.

Sales Representatives and Medical Ears: 'Share-of-Voice' Pressure as a Driving Force on Prescriptions

In 2012, 16,043 sales representatives were responsible for 215,865 physicians countrywide, which means an average of one sales representative for every thirteen physicians.[16] In only one pharmaceutical corporation, Sanofi, 1,927 medical sales representatives were travelling from one general practitioner to the other, at an average rate of 5 or 6 visits per day, to maintain or modify their prescriptive dispositions; and, among them, 633 were dedicated to antibiotics, analgesics and rheumatology.[17] To be sure that these promotional efforts were efficient, marketers relied on data collected by Cabinet Antoine Minkowski, a subsidiary of Cegedim. This private firm was devoted to 'pharmaceutical intelligence', i.e., to the statistical analysis of sales on behalf of pharmaceutical corporations, relying on panels of physicians and considered to be one of the most reliable sources of information concerning the qualitative impact of pharmaceutical promotion on prescribing levels. According to these statistics, for twenty-six antibiotics, only on the French market and for the first semester of 2010, pharmaceutical sales representatives went to see doctors 743,199 times. For some antibiotics, the number of visits were higher than others: in June 2010, doctors were visited 19,605 times for Izilox by Bayer, 26,055 times for Monozeclar by Abbott, 34,470 for Pyostacine by Sanofi, and 4,025 for Zithromax by Pfizer. One category used in these statistical reports, called the 'share of voice', shows that one of the ways to measure marketing activity is not only based on the market share in volume or turnover, but on the *number of times physicians hear about one product when compared to the others*. In June 2010, the 'share of voice' was 12.3 per cent for Izilox, 16.4 per cent for Monozeclar, 21.7 per cent for Pyostacine and 2.5 per cent for Zithromax. In other words, competition is established between pharmaceutical corporations to *capture physicians' listening time and maintain or change their prescriptive dispositions*: Bayer, Sanofi, Abbott and Pfizer, among others, try to prevent competitors from building exclusive links with prescribers.

Other firms, like Glaxo for Augmentin, were not mentioned in these statistics because their drugs were not promoted anymore. The antibiotic market changes rapidly: from 2009 to 2010, some products disappeared, like Haxifal, and others entered the market for the first time, like Texodil.[18] For Pyostacine, even if the overall number of visits declined from 135,514 to 126,026 between the first semester of 2009 and the first semester of 2010, the 'share of voice' slightly increased, from 16.7 per cent to 17 per cent. The level of contact with doctors has been kept: in the small world of French antibiotics, 'Pyostacine voices' remain strongly heard. However, while being heard is one thing, being listened to is another – we may ask whether all these visits are effective? Do physicians prescribe the drug the way they are told to by sales representatives, without considering that these visits will increase the global risk of bacterial resistance? One way to understand this is to focus on a case study, like Pyostacine, a brand name for pristinamycin, and try to explain what indications the marketers target, and if the volumes of prescription evolve accordingly.

From Skin to Lungs: A Promotional Shift for an Old Antibiotic

From 1973 to the end of the 1980s, pristinamycin was used for skin infections and then for ear, nose and throat (ENT) infections, but only occasionally for lung infections. In a promotional clip shown to sales representatives in the 1980s, where an explorer called 'Specy Jones' discovers pristinamycin, the dermatological medical identity is clearly emphasized: by mere chance, the lonesome heroic figure covers a wound with a red-coloured soil sample he has found while running away from Indians in an Argentinian forest – this is how the marketing department was depicting the product at that time. But over the years pristinamycin became so firmly rooted in the market of skin infections and was so widely prescribed by general practitioners for cutaneous indications that its sales couldn't increase any more. It had reached a sort of ceiling, a point of saturation where only a qualitative transformation could reinitiate a marketing progress. Thus marketing managers, relying on their 'chief product managers' – marketers in charge of one product – tried to modify the image of this product. The best commercial leverage was then identified within broncho-pulmonary infections. In order to increase pristinamycin's market, the main strategy was to manufacture a new medical identity. To keep a classical political economist's terms, the new 'use value' of the product had to improve its 'exchange value'.[19] This strategy resulted in a clear progression of broncho-pulmonary prescriptions:

Table 3.1: Structure and evolution of pristinamycin market by therapeutic indication

	2002, Trimester 1		2010, Trimester 1		Increase	
	Volume	Percentage	Volume	Percentage	Volume	Percentage
Total ENT (ear, nose and throat) infections	130,902	41.4%	205,592	42.2%	74,689	57%
BP (broncho-pulmonary) infections	50,172	15.9%	106,634	21.9%	56,462	112.5%
Skin infections	122,510	38.8%	162,542	33.3%	40,032	32.6%
Others	12,390	3.9%	12,717	2.6%	327	2.6%
Total	315,974	100.0%	487,485	100.0%	171,511	54.2%

Source: Intercontinental Marketing Services (IMS) Health, 2010.

This shift of pristinamycin towards a new market, although not finished in 2010, proved successful: from the first trimester of 2002 to the first trimester of 2010, total pristinamycin prescriptions for broncho-pulmonary infections increased by 112.5 per cent – but only by 57 per cent for ear, nose and throat infections and 32.6 per cent for skin infections. Even if other factors may have been important, this result is a good indication that pharmaceutical marketing uses the *scientific plasticity of commodities* as a means to find new markets. But this plasticity is also dependent upon the other related medicines which interact individually on each other and collectively on the whole market, constantly breaking and rebuilding links between infections and antibiotics, diseases and treatments, the art of diagnostic and the power to cure. Of course, long-established images play an important role, too. But they don't remain exactly the same, as marketers tend to renew the slogans and advertising iconographies of even the oldest antibiotics. But antibiotic marketing is not only a science that deals with each medicine individually. On the contrary, the 'strategic plan' elaborated for each antibiotic is profoundly influenced by other products. In the case of the pristinamycin market, for instance, the lives of Ketek and Orelox were interacting.

A Scandal and a 'Patent Cliff' Stimulate an Old Antibiotic

Pharmaceutical marketing is not a professional activity each 'chief product manager' plays individually. It is a collective game: every product has shifting borders that are constantly moved around according to two distinct mechanisms. The first one is due to medical problems that can occur to an antibiotic when strong secondary effects are discovered and hinder the commercial success of a medicine, sometimes after a scandal that can tarnish a drug's reputation forever – this is what happened with Ketek in 2006, after the new drug was found to cause severe liver injury, liver failure and even death, while clinical trials were considered to be 'fraudulent' by the FDA, which impacted global markets. The second one is the result of an economic phenomenon colloquially called a 'patent cliff', i.e., the sharp decline of revenue resulting from a patent expiration, which is what happened with Orelox: its sales plummeted after it lost its protection against competitors. Here, we can see how these two processes can affect the sales of pristinamycin.

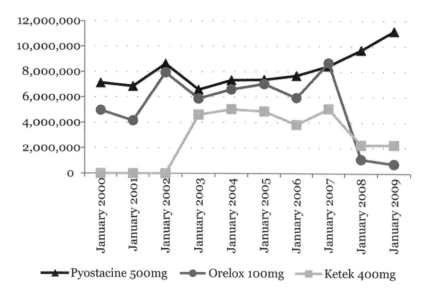

Figure 3.1: Marketing antibiotics: a collective game.

Source: Groupement pour l'Élaboration et la Réalisation de Statistiques (GERS), 2010. Launched on the market in July 2002, Ketek reached 6.4 millions sales in February 2005, before falling down to 1.8 million in February 2008. Orelox, generified, is not promoted anymore, and its sales continue to plummet. Pristinamycin benefitted from these market failures (patent cliff and health-care scandal). It reached its peak sales of above 11 million units in 2008.

For Pyostacine as well as for other antibiotics, marketing tries to change therapeutic indications to fill vacuums created by other products. Over the years, doctors' dispositions, following scientific marketing, may change as they move from one product to another. This mechanism illustrates how, according to Peter Conrad, 'medicalization is more driven by commercial and market interests than by professional claims-makers'.[20] Peter Conrad coined the expression 'shifting engines of medicalization' to describe the role played by these extra-medical influences in transforming medical activities, and the case study of pristinamycin highlights one of these engines, encapsulated in a corporate strategy where therapeutic indications are incorporated within scientific marketing. In this process, although Sanofi's marketing department never considered resistant bacteria as a problem involving fewer prescriptions of their antibiotics, bacterial resistance was frequently mentioned as an issue by doctors and sales representatives in the field.

Second-Line versus First-Line: Two Ways to Prescribe the Same Antibiotic

Criticism of antibiotic overuse is not new. In 1951, the infectious diseases specialist Maxwell Finland was already questioning specific therapeutic usages, such as systematic 'prophylactic use' or 'combined use' of antibacterial agents. He considered the attempt to treat with penicillin 'all people throughout the entire season when respiratory disease are prevalent' to be 'without any value', and opposed the combination of several antibiotics at the same time because of high risks of secondary effects due to uncontrolled drug interactions.[21] Today, these two uses are widely considered inappropriate, but the controversy concerning the definition of misuse hasn't disappeared – it has only been displaced, and lies within new interstices of scientific uncertainties. For instance, it revolves around the opportunity of undocumented or probabilistic treatment in respiratory tract infections, when no rapid diagnostic test has proved the existence of a bacterial origin, and around the choice of a first-line or second-line treatment: many doctors think some antibiotics should be used only when others have failed, so that bacteria will not develop too many resistances. This second question is essential because the misuse of second-line antibiotics as first-line treatment may lead to increased rates of resistance against some antibiotics that should be kept in reserve, just in case other antibiotics are not useful any more. If second-line treatments are not used only *after* another treatment has failed, then a whole collective strategy against resistance that is undermined.

Here, the problem is that the medical guidelines and empiric conceptions of physicians concerning the importance to keep certain antibiotics as second-line treatments often contradict corporate goals. Thus, medical directors within pharmaceutical corporations try to influence guidelines, and marketers often try to convert physicians to a more frequent use of second-line antibiotics as first-choice therapy, telling them their patients would then have more chances to recover promptly. From this standpoint, the issue of resistance is quite flexible and can be used one way or another, in favour of or against second-line therapy. According to a Dutch study, physicians who report seeing pharmaceutical sales representatives prescribe significantly higher volumes of second-choice antibiotics for upper and lower respiratory infections,[22] although these antibiotics should be reserved in case of intolerance or failure of first-choice agents. These results are consistent with our own findings indicating that antibiotic promotion tends to present antibiotics as a solution to resistance.

In December 2010, I collected ethnographic materials while following sales representatives during their working day during two series of visits. These thirteen visits showed me Pyostacine was systematically promoted as a great antibiotic against respiratory tract infections with a lower or even nonexistent resistance rate, and as a first-line therapy, for a short treatment of four days. All these claims were supported by scientific arguments stemming from four new clinical trials conducted in the 2000s targeting pneumonia, tonsillitis, bronchitis and sinusitis – all four based on double-blind, randomized clinical trial, and used as scientific evidence to convince doctors to prescribe antibiotics in these four instances. Most of the time, the second or third sentence pronounced by the representative mentioned first-line treatment: 'I am here for pristinamycin, in first-line therapy, for sinusitis', 'Here is Pristinamycin, for bronchitis, first-line treatment', 'When you have to deal with infectious pneumonia, what is your first choice?' Quite often, the physician would nod, or answer that he was prescribing pristinamycin quite often, as first-line therapy, and the sales representative told me that when she had doubts, she would ask pharmacists in the neighbourhood if the doctor was really prescribing as many drugs as he said he would.

But some doctors were reluctant, not only in their prescribing practice but also in front of the sales representative. One of them raised his eyebrows and asked right away, 'First-line, are you sure?' Another one, when asked by the sales representative, 'Do you prescribe it in first-line therapy, for bronchitis, as a reference?' clearly answered, 'No, not first-line therapy. Second-line'. And when the sales rep said, 'Resistances: for the moment, there are none' the doctor told her, 'For the moment, no resistances, but we'll get some! We are using it more and more, so they will come automatically'.[23] A third physician just crossed his arms and silently shook his head left and right in a clear gesture of disagreement, without explaining anything, as though his interlocutor knew perfectly well she was not telling the truth. Sometimes, doctors would say they were not convinced the drug should be used for tonsillitis, or that four days were often not sufficient, and one of them even mentioned the fact that Pyostacine, as a wide-spectrum antibiotic with a synergistic effect, could be responsible for a high level of co-resistance against other antibiotics even if the rate of resistance against it was seemingly modest. In a nutshell, all scientific claims – for its efficiency against upper respiratory tract infections, low resistance rate, use as a first-line therapy, and short treatment – were challenged by some physicians, and at the end of the day the sales representative told me she had really felt uncomfortable, and still feared she would blush in this type of situation, even after twenty-five years of professional activity.

Although some general practitioners thought such a promotional attitude was consciously deceptive, was this sales representative really willingly distorting scientific evidence? In fact, she was 'doing her job' by applying 'in the field' the strategies conceived by marketers at commercial headquarters, in conjunction with the scientific department coordinating the series of clinical trials on upper respiratory tract infections. And this job consisted of using scientific instability, medical practice loopholes and inaccuracies to make physicians prescribe more antibiotics, even convincing herself that her drug was better than the other ones because its rate of resistance was lower. According to her and to marketers at the commercial headquarters, despite frequent criticism, her arguments progressed. In the course of their discussions with sales representatives, antibiotic prescription appears to be evidence both of physicians' individual autonomy, and of their collective dependence on pharmaceutical corporations.[24]

Even if some of these short medical exchanges are sterile or even counter-productive when doctors do not agree with the use of the promoted antibiotic, they demonstrate the importance of flexible therapeutic use of drugs for pharmaceutical corporations. Repeated several hundred thousand times a year for each antibiotic, the overall effect on drug prescribing and antibiotic resistance is extremely powerful, and doctors will tend to use more pristinamycin for upper respiratory tract infections, as first-line treatment, increasing, in the future, the rate of resistant bacteria without treatment. Their medical 'dispositions' are shaped by scientific marketing, and these dispositions are partly responsible for the emerging epidemic of resistant bacteria. This is one of the reasons why, in the year 2000, public policies targeting doctors were launched by ministries of health or regulatory agencies, to counter-balance the harmful effects of unregulated antibiotic promotion. But in the marketing field, without changing the economic rules of the game, is scientific regulation really efficient?

Scientific Regulation: An Efficient Limit to Free Market Forces?

When a crisis occurs, be it financial or medical, regulation is frequently invoked as a tool to limit the social damages of the free market. However, the term 'regulation' is used in so many situations and for so many purposes that it becomes hard to know what it really means; governments regulate economies, health agencies regulate food and drug industries and world organizations regulate international trade. To avoid confusion, we will define regulation as a 'push and pull' strategy used by governments and public agencies to extend some markets while limiting others for the sake of an economic sector, or for the whole capitalist system to keep its balance. When it comes to pharmaceuticals, regulators protect the markets by providing labels, long-lasting patent protection and regulated prices while excluding undesired competitors. These economic privileges explain why the pharmaceutical sector is among the most profitable ones: it is aided and 'pushed' forward by state regulation.

At the same time, marketing activities have to abide by regulatory rules, which define the boundaries of pharmaceutical promotion and are often described as too heavy a constraint by pharmaceutical corporations, especially in France where 'red tape bureaucracy' is frequently vilipended by top management. For instance, the article L.5122 of the French code of public health prohibits any direct-to-consumer advertising for prescription drugs[25] and the article L.5122–8 stipulates that every pharmaceutical corporation should get an authorization from the Agence Nationale de Sécurité du Médicament (formerly known as Afssaps)[26] before launching any advertising campaigns for medical professions.[27] Moreover, clinical trials should be 'clearly' and 'objectively' presented, the use of 'hyperbolic' expressions prohibited and pharmaceutical sales representative are expected to deliver unbiased medical information. Insofar as this regulation is based on the results of science, it can be called a 'scientific' regulation, often presented as a rational way to protect consumers. But how efficient is such a regulation when the logics of the market lead to an epidemic, when regulators need to change the rules of the game to escape from the medical dead end of resistant bacteria?

Antibiotic Restriction: A Regulation that Goes Back and Forth

To fight against antibiotic overconsumption and its consequence, bacterial resistance, the French Department of Health launched in 2002 a five-year plan called '*plan national pour préserver l'efficacité des antibiotiques*', or 'national plan to preserve antibiotics' efficiency'. The main component of this plan was a public health campaign under the heading 'antibiotics are not automatic' to change the public perception of these drugs. Physicians and laymen had to know, among other things, that antibiotics were not useful against viruses: scientific knowledge, as opposed to popular wisdom, was perceived as an effective barrier to marketing activities trying to extend antibiotic consumption. This campaign had a positive impact on overall antibiotic prescription, which was reduced by 25 per cent.[28] But since then, consumption has been on the rise again,[29] and France remains the highest antibiotic consumer in Europe, behind Greece:

Table 3.2: Antibiotic consumption in Europe: France and Greece at the top of the list (in defined daily dose (DDD) per 1000 inhabitants)

	1999	2000	2001	2002	2003	2004	2005	2006	2007	2008	2009
Germany	13.6	13.6	12.8	12.7	13.9	13	14.6	13.6	14.5	14.5	14.9
Belgium	26.2	25.3	23.7	23.8	23.8	22.7	24.3	24.2	25.4	27.7	27.5
Bulgaria*	15.1	20.2	22.7	17.3	15.5	16.4	18	18.1	19.8	20.6	18.6
Spain***	20	19	18	18	18.9	18.5	19.3	18.7	19.9	19.7	19.7
France	34.3	33.4	33.2	32.2	28.9	27	28.9	27.9	28.6	28	29.6
Greece**	30.7	31.7	31.8	33.8	33.6	33	34.7	41.1	43.2	45.2	38.6
Italy	24.5	24	25.5	24.3	25.5	24.8	26.2	26.7	27.6	28.5	28.7
Netherlands	10	9.8	9.9	9.8	9.8	9.7	10.5	10.8	11	11.2	11.4
Poland	22.2	22.6	24.8	21.4	n.d.	19.1	19.6	n.d.	22.2	20.7	23.6
Czech Rep.	18.6	n.d.	n.d.	13.9	16.7	15.8	17.3	15.9	16.8	17.4	18.4
UK	14.8	14.3	14.8	14.8	15.1	15	15.4	15.3	16.5	16.9	17.3
Sweden	15.8	15.5	15.8	15.2	14.7	14.5	14.9	15.3	15.5	14.6	13.9

Source: European Surveillance of Antimicrobial Consumption, *Yearbook 2009*. * Total use until 2005, outpatient use from 2006. Change of data provider in 2006. ** Total use for the years 2004–8. *** Reimbursement data, does not include over-the-counter sales without prescriptions.

In 2007, after three years of a relatively sharp decline – which was all the more worthy of notice in that it was not observed in anyother country – French antibiotic consumption started to increase again: from 27 daily dose to 29.6, a figure that has increased in the following years. One of the reasons for this setback is the strength of the marketing strategy described above, which maintains, in the absence of continuous training in antibiotherapy for general practitioners, high levels of antibiotic prescription. However, one could argue medical habits are not written in stone, but can be changed. Why, then, did French public campaigns not lead to a permanent change in antibiotic prescribing habits?

Health Insurance Delegates: When Public Policies Conflict with Marketing Objectives

The campaign 'antibiotics are not automatic' did not confine itself to public education. Sure enough, it explained on television and on radio why antibiotics weren't useful against viruses, why resistant rods are dangerous, and why over-consumption could take us back to the pre-antibiotic era of the 1930s. But it went further: regional health security agencies organized concrete door-to-door discussions between doctors and new types of professionals called health insurance delegates, or, in French, 'Délégués de l'Assurance Maladie' (DAM), who were put into operation in 2003.[30] These state-employed health professionals had to give advice and information to doctors, and answer their questions concerning both scientific and regulatory matters. The were 450 of them in the first year and

950 in 2007, and they had to talk about general public health topics such as pregnancy, cancer prevention, sick leaves and antibiotic prescription.[31] During the first three years, they mostly tried to convince doctors they should help the government diminish the public health budget, and had mostly an economic goal. After 2006, they 'medicalized' their discourse and went deeper into scientific argumentation, which was seen by many antibiotics marketers as a threat to their turnover, not only because health insurance delegates tried to fight against overprescription, but also because many of them were former pharmaceutical sales representatives who knew the different angles of marketing, and were considered to be 'traitors' by their ex-employers. In other word, the state, via the public health insurance, was using scientific marketing devices to counterbalance the concept of bacterial resistance disseminated by pharmaceutical representatives.

This counter-offensive was not only communicational: it involved financial incentives for the doctors who decided to follow the guidelines proposed by these state-employed delegates. Among other tasks, since 2008 DAMs had had to talk practitioners into signing contracts called 'Individual Practices Improvement Contracts' – or in French *Contrats d'Amélioration des Pratiques Individuelles* (CAPI) – with the national health insurance. With these contracts, general practitioners committed themselves for three years to diminishing and rationalizing their prescriptions, and to improving the early detection of chronic diseases. For the first time in France, doctors could receive a bonus according to their contribution to state-driven public health guidelines. Two years after CAPIs were introduced, 16,000 doctors had signed them and had received between 1,500 to 4,900 euros a year, at an average of 3,000 euros.[32]

However, this danger to marketing only remained a potential threat, for three interesting reasons. First, 950 health insurance delegates cannot compete with more than 17,295 pharmaceutical sales representatives: the balance of forces remains clearly unequal, and the medical 'share of voice' cannot be controlled by state intervention as long as the number of delegates remains so low. Second, many doctors think the state shouldn't tell them what they have to prescribe, and refused to sign any CAPI, or even to listen to health insurance delegates: caught between two entities threatening their professional autonomy, general practitioners often decided not to choose. Third, this plan was not only implemented for the sake of public health: the idea was also to keep the social security budget low by reducing the amount of antibiotic reimbursement, and from this standpoint it was considered too expensive for the French public services to hire more employees. One of the chief product managers said, during an interview conducted in October 2010 at Sanofi, 'they will spend a million euros on DAMs and CAPIs, and win only a few hundreds of thousands in budget cuts!'[33] From this financial perspective, a high cost initiative to regulate pharmaceutical marketing doesn't seem sustainable, especially in times of economic crisis, when governments intend to restrict public spending.

If these three regulatory pressures – a public campaign, DAMs and CAPIs – did temporarily limit promotional pressures, they did not diminish antibiotic prescription in the long run, not only because they were too weak but also because their objective was not purely driven by healthcare concerns but more fundamentally by budgetary reasons. The systematic use of scientific evidence in favour of antibiotic consumption was stronger, more organized and more financially controlled from the corporations' side. In their attempts to 'push and pull' antibiotic markets to limit antibiotic resistance, regulators didn't clearly succeed in 'pulling' – were they more fortunate when 'pushing' forward antibiotic research and development? Is this other side of the antibiotic market failure more promising? As the attempt to market pristinamycin in the US will show, this is far from certain.

When Multi-Resistant Enterococcus Meets Pristinamycin: A Healthcare Deal at the FDA

Today, regulatory agencies, often under the pressure of infectiologists and physicians who deal with bacterial resistance, try to 'push' scientific research forward by providing pharmaceutical corporations with financial incentives to develop antibiotic research and development, satisfying the industry's demands on prices, legislation, tax reduction and regulatory procedures. Among other measures, to lower the costs of clinical trials, the FDA revised its non-inferiority standards and made the required 10 per cent delta between existing drugs and new drugs more flexible, after pharmaceutical corporations strongly reacted against this clinical trial requirement in 2001–2.[34] Along with the European Medicine Agency, the FDA also published guidelines on prescribing superiority trials against placebos – less rigorous but less costly than non-inferiority trials – for mild to moderate infections.[35] But until now these incentives hadn't given birth to new antibiotic classes.

This concern is not new: since the 1980s and 1990s, the FDA has become increasingly concerned about multi-resistant strains, and some bacteria were more carefully surpervised than others. *Enterococcus Faecium*, for instance, was on the top of the list: it had been found to be resistant to ampicillin in the US in the 1980s and to vancomycin in the following decade. The emergence of vancomycin-resistant *E. faecium* (VREF) in the United States showed the transmission capacities of bacteria and embodied the frightening possibility of a post-antibiotic era for nosocomial infections in critically ill patients.[36] It was first discovered in the Northwest United States, then it was increasingly found east of Mississippi. On its way to the West Coast, the superbug raised more and more concern among clinicians and hospital managers. In 1996, the FDA decided to consider the struggle against resistant bacteria, including VREF, a priority. But the main problem faced by the FDA anti-infective committee in charge of this public health puzzle was the lack of new antibiotics and the very few promising R&D programs conducted by pharmaceutical corporations. It started to look for old drugs that had already been marketed abroad for a long time but had never been approved in the US. These forgotten pills could be of paramount importance in the fight against resistances – and Sanofi's pristinamycin happened to be one of them.

Sanofi, called Rhône-Poulenc at that time, was trying to set foot in the US antibiotic market and had worked on the two molecules of the drug so that it could be both more pure and more effective: the result was a 'new' drug called Synercid, with a mechanism of action extremely close to pristinamycin's, but it could be used in hospital settings. It could therefore be injected into patients suffering from hospital-acquired multi-resistant bacteria, even if the company's market target was of course wider, as it involved pneumonia, skin infections and bronchitis, all therapeutic indications for pristinamycin, as mentioned above. From a purely commercial point of view, it was an opportunity to conquer new customers, and to develop the Americanization of the French company which had started a few years earlier, in 1990, when Rhône-Poulenc bought Rorer Corporation. This convergence of interests between marketing and medicine is at the core of scientific marketing, a hybrid discipline mixing two apparently different armies often fighting two different wars, and trying to find a common ground that may suddenly vanish at any step of the process.

However, contacts were made with Sanofi and a deal was cut: FDA anti-infective committee representatives proposed to consider the classical demands of the firm in exchange for a series of complicated 'compassionate' clinical trials.[37] Here, we refer to 'compassionate' clinical trials as opposed to 'commercial' clinical trials against Vancomycin-resistant *Enteroccocus Faecium*. Sanofi agreed, conducted the series of clinical trials, and presented its clinical results on 19 February 1998 to the sixty-third meeting of the FDA anti-infective committee. On that day, the room was divided into two groups. On one side of the room were the president of the committee and his secretary, eight official members of the anti-infective committee, a consultant, two special guests invited because they had an outstanding experience in this scientific field and five members of the FDA (including the director of the anti-infective department at the FDA). Out of these eighteen people, ten had the right to vote and to recommend whether Synercid should be approved for the US market by the head of the agency. In front of them, a group of executives from the corporation and their allies had to present the clinical results, answer questions and try to convince the board: the director of clinical and regulatory affairs for anti-infectives, a specialist in infectiology from the University of Virginia, the head of the anti-infective department of a medical centre in Portland, a director of clinical and microbio-logical development, a specialist of pharmacokinetics and pharmacodynamics, and an executive from a clinical development department.

Here is how an FDA employee introduced the problem of resistance before evaluating Synercid, depicting desperate clinical situations like this one:

> The patient received a variety of antibiotics, vancomycin to which it was resistant, ampicillin to which it was resistant, minocycline to which it was susceptible, rifampin to which it became resistant, gentamycin to which it was resistant. Some led to tran-sient clearing of the bloodstream, but then [the infection] would come back. The patient also received teicoplanin to which it was susceptible, but the organism devel-oped resistance.
>
> The patient was treated with minocycline for a prolonged period of time and finally discharged, but admitted four weeks later with positive blood cultures and died. Autopsy showed endocarditis with a vegetation of 10cm x 3 x 2, which is a huge vegetation.
>
> This illustrates an organism that could be inhibited. There was minocycline, but this infection, endocarditis, did not respond and the patient went on to die after a six-month illness. [Slide.]
>
> So, what do we do about VRE? The problem again is that the new resistances have been added on to the background of a number of acquired and intrinsic resistances.[38]

Without this worrisome situation, and the risk of a pandemic outbreak, the clas-sical marketing approach may have never succeeded. The FDA had to propose an incentive to the industry, in order to address a public health issue that could not be dealt with only with the federal budget for healthcare. Far from being 'cap-tured', the FDA acts here as a *partner of the industry* and as an institution which is *desperately dependent upon pharmaceutical industry*. The experts' point of view is that healthcare issues, such as bacterial resistance, can only be addressed if industrialists and regulators act hand in hand, and are able to trade despite the lack of an adequate economic model.

But the results of this approval process, based on the analysis of new clinical data for Synercid, were mitigated. First, the series of compassionate clinical trials were hardly evaluable: less than 50 per cent of the patients were evaluable, mostly because of very high mortality rates – 49.5 to 54 per cent, i.e., more than 50 per cent of them, died during clinical trials, which shows that the clinical model of a for-profit drug may not be adequate for complicated healthcare situations where each individual is different, and where the standardized market expectations of the firm are nowhere to be found. In the end, according to the majority of experts, the efficacy of the drug against multi-resistant bacteria was not sufficiently dem-onstrated by the sponsor. Second, frequent and strong secondary effects – venous damage due to injection – were undermining the safety of the drug. Why, then, did the FDA approve the drug? What kind of scientific regulation can approve the marketing of a drug without acknowledging its scientific evidence?

A Paradoxical Approval and the Failure of the White Puma

In the discussion, the firm managers tried hard to convince the FDA experts of the safety and efficiency of Synercid: they invoked statistical demonstrations, public health arguments and biochemical explanations, using a scientific rhetoric similar to the 'demos' used by NASA and Silicon Valley demonstrators when presenting their research to potential employers or investors.[39] But never did they do so successfully; for the most part, clinical studies were not found convincing. Quite paradoxically, the drug was approved nonetheless. The following result of the vote, at the end of the day, shows how politics and scientific evaluations are intertwined when it comes to antibiotics: as the economic incentive for profit was not sufficient for the pharmaceutical corporation to design and launch a drug only for infections involving multi-resistant bacteria, the agency loosened its regulation standards and accepted a drug with a risk–efficiency ratio that was not fully satisfying. But the active chairman of the anti-infective committee implemented the voting procedures nonetheless:

> CHAIRMAN: The question 4(a): Do the data from the studies presented provide evidence that Synercid is safe and effective for the treatment in the sites that have been studied ...? Those who feel that the data support demonstration objectively of efficacy in these sites with VREF, please raise your hand.
> [Show of hands.]
> CHAIRMAN: Three yes. Those who do not feel that efficacy and safety have been demonstrated?
> [Show of hands.]
> CHAIRMAN: Seven. We have 7 no, 3 yes. Part (b): Does the committee recommend approval of Synercid for the treatment of patients with vancomycin-resistant *Enterococcus faecium* infections? Those who feel that we should forward a recommendation for approval for this specific indication, please raise your hands.
> [Show of hands.]
> CHAIRMAN: We need to have all the hands up again, those who wish to recommend approval.
> [Show of hands.]
> CHAIRMAN: Nine.
> Those who do not wish to recommend approval?
> [One response.]
> CHAIRMAN: One. So: 9 to 1 recommending approval for VREF.[40]

This vote is quite puzzling: how can the committee approve a drug (question 4(b): nine 'yes' votes versus one 'no'), and at the same time think the clinical trials conducted by the corporation did not prove the drug was safe and efficient (question 4(a): seven 'no' notes versus three 'yes')? Isn't the FDA undermining its own reputation, based on independence and intransigence,[41] by allowing a drug on the market without sufficient evidence? In fact, this decision is based on the will to send a political 'signal' to the industry: new markets can be conquered if you help us fighting against multi-resistance. The FDA, facing a major health threat that a 'dry pipeline' can't eliminate, manipulated indirect economic incentives to stimulate pharmaceutical research and development. This exchange of clinical trials is an example of a scientific regulation that reveals the powerlessness of the government's regulatory agency and of the medical sphere it intends to represent when facing a shortage of new drugs. Both depend on the industry and on the importance of incentives that could be provided to translate public health ideas into marketing grammar. However, in the end, this drug will turn out to be inadequate to this market: secondary effects on the venous system, combined with poor results on multi-resistant bacteria, will show the inefficiency of this healthcare deal for a drug that was never designed, nor trialled, to fight resistant bacteria.

Conclusion

This short sociology of antibiotic marketing from France to the United States depicts an unintended but dramatic consequence of scientific marketing as a discipline systematically relying on the results of natural and human sciences to build its markets. When it comes to antibiotics, commercial strategies of pharmaceutical corporations simultaneously solve a medical problem and create a new one with the same intriguing commodity. They do so because the arguments that are designed by marketers, and then put forward by sales representatives for each antibiotic – that it is more potent than others, has a lower resistance rate, and is recommended as first-line therapy – favour individual efficiency over general safety. The use of antibiotics for viral tonsillitis, or the prescription of wide-spectrum and first-line drugs instead of narrow-spectrum and second-line therapies, are not irrational or magical beliefs, but belong to a certain type of rationality, which is the rationality of scientific marketing. It systematically tries to extend the use value of antibiotics, even if other competing or contradictory conceptions of the use value are circulating.

In the end, on a global scale, scientific marketing of antibiotics creates bacterial resistances and the use value of all antibiotics tendentially declines: antibiotic overconsumption is involved in a process where the use value of drugs is influenced, transformed, and even tends to be annihilated by exchange value. Around this self-destructive tendency of antibiotics' market value, a triangular game is played between corporations, doctors and governments, where patients are both the objects of healthcare and the targets of marketing, a political concern and an economic failure. We shouldn't be surprised by this process, which is not a distinctive feature of antibiotics. Market obsolescence is even sometimes *programmed* by marketers and, in the case of antibiotics, it would not be a problem if new molecules were found more often or more precisely if the rhythm of drug discovery were similar to the rhythm of resistant strain regeneration. But this is far from being the case because, on the other front line of the war against bacteria, the innovation process is not counterbalancing the effect of antibiotic overconsumption.

4 ADS, ADS, ADS: THE GEPHAMA DATABASE AND ITS USES

Stephan Felder, Jean-Paul Gaudillière and Ulrike Thoms

Printed advertisements have been at the very forefront of the development of modern mass marketing for drugs since the beginning of the twentieth century. Advertisements for secret remedies, which rapidly expanded in the second half of the nineteenth century, were very prominent in the media and in public life and fell under the suspicion that their exaggerated claims misled and cheated patients. These advertisements were criticized against the background of a moral economy that regarded any promotional activity for drugs or medical services as a violation of acceptable behaviour on the part of pharmacists and physicians. Secret remedies, their publicity and the regulation of the latter have therefore raised considerable interest amongst historians and social science scholars.[1] Despite ongoing criticism, print advertisements for drugs did not disappear with the nineteenth century. Not only did they remain, their number kept increasing well into the twentieth century to the point that in Europe, drug manufacturers were amongst the main if not the leading advertisers. As a consequence, publicity remained a target for regulations also well into the century.[2]

Some producers, especially firms that had evolved out of pharmacies, then decided to build on doctors' and the public's negative attitude to advertising and began to position themselves as 'ethical' companies by refusing to advertise or refraining from broad claims so as not to upset their professional colleagues, given that they were responsible for either writing prescriptions or recommending certain products. Though pharmaceutical companies developed a specific style of marketing, which early on comprised distinctive practices such as a system of representatives sent around to address and involve physicians directly and personally, for many decades in the twentieth century print advertising persisted as one of the important tools used to promote new as well as old drugs.[3] Starting around 1900, medical journals as well as newspapers and magazines for the general public were increasingly filled with print advertisements, leaflets and inserts, and even the firms that disapproved of publicity had to advertise their products if they wanted to survive competition on the market, and an entire business of advertising agencies targeting the drug sector emerged from their efforts to organize print advertising. Many of these agencies developed from advertising bureaus that worked as intermediaries between publishing houses wanting to sell advertising space and those who wished to advertise their products and services.[4] In other words, even if by the 1930s other promotional channels like films, hand-outs, conferences, radio and television, not to mention pharmaceutical representatives, could amount to two-thirds of all promotional expenses in large companies like Bayer, Schering or Rhône-Poulenc, print advertisements remained a highly visible tool and an indispensable instrument in the construction of a drug market.

Against this background it is paradoxical that most historical studies addressing print drug marketing have only focused on qualitative approaches by selecting a few ads for one product in a limited period of time. To apprehend the massive amount of print adverts seriously and to analyse it more deeply, one of the approaches of the collaborative GEPHAMA research project was to set up a database that would be representative of this bulk of material. One major aim of the systematic study of ads is to provide a sense of the long duration of advertising campaigns, i.e., to take into account the fact that ads for the same products were repeated in the form of series, that entire classes of drugs were promoted for decades, and that the choices involved in designing, printing and circulating the ads were part of general but changing patterns of the promotional work.

Two other motives for a systematic approach originate in the specific interest of the GEPHAMA project for the emergence of *scientific* marketing, i.e., the complex and massive use of laboratory and clinical research results for promotion. Adverts have certainly had a strong impact on the outlook, structure and development of scientific medicine and its public as they covered an increasing share of the pages in scientific journals. And yet this impact has hardly been acknowledged in the many studies on the relations between the biomedical sciences and the pharmaceutical industry that have been published in the past decades. In most instances, when these studies took any notice of advertisements, they regarded and treated them as external elements that did not belong to the core of medical publications. This way of dismissing promotional copy as unscientific and not medical is a form of boundary work and was echoed in the practice of librarians, who eliminated advertisements when binding medical journals. What was thus eliminated was in fact a major factor in the transformation of collective medical knowledge and of routine prescription practices. Tellingly, the German doctors' bulletin *Deutsches Ärzteblatt* or the French *Concours Médical*, for example, were (and still are) completely financed by the advertisements they ran. We therefore decided to consider ads in bulk and as sources to be studied on a long-term basis.

Methodology

Given the high number of ads, it was clear from the very start that we would have to make a selection of journals and issues to be included in the analysis. From the several hundred medical journals published in France or Germany in the twentieth century, we first chose general medical journals that had – and still have – high circulation and were important mouthpieces of the medical profession. For Germany we decided to include the *Deutsche Medizinische Wochenschrift*, a very successful journal which first came out in 1886, and the *Deutsches Ärzteblatt*, which began its life as the *Ärztliches Vereinsblatt* in 1872 and was renamed *Ärztliche Mitteilungen* in 1900 before it became, in 1930, the *Deutsches Ärzteblatt*, the bulletin of the German physicians' association.[5] For France we selected the *Concours Médical*, which began publication in 1879, and *La Presse Médicale*, published since 1893. Although they were not directly related to professional institutions such as medical unions or the national medical association, these journals targeted the entire profession and, from the early twentieth century on, included in their content clinical reports and advice for daily practice, as well as administrative and legal information.[6]

All four journals were published during the whole time frame designated for the project (1910–80) and all four started well before the big wave of medical specialization that brought about an increasing number of new journals and multiplied the number of medical papers in the inter-war and immediate postwar period.[7] Our journals followed this development as they contained articles on specialities, but their main focus was the general practitioner. They therefore kept track of developments in many fields of medicine, bringing ever-more research results and reports on scientific conferences and meetings to the attention of local physicians, while also discussing professional policies, legal matters and the ethical aspects of medicine. Moreover, advertisements covered a growing share of the space in these journals. As stated by a 1978 report on the situation of the scientific press to the German government, by the end of the century, about 70 per cent of the pages in medical journals were covered with advertisements rather than with scientific text.[8]

Building a drug advertisement database would however face unexpected difficulties in accessing the advertisements. Even though, from an historian's or a linguist's point of view, advertisements can be seen as indispensable sources, as mentioned earlier, librarians usually removed the advertising sections from the volumes before sending them to be bound. Journal publishers on their side made this easier by placing the ads in separate sections or on the front and back pages of an issue, which were also removed before binding. What a reader usually finds in scientific libraries is therefore volumes without any advertisements. It is only in the oldest issues of the nineteenth and early twentieth centuries that ads were kept because they were scattered throughout the issues with no clear differentiation between text and advertising sections.[9] It took considerable effort and time to identify volumes of the journals containing all the ads for our investigation, especially as publishers very often made the same choice as librarians when creating reference collections of their journals. The main consequence of such limitations in the establishment of continuous and representative series was to restrict the present exploitation of the database to two rather than four journals, those for which most issues could be found with their advertisement sections, namely the *Concours Médical* (*CM*) in France and the *Deutsche Medizinische Wochenschrift* (*DMW*) in Germany.

A second difficulty was the massiveness of the source. For instance, according to our estimates, the full number of ads to be analysed for the *DMW* would have amounted to over 200,000. We therefore decided to use the methods of modern communication science to extract a representative sample from this body.[10] This led us to collect the advertisements for every fifth year from 1910 to 1980.[11] For the case of Germany – where many more ads were published than in France – the number of ads would still have been far beyond anything manageable. We therefore further limited their number by including only every seventh issue from the fifty-two yearly issues to bring down the amount of ads to a manageable level comparable to the corpus originating in the sampling from the *CM*. This choice was distributed equally over the years, thus covering seasonal variations. One additional caveat to be mentioned is the question of inserts. We simply had no instrument to know for sure whether inserts had been removed, which had disappeared or for what reason, whether by the archivists, by an interested reader who wanted to take an insert home, or because the inserts had fallen out of the volumes during their travel to the final stocks.

In spite of these limitations, the result was a representative collection covering the decades between 1910 and 1970 in a comparable manner for both countries, and for another decade in the German case, allowing the identification of trends and their quantitative evaluation, even though deep statistical accuracy was not possible. It was actually reassuring to see in the early stages of exploiting of the database that even a first and cursory glance revealed striking changes, so we deemed that it was justified as well as rewarding to invest a massive amount of work in the analysis of their appearance, i.e., of their formal, visual and textual composition.

As Richard Pollay has pointed out in his descriptive analysis of print advertisements, the focus of advertising histories 'has been primarily on the politics of the profession, rather than on its product, the advertisements themselves'. Existing work has thus been 'more concerned with sociological analysis, coffee table varieties, social portrayals and criticism than with techniques and tactics' of advertising.[12] In contrast, our approach would help shift the perspective from the theory to the products of advertising and to the role they play in the construction of pharmaceutical markets.

Two levels of comparison were envisioned. The first, longitudinal and across time, aimed at sketching out general trends in advertising, such as use of colours, changes in layout, use of visual techniques and type of information included. The second level of comparison was between the developments in the two countries under study, based on the idea that commonalities would be robust markers of general changes in drug marketing practices. Moreover, national differences might not only reveal different regulatory frameworks but, more importantly, could be envisioned as reflections of local therapeutic and medical cultures. One pressing question was in this respect the role advertisements played in triggering changes in medical categories and definitions of diseases.[13]

As drug treatment differs enormously depending on the disease and the pharmaceutical market is highly diversified into different submarkets, we concentrated our in-depth analysis on specific therapeutic classes: sleeping pills, antidiabetics, sex hormones (including contraceptives), painkillers and psychotropic drugs.[14] Assignment to these classes was based on references to certain symptoms, effects or disease categories in the key words or key symbols of the advertisements.[15] In order to manage the many ads we developed a reference Excel data sheet to record their different characteristics. Its framework distinguished three main fields: formal, textual and visual elements. The 'formal' section collected basic information on the source such as the date of publication, name of the drug and manufacturer. Under 'textual' we included the different written elements in the ads, for instance the symptoms or indications mentioned, the slogans used and the naming of side and adverse effects. Under 'visual' we recorded whether the ads contained pictures, graphs or photos, whether these were in colour or black and white, whether they displayed patients and/or doctors, and whether the diseases were visually represented. Our intentions were to first grasp the formal changes, then to understand the changes in the way information was presented and, third, to consider how the firms referred to the potential uses, purposes and applications of the different products. All this was intended to improve our understanding of how the construction of the drug market (and of the respective sub-markets) worked in practice. In order to reflect on these differences in an appropriate way and to respect the limited space available here, the following presentation of results and analysis concentrates on ads for psychotropic drugs from the *DMW* and the *CM* only as a means to illustrate the potential of the database.

Psychotropic Drugs: Number and Size of Advertisements

This group of pharmaceutical drugs includes all the products associated with psychiatric or neurological disorders, but also – in order to establish a long-term series – the drugs associated with calming and sedative effects beyond the well-known post-war palette of neuroleptics, antidepressants and tranquilizers.

At first glance a comparison of the absolute figures for France and Germany seems to prove that there were many more adverts for psychotropic drugs in France.[16] Nevertheless, we have to remember that the German figures are derived from a sampled body of data. This number needs to be multiplied by 6.25 to make a reasoned estimate of the total number of existing ads and results in approximately 2,580 ads for psychotropic drugs in the German journal, which outnumbers the French advertisements and reflects the more general massive input of publicity in the *Deutsche Medizinische Wochenschrift* (*DMW*).

Table 4.1: Number of ads per year (absolute figures)

	Concours Médical (*CM*)	*Deutsche Medizinische Wochenschrift* (*DMW*)
1913–15	5	64
1920	37	1
1925	62	3
1930	77	18
1935	46	0
1940	30	1
1945–8	21	20
1950	38	1
1955	61	4
1960	69	67
1965	67	77
1969–70	80	75
Total	593	331

Source: GEPHAMA database.

In spite of all the shortcomings due to the mix of sources, some general trends became very visible. First of all, in contrast to what might be expected on the basis of the existing historiography of the therapeutic revolution in psychiatry and mental health, advertisements for drugs targeting mental or nerve disorders were abundant long before the 1960s. This was especially true in the French case, where the number of advertisements took off during the 1920s and 1930s. This must be seen in the context of the general development of advertising, which was massively used to overcome the economic problems of the 1920s, when advertising began to be institutionalized.[17] Companies set up special 'propaganda' and advertising departments; new specialized journals were founded like the German *Medizin und Werbung* in 1932; and educational institutions for advertisers and specialized advertising agencies were created.[18] During the 1940s, the number of ads dropped sharply, especially in Germany, mainly due to the war, as especially shown by the 1941 *Stop-Verordnung* (Stop Decree) that prohibited the launch of any new product, and also to the cutback in the number of pages in scientific journals. Advertising was ultimately totally banned in 1943. After the end of the war, it was quite a while before advertising developed again because the firms first had to solve basic problems of production, the supply of raw materials and transportation.

Starting in the late 1950s and early 1960s, the number of advertisements grew enormously in both countries. In the 1960s and 1970s there was a second wave of professionalization in pharmaceutical marketing, which was rooted in the general growth of the drug sector, in the convergence of in-house clinical research and promotion, and in the development of communication on scientific and market research.[19] This development led to the implementation of new theoretical models, to the release of new, specialized textbooks and to the creation of new journals.[20]

As firms were increasingly willing to spend money on advertisements in journals, the number of ads, as well as their size, grew. Until 1955 the majority of ads were smaller than half a page; after 1960, this was inverted. Smaller ads became the exception. As for full-page advertisements, before the 1950s they occurred rarely in the *DMW*, while they made up nearly one-fourth of all the ads in France. Post-war growth is then striking: until 1970 more than 60 per cent of the ads in the *Concours Médical* (*CM*) covered a full page or more. Development in Germany was similar although with a ten-year lag. An interesting question arises as to whether and to what extent this development was a reaction to the changing regulatory framework, which required that advertisement copy include a growing number of different types of information, but obviously this alone does not suffice to explain this development as the alterations were also linked to changes in visual techniques.[21]

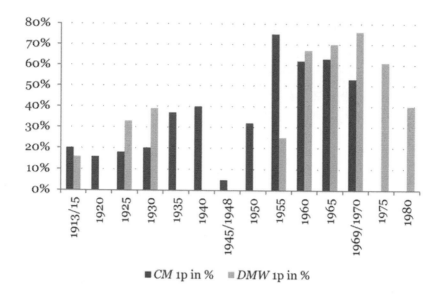

Figure 4.1: Percentage of ads covering a full page or more.

Source: GEPHAMA database.

Parallel to this development, the firms increasingly abstained from advertising more than one product in a single ad. This had been rather common practice up to the 1930s, when the scientific reputation of the firms and of the brands as such was very much at the core of their advertising strategies.[22] Ads with multiple products pointed to the scientific potency of the producing firm rather than to the uniqueness and singular properties of a product. Post-war, the markets became more centred on blockbusters, and the massive use of specific drugs came to the foreground, with single products gaining visibility. Remarkably enough, the multiple products strategy was stronger in the ads from the *DMW*. This must be seen as a reflection of the initial domination of large companies in Germany, companies that invested early in image building with special emphasis on the idea of a research-based company.

In 1925, 67 per cent of the ads in the *DMW* presented more than one product; in 1930 this percentage was in the same range, at 50 per cent of the ads. In contrast, this was only the case for 34 per cent of the French ads in 1925 and 22 per cent in 1930. In 1955 the *DMW* still had 50 per cent of such ads, while the respective figure for the *CM* had already gone down to 18 per cent. At the end of the time period under investigation, the situation was, however, almost the same in both countries. Already, in 1970, the percentage of ads promoting several products had gone down to only a few per cent in the *CM*, and these disappeared entirely from the *DMW* in the 1970s.

Psychotropic Drugs: Visual Elements and Strategies

Visual elements are very important parts of adverts, as they condense information and are thus an answer to space limitations. Moreover, they use emotional channels to convey subtext, especially through colours and pictures. Works in the history of advertising have rightly stressed the growing importance of illustrations in ads starting in around 1900.[23] Our sample shows a marked and constant increase of the share of ads illustrated with pictures.[24] By 1913–15, 16 per cent of the ads from the *Deutsche Medizinische Wochenschrift* (*DMW*) were illustrated. By around 1955 the percentage of these ads had reached 50 per cent, while already two-thirds (59 per cent) of all ads in the *Concours Médical* (*CM*) were illustrated. In 1970 this number was close to 90 per cent. Ten years later, there was not a single ad in the *DMW* with no illustration.

We then tried to differentiate which visual strategies and representations were used by the agencies and how their use changed over time. What we found was a marked increase in the number of visual techniques elaborated since 1900, when graphic arts emerged.[25] Sometimes created by artists like Toulouse-Lautrec and Hans Hohlwein, they began to play an important role in the aesthetics of advertisements, especially posters. This development then swept over first to magazines and then to newspapers. Firms had previously relied on their own advertising departments, but now began to cooperate more closely with graphic artists, and later with agencies, which were professionalized, as shown by the foundation in 1924 of the prestigious German journal *Gebrauchsgraphik. Monatszeitschrift für visuelle Communication und künstlerische Werbung* (*Applied Graphics: Monthly Journal for Visual Communication and Artistic Advertising*). This development resulted, for instance, in the creation of pretentious brand signs and in building the corporate image of pharmaceutical firms as well as the identity of certain products. Firms increasingly chose firm and brand colours and developed sophisticated colour concepts for their product palette as well as for single products.[26] These were planned and developed to create visual references between packages, ads and other promotional material.[27]

The rise of visual elements stretches over the entire period of our investigation. In comparison to developments in other industrial sectors, this change took much longer in the pharmaceutical industry. This was less due to the development of printing techniques and more due to a question of the design and conception of medical-scientific journals. In contrast to mainstream magazines, the publishers of journals for medical professionals came late as they kept their graphic design rather plain for a long time. Nonetheless, schematic or even idealized drawings in black and white played an important and increasing role. In fact, until 1930, all ads in the *DMW* were in black and white and remained so during the first decade after World War II. From then on, coloured graphic elements were to be found here and there in single ads. This development accelerated during the 1950s. In 1960 the share of coloured ads stood at 50 per cent in the *DMW* and continued to grow to nearly two-thirds in 1970 and to three-quarters by 1975.[28] French adverts in medical journals seem to have resorted to colour earlier. In the *CM*, 8 per cent of the ads were coloured in 1950 and their percentage grew quickly to 49 per cent in 1965, which was similar to the German percentage of 45 per cent. They then outgrew the *DMW* pattern with a stunning 89 per cent in 1969. On the other hand it took a particularly long time for photos to be integrated into the graphics toolbox of pharmaceutical advertisers. In 1930 only 10 per cent of the German ads in the psychotropic subset of the database contained a photo. This percentage grew to 30 per cent in 1960, while drawings still remained important. In 1980 one-third of the ads in the *DMW* still contained drawings, but 56 per cent of the ads contained photographs.

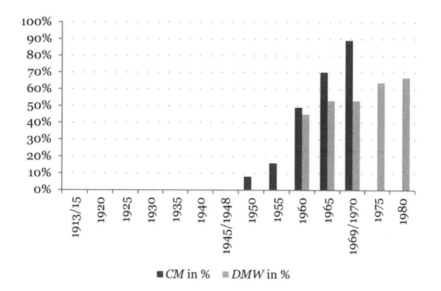

Figure 4.2: Percentage of colour ads.

Source: GEPHAMA database.

In contrast, German ads were quick to include brand signs and firm logos as central elements to relate a product to the firm's image. This was an especially sensitive issue in the case of pharmaceuticals, for which branding had been associated with their industrialization, with their departure from preparations made in pharmacies, and during their early history as branded products.[29] By 1925 one-third of the German ads already contained a logo; five years later the share stood at nearly 75 per cent and continued to grow. In contrast, only 11 per cent of the ads in the *CM* displayed a logo in 1930. The figures 'exploded' after World War II and by 1955 had already reached 50 per cent. What accounts for this huge difference? One plausible explanation is that the German pharmaceutical industry was already more concentrated, with large firms trying to generate trust in the company rather than in a pharmacist's name, and therefore trying to build a firm image. In France, the production of many products remained limited to small firms owned by individual pharmacists. As we will see below, French ads tended to focus on the products, the composition of the drug and its effects.[30]

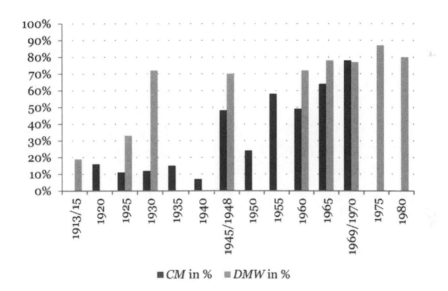

Figure 4.3: Percentage of ads containing company logos.

Source: GEPHAMA database.

This raises the question of whether the use of a logo replaced the products as such, or what role the products played at all as elements of the ads, where they could be shown as pills, powder or other preparations or where they were represented by a package. The share of ads displaying the advertised products was surprisingly low. Standing at 15 per cent during the first years, it climbed to nearly 20 per cent in 1960 and to 30 per cent in 1980. It is interesting that the German ads showing the products did not increase in the case of psychotropic drugs but instead declined after the 1970s, whereas they grew in France. Here, the percentage outnumbered that in the German journal in all years investigated.

Similarly, the ads from the German *DMW* did not often use the technique of representing drug effects. In 1948 only 5 per cent of the German ads pointed to effects; in the 1950s, this practice was not found at all but then rose to a maximum of 33 per cent in 1965, which was followed by an intriguing decline in this trend in 1970 and in the following years.[31] In contrast to this, the French data show a marked increase from 0 to 13.5 per cent in 1920, with a subsequent decrease. During the post-war period in France these shares increased permanently and continuously to 51 per cent in 1970.

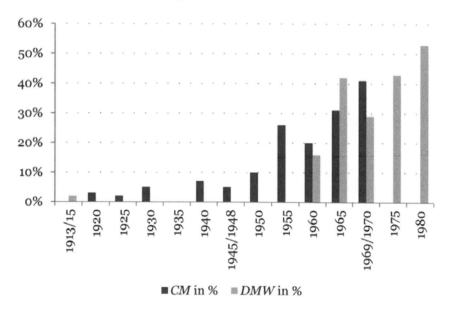

Figure 4.4: Percentage of ads showing the patient.

Source: GEPHAMA database.

Patients – though they are the target of all medical activities – were not often represented in the advertisements of our corpus during the pre-war period. In the case of the *DMW* the share of ads including images of patients reached 16 per cent in 1960 and 42 per cent in 1965. Although it went down to 29 per cent in 1970, this seems to be incidental as the shares later stay higher than 40 per cent. This massive presence was all the more interesting as the new drug law of 1965 had banned the representation of patients and doctors in advertisements targeted to laypeople, whereas they were explicitly allowed in adverts in scientific and medical journals directed to experts.[32] In France, the patient is also present in a small number of ads during the pre-war period, with figures rapidly increasing after the war to reach 25 per cent in 1955, 31 per cent in 1965 and 41 per cent in 1969.

In contrast to the rising visualization of patients, doctors were rarely represented. They never surfaced in the French corpus, while in the German ads for psychotropic drugs, they show up only in 1970 and 1980. This may originate in the fact that physicians are the target group of the ads but not the end-users of the drugs. Doctors are addressed in their professional role, which somehow conflicts with advertising. The firms may have assumed that doctors preferred to not be 'used' or shown in ads at all.

Otherwise, there was a clear increase in the display of symptoms from which a patient suffered – but again, there are national specificities as in the *DMW* not a single ad representing, instead of just mentioning, symptoms can be found before 1960. This is definitively due to the Nazi decree of 1941, which prohibited showing either the patient's suffering or raising fear.[33] Although the French figures indicate a certain inhibition in using such pictures, which would point to an unwritten moral code, the French advertisers were less reluctant than the Germans. Already in 1955, 36 per cent of ads represented the symptoms. This number increased to a maximum of 39 per cent in 1965. German ads caught up during this time: beginning with 6 per cent in 1960 (when the French figure was at 25 per cent), to more than 12 per cent in 1965 and 19 per cent in 1970. These figures are by and large 5 per cent higher than those for the entire data set of all German ads.[34] After a new plunge to 6 per cent, the figure for the German ads reached 33 per cent in 1980, when the overall figure was at only 18 per cent. This points to the need felt to visualize the symptoms in order to create an impression of patients suffering from stress, whereas in other diseases like diabetes the medical risk of going untreated meant that this would be unnecessary. All in all, the French percentages are several times higher than the German ones due to different regulations and, perhaps, different habits of advertising firms. Interestingly enough, the binding power of the 1941 decree was reduced under the pressure of on-going developments. Even the regulation of the 1965 law which once again prohibited producing fear in laypeople was obviously disregarded.

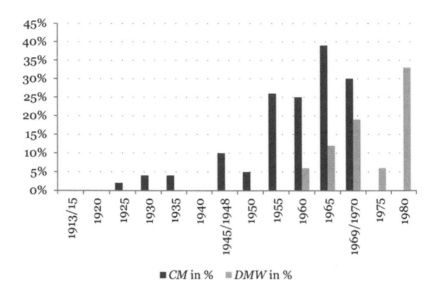

Figure 4.5: Percentage of ads displaying the target symptoms.

Source: GEPHAMA database.

Finally, representation of the anatomy, i.e., of diseased bodies and body parts, shows an opposite pattern. It was a widely used technique in the post-war set of *DMW* adverts but remained less important in the French case over the same time period since it did not increase above its pre-war level of 4 to 8 per cent.

Psychotropic Drugs: Textual Elements

For reasons of space, it is not possible to document or discuss in depth all the textual elements included in the ads and the way they changed over time, but to give a sense of how the database can be used in this respect we shall discuss slogans and effects briefly in order to concentrate on the question of indications.

Slogans, in the sense of catchy phrases, are important components of promotional copy as they seek to emphasize the characteristics and/or the effects of drugs. In the case of the French ads for psychotropic drugs, slogans were used from the very beginning of our period, while evidence of use is scarce in the early decades of the German sample. In both countries the inclusion of a slogan became a massive practice after World War II, although the German figures remained somewhat variable, oscillating between 10 per cent in 1945–8 and 52 per cent in 1970. Whether this might be explained by industrial self-regulation, i.e., the firms having possibly chosen to represent themselves as serious, scientific entrepreneurs keeping away from 'high claims', is an open question.

Effects were not systematically addressed in the German ads, while they were in more than half of the French ones over the entire period, and especially after World War II, when their number grew from almost three-quarters of the ads in 1965 to 92 per cent in 1970. During that same year, only 32 per cent of the *Deutsche Medizinische Wochenschrift* (*DMW*) ads for psychotropic drugs described effects. Although the figure doubled to 67 per cent in 1975, this seems to be incidental as the following year numbers were down to 43 per cent. One interpretation of this difference may be, once again, the propensity of French drug advertisers to push the products in a stronger, more aggressive way than their German counterparts. In any case, the pattern with side effects is consistent with this assumption since the information on side effects is more often included in *DMW* ads than in those of the *Concours Médical* (*CM*). That this difference is not a direct outcome of stronger regulations after World War II is evidenced by the fact that the *DMW* pattern was already established in the 1920s when one-fifth of all the ads provided information on side effects. This number rose to a peak of 50 per cent in 1955, then, for reasons unknown, was halved over the next five years to reach a minimum of 13 per cent in 1970. Obviously motivated by the preparations for the new 1978 drug law, the percentage reached 37 per cent in 1975, while it was at almost 70 per cent in 1980.[35]

Textual information on the indications was present in an overwhelming share of the French ads from the very start, which may be due to the relatively strong French regulations on drug advertising and the obligation to include this information. Before the 1978 drug advertising law there was no regulation in Germany, that is, no list of elements that a production firm had to include in its ads. The Germans therefore had somewhat more freedom. Nevertheless, the overall development – and even more interestingly, its result – was almost the same: information on the indications of a drug was almost always included, and especially so in the case of Germany starting in 1970, when all ads had this element of information. The situation is somewhat different for the composition of the drugs, which was not systematically given. In the case of French ads, the percentage was nearly 100 per cent as early as 1913–15, when it stood at only 48 per cent in the German case. Surprisingly, this share went down, though much more in France than in Germany. Nonetheless in France, starting in 1965 almost all ads provided the composition; in 1970 Germany joined in this practice. The 1978 regulations were, however disregarded, as these percentages went down once again to 80 per cent in 1980.

Changing Indications: Emerging Markets for Psychotropic Drugs

Indications play a unique role in the construction of pharmaceutical markets since they provide a direct link between the properties of a given product as the manufacturers define them and the doctor's prescription practices leading to purchase and consumption. We therefore recorded all the indications mentioned in the database advertisements. In the case of psychotropic drugs, we expected to find marked changes in the lists of indications, with for instance the development of submarkets associated with the post-war diversification of psychoactive agents. The question of which category – i.e., symptoms, diagnosis or indications – should be used and lumped together to follow these changes is complex, as we know all diseases and illnesses are historically and socially constructed.[36] The problem might however be less acute when giving up the idea that there is a 'hard core' of stable medical reality to be identified and followed behind the shifting vocabulary of medical texts and pharmaceutical adverts, in other words, by identifying a series of key terms that – in spite of their shifting specific definitions – have been used for decades to signify markets in the general domain of mental health and psychiatry. In our case, this selection was based on two resources: the very significant historiography of the domain, that of psychotropic drugs in particular, and systematic recording of the terms used in the advertisements. Of course, a proper interpretation of how ads shape medical categories cannot be based only on an analysis of the ads themselves; it needs proper contextualization and other sources related to marketing campaigns, company strategies, professional expertise and doctors' practices in order to identify developments in industrial and university research and to seek the scientific, cultural, social and political response to the research findings.[37] But even at first sight it is remarkable that early ads for psychotropes such as the ad for Neuronal from 1912 (Figure 4.6) do not mention diagnosis or target symptoms at all. The following remarks do not so much give a history of the change in psychiatric disease category. They are more limited, and simply mean to open a window on these developments in order to highlight interesting entry points for further research.

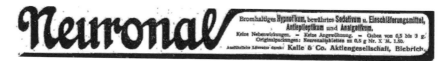

Figure 4.6: Advertisement for the bromide, Neuronal; image reproduced by kind permission of Deutscher Ärzte-Verlag GmbH.

Source: *Ärztliche Mitteilungen*, 13:2 (1912), p. 22.

Following the incidence of the word 'neurasthenia', for example, we find that this was an old concept of nervous disease that had already lost its commercial importance before the end of World War II, although its incidence in related ads was rather high at the beginning of the twentieth century, especially in France, where 35 per cent of all ads for psychotropic drugs mentioned it in 1920 and 43 per cent in 1925. By 1930 this figure had gone down to 27 per cent, and a further decrease followed. Such figures were never reached in Germany. Though the percentage of ads citing neurasthenia was 30 per cent in 1913–15, it subsequently plunged. It was only in 1930 and in 1948 that any ads mentioned neurasthenia at all, but at the low percentages of 12 and 3 per cent, respectively. This striking difference mirrors the different constructions of madness in the two countries, with French doctors specifically interested in the neurophysiological understanding of mental disorders.[38] It is therefore not surprising that the subgroup of 'nervous weakness', under which we gathered a series of categories ranging from *asthénie* in French to *Nervenschwäche* (neurasthenia) in German, shows a similar picture. Very few German ads mention these terms, and interestingly, do so mostly during the troubled times of World War I and the post-World War II period. In contrast the vocabulary of 'nerves' was a constant in France, stretching out over the entire time period with peaks at 17, 13 and again 13 per cent in 1930, 1955 and 1965, respectively, while the figures otherwise oscillated between 4 and 9 per cent.

The long-established diagnosis, 'epilepsy', shows a different pattern. It was initially fairly equally shared in both countries with high figures peaking at 26 per cent in France and 33 per cent in Germany. The diagnosis disappears earlier in Germany than in France. This may be interpreted on the basis of the fact that epileptics were discredited as suffering from an inherited pathology during the Nazi era and were therefore prosecuted and murdered.[39] It would not therefore have been wise to underscore this disease in advertising. Even though the indication still played a role in France and accounted for a 17 per cent share in 1940, it became a marginal entry in the post-war years, amounting to only 7 per cent of the ads in 1960 and with not a single ad referring to epilepsy showing up in 1965. This pattern is not only related to changes in psychiatric classifications and the rise of psychodynamic explanations, but also linked to the history of barbiturates, which had been considerably used in epilepsy since the turn of the twentieth century but had lost ground in the context of the 'therapeutic revolution' in psychiatry when other drug classes with fewer side effects were introduced.

The status of sleeping disorders is different as this indication is not linked to etiological but to symptomatic entries. Sleeplessness is actually a very common complaint and reference to the absence of sleep or troubled nights is a very common feature in the ads. Again, such problems appear more often in French ads, but are by no means absent from the German ones. In France, figures show two phases. The first phase saw an increase until World War II, with results peaking at 40 per cent in 1940. In a second phase, World War II brought about a sharp decline which may be viewed as a consequence of more pressing and acute needs. Reconstruction restored a level of 20 to 25 per cent in the 1950s. The general growth of psychotropic drug consumption in the 1960s is obvious, with an increase to 39 per cent in 1965 and 35 per cent in 1970. In Germany similar values were only reached in 1930 (24 per cent) and 1955 (40 per cent). Unfortunately, the missing figures for 1935 and 1940 mean that developments under the Nazi rule cannot be examined, which would have been particularly interesting as the system restricted the use of narcotics massively, and this may have had some impact on the long-term consumption of sleeping pills. However, with the exception of 1955, when for unknown reasons the share reached 40 per cent, adverts in the *Deutsche Medizinische Wochenschrift* (*DMW*) scarcely address this use as, after that, the figures remained at a low 7 to 15 per cent.

The existing figures for sedating medications plea for an increase in the German figures before 1945, which then went into continuous decline from the relatively high share of 35 per cent in 1945–48 to 10 per cent in 1965, while in 1975 and 1980 there was not a single ad for this product group, something that may have resulted from the massive propaganda against sedatives.[40] Given the generally higher incidence of psychiatric diagnoses in the French sample and the overall trend to use such pills in France, one would have expected higher shares in France, but the opposite was true. A first peak was reached at 29 per cent in 1925, and then it was followed by a continuous increase in the pre-war years. In the French case there were no such ads in 1945–48, while the share moved once again up to 26 per cent in 1950, then into continuous decline, ending at 9 per cent in 1970.

The case of anxiety and anxiolytics is important as the latter became major drugs of the post-war era and the most frequently prescribed of all psychotropic drugs, typically in the context of general practice rather than of specialized psychiatry and hospitals.[41] In the pre-war years the German *DMW* contained only a few ads for drugs targeting anxiety, reaching a peak of 12 per cent in 1930. Again, this may well be due to the 1941 decree, which strictly prohibited using fear in advertising. Whether this really covers anxiety as a general state is debatable, though possible. Nevertheless, it seems more probable that it was impossible to highlight fear during the Nazi era – and in its aftermath – when the population was educated systematically not to show fear at all and to contain all emotions. This was different in France, where anxiety surfaced early, even before the launch of major post-war tranquilizers like Valium and Librium. The French figures show that in the 1930s already more than one-third of the ads for psychotropic medication included anxiety as motive for use. It is all the more significant and unexpected that during the post-war era, the French figures rise continuously from 16 per cent in 1950 to 36 per cent in 1970, thus barely matching the pre-war level even when tranquilizers were introduced to the market. There is no comparable development in Germany. German manufacturers and physicians obviously did not see or name anxiety as a specific and major problem for a rather long time. If anxiety occurred in ads with a maximum share of 19 per cent in 1960, this seems to be of little significance since in the following years the figures dropped to 4 per cent in 1965 and 8 per cent in 1970. It was only in 1980 that the level reached 21 per cent, which is comparable to the French numbers. This data thus raises interesting questions regarding the local specificity of minor psychiatric ailments and their treatment, with for instance the possibility that in France, the more biological culture of psychiatrists resulted in an early translation of diagnoses like neurasthenia or asthenia to anxiety as a way to characterize patients coming to general practice with minor but multiple and shifting complaints. As Figure 4.7 shows, the ads differed massively from the ads from the 1920s as they envisioned the target symptoms from which the patient suffered in a very impressive manner.

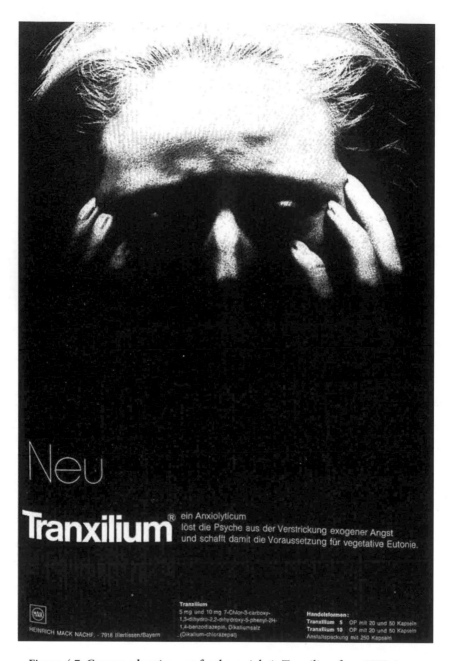

Figure. 4.7: German advertisement for the anxiolytic Tranxilium from 1970; image reproduced by kind permission of Deutscher Ärzte-Verlag GmbH.

Source: *Deutsches Ärzteblatt*, 27:2 (1970).

To check this interpretation we also examined the specific use of 'tranquilizers' in the ads. The first result was that in spite of their massive visibility in medical history, their incidence in the ads is surprisingly low, and especially so in comparison to the much higher figures for sleeping disorders. Of course, banal disorders are more frequent and as the market was filled with many different sleeping pills, competition through marketing was intensified. Yet even when tranquilizer sales boomed in Germany and France, their visibility in ads never exceeded 7 per cent (1969–70) in the *DMW* and displayed only slightly higher shares in the *CM*. Here the enduring dominance of 'old drugs' discussed by Nils Kessel in his contribution to this volume had considerable impact.

The case of depression provides some clues to this situation, showing a similar contrast between France and Germany. While there was a long-standing history of this indication in France, with one-third of the ads for psychotropic drugs in the *Concours Médical* (*CM*) mentioning it (13 per cent in 1930, but 29 per cent in 1935 and 27 per cent in 1940), it was absent from the ads in the *DMW* before 1960. The German situation thus reflects what might be expected on the basis of the historiography of antidepressants. The French point to a situation where various forms of mood and emotional disorders were recognized and considered a legitimate topic for therapeutic intervention. The motives of this visibility remain to be investigated. One should however remember that the meaning of depression in the 1920s and 1930s was very different from our present understanding of depression as a mass, relatively mild condition, most cases of which do not require treatment in hospital but can be handled in general practice.

Finally, a category needs to be mentioned for which the trajectory stands out from all the previous ones since it only appeared in 1960: namely, stress. Stress emerged as a topic of medical concern in the US medical literature in the 1940s, but became a pharmaceutical indication only with the development and mass sale of corticosteroids.[42] In our corpus, stress surfaces in 1960 in the *CM*, though as a marginal item, and then quickly disappears. In the German *DMW*, this indication shows up in 1969–70 and thereafter remains present at a stable 7 to 8 per cent. This finding leads to the interesting question of whether Germans tend to be 'stressed' where the French experience 'depression', in other words, whether a different moral economy of work was at play in the definition of these marketing targets, with a German industrial culture leading to the idea of the stressed white-collar worker as an icon of the side effects of growth and progress.[43]

Conclusion

To conclude we would like to return to the two components of the database, namely the formal aspects of pharmaceutical ads on the one hand and the medical information they use and represent on the other. The first dimension clearly documents the quantitative rise of advertising and its growing sophistication. In this respect, the trends toward larger, coloured and illustrated ads including brand logos, slogans and information on indications run parallel in both France and Germany. They strongly testify to the professionalization of drug marketing, even if this was by no means a simple linear process, and though the temporality may differ between the two countries. Differences appear much more significant when considering not only the rise of visualization and technical sophistication, but also the choice of elements represented. Thus, the ads in the French *Concours Médical* (*CM*) show a strong and early commitment to the visualization of effects and symptoms, which appears as a late phenomenon in the German *Deutsche Medizinische Wochenschrift* (*DMW*). This can be interpreted on the basis of different industrial structures (the importance of small firms with few products in France) and regulatory patterns (the more stringent 1941 German law) but it also points to the mounting visibility of the technical and medical information in the advertisements included in the database.

This decisive feature in scientific marketing had important consequences because ads became increasingly dependent on local medical cultures, a phenomenon reflected in the differentiation of indications in our corpus. This may be counter-intuitive when taking into account the links between the twentieth-century transformation of pharmacy and the development of scientific marketing. Post-war industrial pharmacy is usually associated with the growth of research and development, the changing scale of the market, and its internationalization. This can be expected to result in an enlarged circulation of medical knowledge as well as of therapeutic agents, and to convey more homogeneous – transnational – indications and categories. What the database indicates is not only that there was a persistence of 'old' differences in marketing targets but also a making of 'new' ones.

As discussed above, such an evaluation is predicated upon the possibility of comparing the medical vocabulary in our two national corpuses. This is no simple issue as there is, for instance, no previous evidence that the French '*asthénie*' can be rendered in the German '*Nervenschwäche*'. The solution adopted in the construction of our groups of indications was twofold: first to rely on terms like neurasthenia or stress, which were taken to be similar in medical dictionaries of the time and, when this proved not possible, to include a whole palette of synonyms rather than single nouns (including for instance '*faiblesse nerveuse*' (nervous weakness) in the French count of '*asthénie*').

Once this is deemed acceptable, the use of certain indications appears relatively constant and comparable in both countries, a feature that seems to testify to stable market niches addressing recurring, often minor, complaints such as sleeping disorders. In contrast, major diagnostic categories like neurasthenia show a highly contrasted fate and great variability of occurrence, most probably because of the periodic reconstruction of medical classifications and nosography. The main feature is however that more recent categories like anxiety, stress or depression, which are associated with the post-war therapeutic revolution in psychiatry, reveal equally contrasting patterns in the ads of the *CM* and the *DMW*. What made depression and anxiety so visible in France rather than stress cannot be properly discussed without further inquiries using other sources – industrial as well as medical. It is, however, a merit of the database to signal such differences, as well as point to the specificity of national medical cultures and beyond, to the different pictures of the sane/insane body that have prevailed in France and Germany.

5 MARKETING FILM: AUDIO-VISUALS FOR SCIENTIFIC MARKETING AND MEDICAL TRAINING IN PSYCHIATRY: THE SANDOZ EXAMPLE IN THE 1960S

Christian Bonah

Introduction

The goal of the present volume is to study, from the angle of promotional strategies, the evolution of the relationship between industry and pharmacy, physicians and patients, resulting from the industrialization of drug research, development and distribution during the twentieth century. It is pursued in this paper from the perspective of a specific corporate communication tool: the production and distribution of audio-visuals. More specifically, this paper aims to investigate the role of medical films in the transition that is central to this volume, which may be characterized as leading from advertising to scientific marketing between 1940 and 1970.

Scientific marketing in the pharmaceutical sector may be defined along three major lines. First, and in contrast to advertising, scientific marketing communicates scientific and technical information to a professional addressee, in general a prescribing physician. Referring to the 'scientific' in scientific marketing, the information usually deals with a specific substance and its effects, intentional or unintentional, its use and its usual dosage. In other words it contains and involves professional information. Second, there is 'marketing' in scientific marketing. In a general economic and commercial context this refers to an allegedly American post–World War II model in which marketing practices were framed and informed by the social sciences psychology and economics.[1] The practices were based on the paradigms of market research, systematic market observation and customer surveys on the one hand, and experimental psychology and behavioural studies of (customer) persuasion on the other. Third, in the context of investigations in this book, scientific marketing may be conceived as a multitude of practices that are intended to entangle research, drug evaluation and promotional strategies. Scientific marketing thus establishes a kind of seamless web between substance evaluation, medical information and industrial promotion. The present paper argues that these three defining elements – scientific content, empirical social science–based promotion and intentional blending of professional and promotional aspects – can be observed not only in research settings including controlled clinical trials, but also well in a second arena, which in the 1970s and 1980s became identified as postgraduate professional training.[2] It will be argued here that similarly to drug testing and evaluation, medical postgraduate education organized by the pharmaceutical industry provided technical and scientific information to physicians, monitored reception and entangled postgraduate training with drug promotion, a concept framed in the late 1960s as 'promotional information'.[3]

The beginnings of 'scientific marketing' took root in Germany after World War I and later in France, where implementation seems to have started after World War II.[4] As illustrated by Jean-Paul Gaudillière and Lucie Gerber's contributions in this volume, the period after 1945 combined instruments for systematic market observation and customer surveys with particular forms of conveying information in which the scientific dimension of pharmaceutical companies' activities and products was emphasized. In contrast to traditional product advertising, in scientific marketing 'promotional' information mimicked academic journals and publications, invested in professional meetings and scientific seminars, and used sales representatives for drug presentation, all of which were targeted at prescribing physicians in their professional culture. The pharmaceutical industry also sponsored medical films, as suggested in the editorial of the French medical film periodical *Cinéma/Médecine* in 1972:

> The general idea of this [medical cinematographic] production – which is essentially linked to the pharmaceutical industry – consists in reaching practicing physicians: by participating in their information and their training, in return they offer a better opportunity of commercial profit through their prescriptions.[5]

This paper will thus argue that analysis of scientific marketing should also refer to practices including medical and scientific films.[6] It will highlight a transformation in which early product advertising films for general audiences were supplemented, starting in the inter-war period and increasing significantly after World War II, with scientific information and professional training films to be used for marketing purposes with professionals. Our central claim will be that marketing films echoed the general transition to scientific marketing and may be seen as the fourth component of scientific marketing, alongside promotional research, sales representative systems and written 'scientific information' published in journals. As concluded in 1969 by the editor-in-chief of *Cinéma/Médecine,* Philippe Chantelou: 'Medical films basically belong to the pharmaceutical industry, which has given these films a promotional function.'[7]

In advertising and marketing corporate messages are addressed to professionals who are often self-conscious about their status and self-image as liberal professionals, not businessmen with commercial concerns. For many, this difference symbolized a divide between charlatanism and orthodox medical practice, and throughout the twentieth century physicians were generally uncomfortable about being directly associated with commercial practices.

Promotional departments within the pharmaceutical industry originated in the inter-war period as 'propaganda departments' in corporate organizational charts. The negative connotation of propaganda after 1945, associated with National Socialist indoctrination practices and deceit, generated the need after World War II to dissociate corporate promotional 'propaganda' from political totalitarian propaganda. The pharmaceutical industry's intention to remain clear of charlatan advertising on the one hand and of the post-1945 negative connotation of propaganda on the other metamorphosed its existing promotional structures in the 1950s from '*Propaganda Abteilungen*' to 'departments of information, communication and marketing'.[8] At the heart of this reorientation was science as a practice and as an 'objective' and supposedly value-free expertise suggesting professional and moral value. For the above-mentioned reasons, corporate 'communication' in the post–World War II era became 'scientific' marketing.

This contribution will thus turn to one specific 'scientific marketing' tool and practice that has not received much of attention: industry-commissioned medical films. Historians' relationships with images are always somewhat troubled, and this is especially true for moving pictures. Little has been studied with respect to corporate films that were produced as marketing tools in the pharmaceutical sector.[9] Yet as the following will show audio-visuals were and are significant tools for scientific marketing. In a first step the paper examines the origins of film advertising in the pharmaceutical sector and the institution of advertising films in a production setting analysed as the 'advertising-film triad'. A second step will highlight changes that occurred after World War II and materialized in a setting where film had become part of scientific marketing. 'Film marketing' suggests in this context on the one hand the utilization of scientific, research and training films in a so-called multimedia alliance (*Medienverbund*) of corporate communication strategies defined as a 'network of competing, but also mutually interdependent and complementary media or media practices'.[10] In this process a new category of scientific advertising and promotional information film established itself, characterized by its more vocational and less direct product advertising–oriented nature. This transformation was matched by a second one that gave a second meaning to 'marketing film'. Medical and scientific film directors of the 1950s and 1960s engaged in a strategy to enrol medical opinion leaders and, through them, pharmaceutical companies, to finance the production of medical and scientific films otherwise impossible to make. In this second sense, film directors pitched scientific and medical films that they wished to shoot to the pharmaceutical industry and in the process imposed their desire to ban specific product promotion from their films.[11] Analysed in this second step as the 1960s 'film-marketing triad', the constellation describes this meeting of mutual interests where film marketing implied that the independence of film directors was the very basis for investment in their films by pharmaceutical corporations as part of their scientific marketing strategies. In a third step, the paper will present this film form of scientific marketing by using a specific example.

The Origins of Pharmaceutical Advertising Films

Visual and film studies have recently devoted increasing attention to a category of films that for a long time were considered marginal, uninteresting or even simply lost.[12] What these films have in common is that they were quantitatively of utmost significance in terms of film production on the one hand and that they were produced and screened in industrial, educational or not-for-profit organization settings, far from commercial film channels.[13]

Not only are these so-called sponsored 'utility' or 'ephemeral' films an important source for medical film history, they may also be used to appraise the scientific marketing strategies and activities of pharmaceutical industries from a different angle.[14] These films were made by a particular sponsor for a specific purpose other than as a work of art. Films were designed to serve a specific pragmatic purpose for a limited amount of time.[15] Film archivists estimate that the industrial and advertising film genre alone accounts for more than 400,000 films produced between the 1910s and the 1960s in the US and, as such, is the largest genre of films known today.[16]

A new era of pharmaceutical communication began in the 1920s when industrial corporations of the petrochemical and pharmaceutical sector initiated film production and set up their own independent film units, as was the case, for example, in Great Britain for the Shell Corporation Film Unit.[17] In Germany the Pharmaceutical Research and Serobacteriological Department of the IG-Farbenindustrie formed a working association with the Universal Film Aktiengesellschaft (UFA) supported by the Rothe Institute for medical film in 1925.[18] According to accounts of the time in the Bayer in-house journal for mainstream advertising, the 'particular requirements of the pharmaceutical industry' identified as 'the inconsistency of demand in the pharmaceutical sector' made it necessary to organize medical film work, and just a year later, in 1926, the pharmaceutical company

Hoechst in association with Bayer established the Hoechst film unit (*Filmstelle Hoechst*).[19] The same year, film director Oskar Wagner left the UFA to organize film production for chemical and pharmaceutical companies in their newly created film units. An independent film department, the 'Filmzentrale Bayer Leverkusen' eventually appeared in the Bayer organizational charts in January 1934. The unit was responsible for mainstream and scientific film production under the direction of Dr Spielmann. Over the next two decades the Bayer Film Unit produced close to 100 films, often in cooperation with the UFA.

Starting in the inter-war years, industrial corporations engaged heavily in the production of advertising films. Bayer for example produced five Cafiaspirina (an Aspirin association made for Latin America) 'propaganda shorts' – *Falstaff, Sinbad der Seefahrer, Der besiegte Zauberer, Don Pancho* and *Stierkampf* – which were produced by the leading German advertising film director and producer Julius Pinschewer.[20] Beyond these series of outright product-related short films equivalent to newspaper ads, longer 'scientific' advertising films intertwined research and educational film elements with product-specific advertising.[21] Similar film production in Great Britain can be related to John Grierson, who in 1930 established the Empire Marketing Board Film Unit that in 1933 moved to the General Post Office. Grierson also convinced the oil company Shell International to establish its own film unit under the direction of Edgar Anstey. [22]

Typical of productions of the time was a series of German malaria films coproduced by the UFA and Oskar Wagner.[23] Technically up-to-date, the motion picture *Malaria*, for example, staged for more than half of the film a medical and public health–oriented description of the disease and displayed in the last part of the film some recent products developed by Bayer, including Plasmochin, Atebrin and Resochin tablets and their dosage and treatment schemes. Not only did these scientific advertising films (*Wissenschaftlicher Werbefilm*) differ in content and length from conventional advertising shorts, but they were also aimed at a distinct audience: Plasmochin, Atebrin and Resochin prescribing physicians.

Scientific advertising films thus established a triad where a pharmaceutical company wished to address a specific message to physicians as an audience and as potential drug prescribers. Using film to do so, the company could use internal film production facilities and teams or mobilize external filmmakers. For prestigious projects, companies turned to film directors of considerable reputation like Julius Pinschewer or Walter Ruttman, who under contract would put their artistic know-how at the service of the sponsor's message.[24] In practice, there was some tension between the film directors, who intended to remain the authors of their films beyond the sponsor's intentions, and the financing corporation's messages, orders and authority, to which film directors were not accustomed, especially outside film directors who were hired.

Gradually, between the 1920s and 1940s, a number of film directors came to specialize in institutional films and set up their own specific film companies, as indicated by Jean Benoit-Lévy's studios and his *Édition française Cinématographique* in France or the *Eastern Film Corporation* set up and directed by Frank A. Tichnor in the US.[25] Starting in the 1930s pharmaceutical companies increasingly began setting up their own film departments and hiring their film production staff directly, as illustrated above in the Hoechst and Bayer cases. Internalization of film production had the advantage of being able to control the film production and the conveyed messages closely and to make the hired film directors directly aware of corporate culture and needs. The intimacy of hired film directors with corporate objectives and identities was offset by the fact that companies depended on the individual film director's artistic and personal film style. The corporate promotional films of the pharmaceutical industry of the inter-war years, whether short promotional films or longer educational and scientific advertising films, generally included sequences of direct product advertising. As such, film production was equated with pharmaceutical advertising practices, be they directed at physicians or at the general public.

Marketing Medical Film

The 1950s and 1960s were witness to a hitherto unknown development of medical corporate films.[26] According to the film scholar Gérard Leblanc the 'extraordinary period of the 1960s' was less about medical films as such than about a golden period for industrial filmmaking in general related to the generalization of corporate films.[27] In the late 1950s the Swiss pharmaceutical company Sandoz decided to set up a film library for medical films, the Cinémathèque Sandoz. The French writer and translator Michel Breitman (1926–2009), known as the translator of the writer Dino Buzzati and the author of popular novels including *Fortunat* and *Sébastien* published at Gallimard, but also as a screenplay writer and film connoisseur, became the director of the film library. Contrary to what its name suggested, the Cinémathèque was not just a place for the distribution of films with medical content; it was also the initiator of a new corporate film production strategy by Sandoz. It financed, created and distributed free copies of medical films produced by Sandoz for physicians. It was therefore as much a film production 'company' as a film distribution library. Assisted by Jean-Charles Gaspard, Breitman commissioned for Sandoz films such as *Le Horla* (1967) or *L'Ordre* (1973) directed by Jean-Daniel Pollet, which today belong to the classics of documentary film.[28]

Sandoz's 1969 catalogue of medical-scientific films indicates that the library had 116 films on offer for free that were produced by Sandoz between 1958 and 1969, meaning an average of ten films produced or sponsored per year. Amongst the authors and production companies in the catalogue, one specific company and its director stand out: ScienceFilm, a company set up in 1946 by the French film director Eric Duvivier. Fifty-eight out of the 116 films sponsored by Sandoz were produced by ScienceFilm, i.e., 50 per cent of production. We have defined a more restricted film corpus to be studied in the following analysis, which will focus on pictures related to and listed under one specific disease category heading: psychiatry. Psychiatric films alone account for roughly one film out of five produced during the first ten years of the Cinémathèque's existence.[29] In terms of numbers this is the most outstanding subject in the films produced. Twelve of the twenty-six films listed under the 'psychiatry' heading in the catalogue are creations of ScienceFilm and its director. The choice to investigate films in the field of psychiatry may be further justified by the fact that psychoactive substances were of particular interest to the company that had been associated in the 1940s with the invention and development of LSD, and in the 1950s with the psychopharmacological revolution of neuroleptics, tranquilizers and antidepressant drugs.[30] Psychiatric films occupied a significant part of early Sandoz film production and played a significant role in the company's strategy to distribute and show these films in special events organized for physicians and at professional scientific meetings.

The man behind ScienceFilm, the film company specializing in medical films, was Eric Duvivier (1928–). Duvivier was the nephew of the better-known film director Julien Duvivier (1896–1967).[31] Growing up in a filmmaking family environment – his father worked with his uncle – Eric Duvivier began to study medicine immediately after World War II and, bridging interests, organized a film club for medical students. He eventually dropped out of medical school and devoted himself entirely to filmmaking.[32] Duvivier soon set up his first production company in the late 1940s. Initially the company thrived by copying 16mm and 35mm films for major film studios in Paris, a rather lucrative activity immediately after 1945. At the same time, Duvivier mobilized his uncompleted medical education to start producing medical and scientific films for professional audiences. The first medical films he directed involved mainly anatomical subjects, such as his first film, *L'os temporal, Le péritoine* or *Anatomie de l'épaule/hanche/genou*. Well established in the field by the late 1950s, he became a natural partner for the Sandoz film library project and directed his first film for Sandoz in 1959, *Le cycle du fer dans l'organisme*. The production catalogue of Duvivier's film production company contains a list of more than 700 films produced between 1950 and 2000. Given the 596 sound-and-colour films that are listed in the 1988 ScienceFilm catalogue, Duvivier sustained an average production of fifteen films a year for over forty years. The place of psychiatric films in the Duvivier film corpus is significant. The 100 films with psychiatric subjects made between 1950 and 1988 account for roughly one-sixth of the film director's activity.

Amongst them there are titles like *Sémiologie psychiatrique: cinq observations* (n.d.), *Le métoclopramide* (n.d.), *Dépression d'automne* (n.d.), *Syndrome hébéphréno-catatonique* (1971), *Expérience délirante primaire chez un adolescent* (n.d.), *Psychose alcoolique* (n.d.) and *État démentiel: maladie d'Alzheimer* (n.d.).[33] These titles clearly connote the professional and medical-training orientation of the films produced by Duvivier and his company. The films were commissioned and produced for pharmaceutical industries like the Sandoz film library. At the same time rather unexpected titles – like *La femme 100 têtes* (n.d.), based on a 1929 novel by Max Ernst, *Les années folles de Sylvain Fusco* (n.d.), a French painter who had been committed at the mental institution Asile départemental du Rhône, *Ces maladies qui nous gouvernent* (n.d.), a critical appraisal of diseases from which leading world politicians suffered, *Images de la folie* (n.d.), *Images du monde visionnaire* (n.d.) and *Autoportrait d'un schizophrène* (1977), presenting subjective audio-visual and written testimonies of patient views – also appear in the film catalogue, triggering the historian's attention. Indeed, the films produced by ScienceFilm and Duvivier in the field of psychiatry can be divided into two sets. One is clearly established as a set of teaching films for postgraduate physician training including for instance films on psychiatric clinical symptoms (*Sémiologie psychiatrique: cinq observations)*, disease descriptions (*Syndrome hébéphréno-catatonique*) or new drugs (*Le métoclopramide*). The other set involves a highly intriguing production of rather avant-garde experimental films with titles like *La femme 100 têtes* or *Images du monde visionnaire* (see below), entailing further investigation. How did cooperation between a pharmaceutical company and ambitious, marginal and experimental documentary filmmakers actually work?

Eric Duvivier, ScienceFilm and the Sandoz Medical Film Library

The ScienceFilm catalogue reveals a significant detail that leads to a better understanding of company strategies in medical film production. Films are listed according to subjects and medical disciplines and, most interestingly, titles are followed by names of prestigious professors of medicine and their city of activity rather than by the identity of the sponsoring pharmaceutical company. A 2012 interview with Duvivier revealed that from the film director's perspective the 'advertising film triad' was transformed in the 1950s and 1960s into a 'film marketing triad'.[34]

The scientific advertising film triad of the 1930s is a corporate communication tool with which the company intends to address a promotional message to an audience of physician prescribers. A film commission is issued to a film director or to a film company specifying the central message, and sometimes a detailed scenario. Film directors translate the message into their own film language and expression. Tensions arise between the intentions and messages of the corporate film and the film director's views. In the film marketing triad of the 1960s the medical film director and his film company enrols medical professors as opinion leaders to identify medical training subjects. Film projects are jointly presented to corporate communication bodies like film libraries. The pharmaceutical company commissions a film from a film director or a film company on the basis of an association between the film director and a medical professor. Physicians are conveyed as audience and prescribers to medical film events where corporate messages on individual products are additionally presented off screen. The film-sponsoring pharmaceutical companies are included only in the film credits.

Duvivier followed a strategy according to which the medical film producer and his production company first identified a medical expert receptive to film and approached him to suggest producing a film with a topic of his choice. From there on, the physician-professor became the 'producer' of the film in terms of its content. The credits in these films display revealing ambiguities, with films credited as directed by the medical authority and produced by Duvivier and his company. Contrary to usual practices in the film world – where a film producer is the arrangement and financing authority of the production of a film, the film director is the artist making the film and a screenplay writer may produce a script – in the medical film marketing world it was the content-providing physician-professor who was designated as the film director, and Duvivier, who in the regular film world would have been the 'film director', became the film producer. Where 'a film by Eric Duvivier' would not have been identified by practising physicians, 'a film by' Professor Jean Delay, Marcel Bessis, Jean Bernard or Jacques Chretien, for example, worked as a signal in the social world of physicians.

With a subject at hand, Duvivier then approached a pharmaceutical firm relevant to the professor's medical specialty. In this medical film marketing triad, Sandoz is just one amongst many pharmaceutical companies with which Duvivier and ScienceFilm produced films. For the physician, the production of a film allows public representation of himself or public display of his specific working topics and theories. This had been an old tradition of medical filmmaking since the early 1900s, when Eugène Doyen produced his first surgical films mixing the intention of improving surgical techniques through film observation with public representation and publicity for the medical or surgical author of the film.[35] For Duvivier this two-step strategy consisted in first ensuring the interest and collaboration of a high-profile medical expert. Identified as an opinion leader by the profession and the pharmaceutical industry, his/her symbolic capital was then transformed by Duvivier into film production budgets from the pharmaceutical industry. The industry calculated that medical opinion leaders could be portrayed as pharmaceutical opinion leaders in fields of specific drugs.[36] Film producers mobilized high-profile physicians as incentives for the industry to finance production of the film. Sandoz would not have sponsored a film by Eric Duvivier, but would do so, and did, for a film 'by' Jean Delay and Henri Michaux (see below). Leading physicians engaged in film production with a film professional on a medical subject. Leaving financial aspects to the production company, they apparently stayed clear of pharmaceutical advertising and promotion, a subject always potentially controversial to them.

Once the budget was allocated, the film director and the production company requested written content from the physician then established a working space for the film director almost entirely at his discretion. This way the marketing film triad ensured significant financing for prestigious film projects and at the same time maintained room for the film director's creativity and his possibility of arguing for limited corporate control by the financing pharmaceutical company over the structure and content of the film. In practice, this meant that all of the more than 700 films produced by ScienceFilm started with a company logo such as 'Sandoz presents ...', but then no further mention was made of the company. A total absence of product-related promotion was characteristic of these films. Directors like Duvivier had always been eager to protect their filmmaking freedom from the promotional mission of their films. This meant that promotional intentions were relegated to how the sponsors then used the films rather than stated through messages embedded directly in the films. Films were used during events, with their screening part of multimedia alliances in which product promotion was an element of the surrounding organization, i.e., performed by company employees and through stands at the events. The 1960s and 1970s medical filmmakers' attempt to distance themselves from specific product advertising in their commissioned film work may have later been echoed in culture-sponsoring practices. Criticism at the time, however, observed something else, as mentioned in continuation of the above-cited editorial:

> The general idea of this [medical cinematographic] production – which is essentially linked to the pharmaceutical industry – consists in reaching practicing physicians: by participating in their information and their training, in return they offer a better opportunity of commercial profit through their prescriptions.
>
> This perfectly admissible idea has been hidden for a long time behind the sponsoring culture (*mécénat*) aspect, but it has increasingly become publicly admissible.[37]

To get a better understanding of this three-way collaboration between medical film producer, pharmaceutical company and physician we will turn to an exemplary case study of a film and analyse its intrinsic film elements as well as the film screening as part of a promotion scheme.[38]

Visions from a World of Fantasy (1963)

In 1963, Duvivier produced the film *Images du monde visionnaire* (*Visions from a World of Fantasy*) described as 'a film by Henri Michaux (1899–1984), a French-Belgian poet and artist affiliated with the lyric abstraction movement and having experience with illicit drug consumption'.[39] Under the influence of mescaline, a psychoactive substance, Michaux produced the 'mescaline drawings' at the heart of the film. Directed by Duvivier, the thirty-four-minute colour film shows, in two parts, the images seen by a normal person submitted to two successive experiments.[40] In the first he is under the influence of Hallucinogen A (mescaline), and the spectator sees trembling, coloured configurations with no apparent coherence, constantly changing and differing shapes of imaginary creatures or unidentifiable objects or substances permanently in the process of becoming something else.

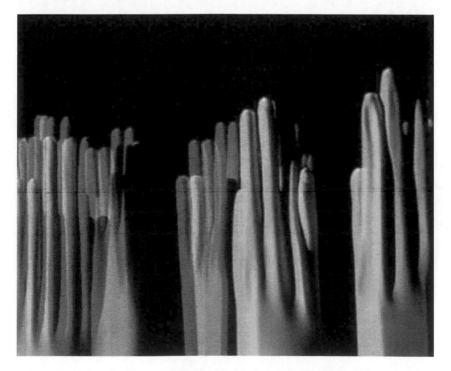

Figure 5.1: Mescaline vision in the film *Images du monde visionnaire* (France, 1963); image reproduced by kind permission of E. Duvivier.

In the second experiment, with Hallucinogen B (hashish), known objects become visible on the screen for the spectator, but they are deformed, bizarre and in strange positions and situations. A sense of open or suppressed commotion and disturbance is evident. Everything seems tend to be torn away from the earth or from its normal surroundings. A bridge rises dizzily high into the sky. A head is separated from a trunk by a sword. Through the gaping wound in the neck thick vapour ascends from the motionless body.

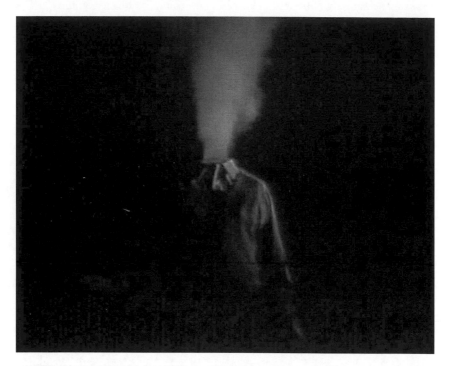

Figure 5.2: Hashish Vision in the Film *Images du monde visionnaire* (France, 1963); image reproduced by kind permission of E. Duvivier.

Henri Michaux indicates in a written preface to the film that the:

> purpose of this film is to show the kinds of thought images [*images de pensées*] which pass, with intense clarity and without any act of volition, through the mind of a person who has been subjected to the action of certain psychotonic substances, and the special way in which they appear and vanish. Two types of images correspond to the two hallucinogenic substances, and their differences rather than their similarities have been stressed here.[41]

Today's audience might find it difficult to make sense of what is basically a strange experimental film and to imagine why Sandoz would have produced such a film and to whom it was addressed and shown.[42]

The missing link of interpretation comes from the on-screen foreword to the film, explaining that '[w]ith extraordinary lucidity and incredible precision,

Henri Michaux has been capable of fixing in his memory these or those images of the visionary world that appear under this or that hallucinogenic substance'.[43] The medical advisor to the film underscores that the great scientific value of Michaux's 'mescaline visions' justifies the medical perspective of this film produced by Duvivier. In the ScienceFilm catalogue the picture is associated with none other than Professor Jean Delay. Delay, one of the founding fathers of the introduction of chlorpromazine in the psychiatric wards of the Sainte Anne hospital in Paris in the 1950s, presented the film in 1963 to a medical audience and justified his interest in the undertaking as follows: 'The analogy or the identity of these [psychoactive drug–induced] experimental states, which can be produced and reduced within a few hours, with certain states of mental alienation are at the origin of current research on the biochemical pathogenesis of psychoses.'[44] General physicians are shown a self-experiment with mescaline and hashish. For thirty-four minutes, they become silver screen scientists observing self-experimentation and are visually exposed to its consequences; they become movie theatre armchair psychiatrists exploring the insides of psychotic sensations. They are familiarized with impressions and perceptions that it is suggested psychotic patients have and with how the new psychoactive drugs might make them disappear and appear.

What the psychiatrist expert Jean Delay expected from the film was to communicate to a wider public of physicians the underpinnings of the psychopharmacological revolution of which he was a leading figure. For the film director Duvivier, collaboration with Michaux and the subject of a film on visual perceptions under the influence of psychoactive substances offered the possibility of an experimental film with no narrative or plot; simply an arrangement of visual effects and perceptions in a (movie) world of visions. Public representation of the medical opinion leader, a broad dissemination of the new psychopharmacological gospel and the corporate interests of a firm with a strong standing in research on psychoactive drugs – including LSD – were the benefits aligned by the filmmaking triad in the specific case of the 1963 film described here. The three-way alliance between a film director (wanting to produce an experimental film on drug perceptions), a psychiatrist expert (wanting to communicate his theories and conceptions on psychosis and its treatment) and a pharmaceutical company (researching and distributing psychoactive drugs) thus combined what at first glance was hard to situate or understand: an experimental film entitled 'Visions from a World of Fantasy' produced and distributed through the medical film library of a pharmaceutical company: Sandoz.

But what was a physician to do with an experimental film in a library? This is precisely where the medical film screening scheme enters our analysis. Films like the one described here were brought into evening film programmes organized by Sandoz in major towns and cities throughout the country and beyond. Sales representatives convened prescribing physicians. Art films were good selling attractions in these ambiguous situations placed somewhere between entertainment (an artistic experimental film) and scientific information (what's new in psychosis and its treatment). These evening events were announced as an 'evening for physicians' cast in professional terms as a meeting on 'clinical features and news' in the field of psychiatry. Medical experts like Delay served as leading clinicians. In the world of medical film, scientific figures became attractions just like movie stars in general entertainment. The attractive value of these social gatherings designed for physicians thinking of themselves as a highly cultured part of society was furthered by completing them with services ranging from refreshments to complete evening dinners. During these social gatherings, scientific films were accompanied by leaflets, hand-outs and the like containing specific product information messages not included in the films, and sales representatives could establish close and relaxed relationships with the physician-prescribers they were to visit in their office.

Recruited in 1964 by Henri Clouzot (who had acknowledged Duvivier's 1963 film *Visions from a World of Fantasy* discussed above), Duvivier produced the special effects for Clouzot's uncompleted film *L'Enfer* (Hell). The footage of 'hallucinatory sequences' with Romy Schneider were reused in the film *Une psychose en enfer* produced by Sandoz, directed by Duvivier and presented by Dr Patrick Lemoine, head physician of one of the major French psychiatric hospitals, Le Vinatier in Lyon. As indicated in the invitation, 'lunch [would] be served at the end of the film screening'.

Added value for the corporations was that the films, because they did not feature any ads for specific products, were also included in wider distribution circuits including those of the Ministry of Foreign Affairs, which in the early 1960 established the audio-visual catalogue of the Saint Antoine hospital, a catalogue destined to the cultural sections of embassies throughout the world.

Visions from a World of Fantasy was thus translated into English and travelled to embassies, which organized screenings of avant-garde cinema, movies on French science and, in passing, some publicity was made for the pharmaceutical company that had sponsored the film with no apparent commercial agenda, just for the sake of supporting science, culture and the arts.

In a closing remark let us return to pharmaceutical companies and their interest in setting up a film library like the one operated by Sandoz. The scientific film marketing strategy pursued by the company consisted in the fact that pharmaceutical companies would buy into the film producer's strategy to use high-profile medical physicians or scientists for the visibility and distribution of their films. Sandoz's prestigious production policy granting film directors considerable space for authorship and film expertise, as well as excellent working conditions, led to high-quality film production, which turned the Sandoz film library itself into an opinion leader amongst pharmaceutical companies; similar film production was quickly imitated by other companies including Rhône-Poulenc, Lagrange, Beaufour and Ciba-Geigy. The concept of scientific film marketing became generally accepted in the 1970s.

An interesting point is that in this trade-off, filmmakers and artists fared quite well. A number of the films were experimental in nature and would have been impossible to produce in official production circuits that depended on paying audiences. Furthermore, many of the films adopted a resolutely patient-oriented perspective, which was in tune with *cinéma direct* in which directors attempted to get audiences completely immersed in the world that was filmed.[45] Off-screen voice commentary was very limited when not completely absent from the films, and patients often gave their point of view. In this sense, film directors to some extent subverted the pharmaceutical intentions of their sponsors. They kept control over what in the end remained their film. What was being sold to the pharmaceutical industry was the film and its use more than the content and craftsmanship of the film. As these films were coproduced by a physician for the content and a film director for the images, they were basically attractions, whether scientific or educational.

Conclusion

In contrast to earlier advertising films of the 1930s, film marketing of the 1960s established a divide between the film and the promotional object. Film directors were delighted by this trade-off that allowed them to serve commercial interests less visibly. Physicians welcomed the illusion that the films and film screening events were professional and of a purely cultural or scientific character, as suggested by the films. No direct drug promotion appeared in these films. Pharmaceutical corporations concentrated on off-screen hosting and assistance to develop promotional activities that they could adapt and control very efficiently under the direct supervision of their personnel.

The transition from 1930s advertising films to 1960s film marketing may be illustrated by the fact that although specific product-related ads did not disappear altogether, the films described here did completely ban them. In the 1960s, Sandoz's film marketing product-related scientific information was not delivered in the films themselves but in accompanying events and brochures. That is to say, the 1960s films were corporate marketing films as part of an overall strategy scheme, not as films in themselves. Compared to the Bayer malaria drug, Resochin, advertising film discussed earlier, what the 1960s films lost in terms of specificity and identity as promotional tools they gained in flexibility and multifunctional use. How they were integrated in other modern marketing practices remains to be investigated in the corporate archives of information and communication departments of the pharmaceutical industry.

With respect to the definition of scientific marketing used throughout this volume, the films analysed here are not so much a mix of clinical evaluation, research and marketing as they are entertainment and education for physicians. My concluding argument is that scientific marketing of the 1960s and 1970s should be defined along two lines. One is the line of clinical forms of scientific marketing entangling drug research and clinical evaluation practices. The present paper argues that there is a second line establishing a continuum between a professional's social life – entertainment – and his professional requirement of continued postgraduate training and education. What characterizes the two lines of scientific marketing is the hybrid nature of objects and practices on the one hand and the ambiguity or multidimensionality of the objectives and tools employed on the other. In both cases, a space of practices emerges where pharmaceutical companies become much more than simple providers of scientific and medical information in the guise of evaluation tools and results. Companies harnessed apparently neutral and objective practices to their promotional activities. This was the other, hidden, face of 'scientific' marketing starting in the 1950s.

The present analysis suggests that the designation of 'scientific marketing' should include another of these complex spaces of exchange between pharmaceutical corporations and their direct or indirect interlocutors and 'customers'. A field of practices that has not drawn much interest amongst medical historians emerges from a different historical source – corporate medical films – and may be considered as a significant piece in the puzzle of scientific marketing.

It is a general assumption that the world of physicians may be characterized by its troubled relationship with marketing and commercialization. If this is so, then maybe the Sandoz film library became a successful enterprise precisely because commercial aspects were distanced – whether by film directors, by the pharmaceutical company itself or by both – from events that were organized to stir up attention and encourage a good time. A specific economic context of significant promotional investments in a flourishing industrial branch (pharmaceuticals), the acknowledgement of film as a significant vector of information, education, research and promotion, and a pharmaceutical company's engagement in prestigious film production as a means to promote a corporate image and individual products to physicians together gave birth to a hybrid form of education/entertainment that produced attraction. The broader film-based promotion scheme – where and how films were screened – was organized through periodicals (*Médecine/Cinéma*), with lunch or dinner film screening events alongside pharmaceutical sales representatives, and by renting films out to physician gatherings and teaching classes.[46] It was the schemes in which the films were set which were promotional and commercial.

What that leaves us with today is a series of astonishing films. Viewed from the perspective of film producers and directors, Sandoz film production and distribution was a courageous experiment. A major corporation provided budgets and distribution for experimental and documentary films that were marginal to mainstream entertainment but highly significant for documentary and auteur cinema. The Cinémathèque was an undertaking that was original, clearly not completely thought through from the beginning in strategic marketing terms and probably hardly imaginable in the world of marketing after the 1990s. It became part of the scientific marketing practices of the 1970s and 1980s and perfectly illustrated the move from advertising to scientific marketing. Last but not least, the promotional events organized for medical and scientific film screening may be seen as seminal and 'ancestral' forms of postgraduate medical training. Conceived in the framework of pharmaceutical scientific marketing, these origins go a long way to explain persisting links between postgraduate medical training and the pharmaceutical industry throughout the second half of the twentieth century.

6 IMAGES, VISUALIZATION AND THE PRACTICES OF SCIENTIFIC MARKETING IN POST-WAR FRANCE

Anne-Sophie Mazas

What is at stake here – and this must be the starting point – is the physician's situation when facing a specific therapeutic problem for which he needs a product ... The person we are addressing is the attending physician who has had a number of solutions at his disposal, which might not all have been fully satisfactory so far. So let us put ourselves in his place; let us try to become part of his reasoning at the spot where there is a flaw ... Advertising is all about popularization.[1]

One of the major transformations of drug promotion practices in the post-war era has been, as outlined in the introduction to this volume, the development of scientific marketing. For the purpose of this paper, scientific marketing will be defined as a combination of three different moves: (1) the professionalization of advertising as illustrated by the rise of specialized advertising firms and the introduction of marketing courses in business schools; (2) an extended mobilization of biomedical research results for the purpose of market building; and (3) the development of marketing as a research activity beyond just analysing sales figures in the context of the planning and organizational development of large firms.

As a consequence of this conjunction, there was a rapid extension of the palette of promotional media and marketing techniques used by the largest firms operating in the markets, which in most European countries were definitely growing. This is explained in *Corporate Diversity*, a book on Geigy's advertising and design sponsored by the firm in the 1990s to memorialize this transformation.

Physicians were addressed using the following media: direct mailing, advertisements in professional journals (scientific publications with advertising inserts), sample packages, promotional gifts, talking material, clinical works and reports, conferences and medical films. Sales representatives' calls on doctors were also part of this coordinated mix of media, but representatives did not report to the propaganda department. These diverse means of advertising were rolled out over time in order to hold the physicians' attention.[2]

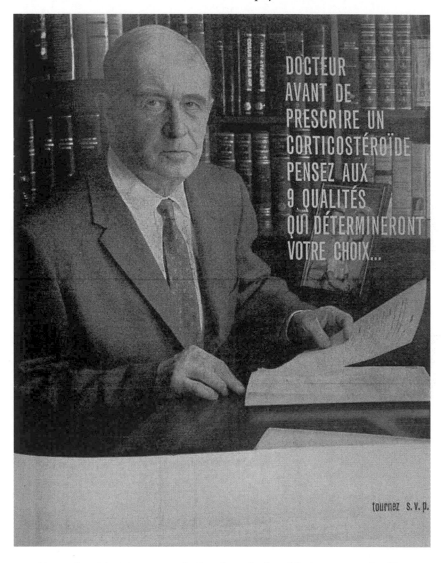

Figure 6.1: Advertisement in the French medical weekly *Concours Medical* for Triamcinolone, a corticosteroid from Squibb .

Source: *Concours Medical* (September 1960), first page.

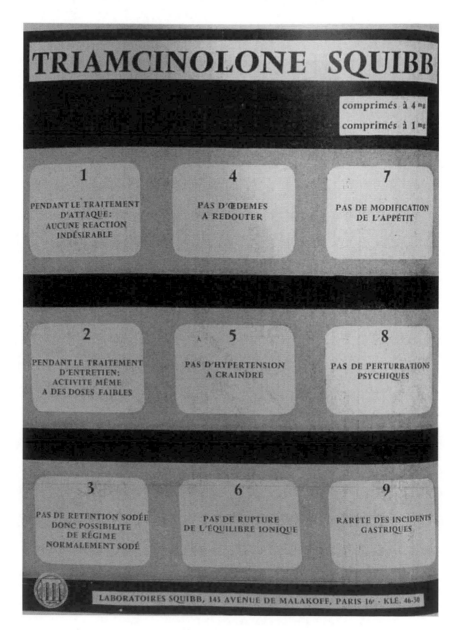

Figure 6.2: Advertisement for Triamcinolone.

Source: *Concours Medical* (September 1960), second page.

This paper approaches this complex perspective from a specific vantage point, which is the new position given to scientific information and the way permanent reference to research results was incorporated, translated and used in advertisements for physicians, in other words to define the usefulness and uses of drugs and shape prescription practices.[3] The magnitude of the shifts at stake can be illustrated by comparing advertisements from the *Concours Médical*, one of the two periodicals read by most French practitioners from the 1930s on. In these visuals, although superficially the technique used – a printed ad spread over two pages published in a professional journal – seems to be the same, it is radically different and does not serve the same purpose at all. Before the war, different boxes simply placed side by side introduce different products; they do not belong to the same therapeutic class nor do they address the same disorder, but they are produced by the same company. The laboratory was thus promoting its name and the diversity of its catalogue. In contrast, in the 1960s (Figures 6.1 and 6.2) the double-page technique is concentrated on a single product and a single medical target and – this is critical – it is bursting with scientific information. The information does not only refer to the properties of the product; it focuses on its clinical value and the proper way of prescribing it: pathological targets, symptoms to be taken into account, dosage and forms of administration, possible side effects and causes of adverse reactions. All of this had become part of what good promotion should include. Although medical science and clinical research were centre stage, in its form and content this material was not a scientific article, it was a marketing tool and was designed and read as such.

The question we wish to address is therefore part of a puzzle: How did postwar scientific marketing work? How did it articulate, in practice, research and promotional techniques? Articulation in this context has two dimensions that are only contradictory if science and the market are considered as ontologically distinct. On the one hand, scientific marketing is about making links – i.e., combining research results – and about translating company-based knowledge into advertising components in order to establish the identity of a product. On the other hand, the scientific marketing of drugs is about setting boundaries because to be successful, given that they are above all addressed to professionals whose expertise must not be challenged, information must be recognized as such; it must find a way to be distinct from advertising and purified of it or, better said, of the most obvious marketing devices such as slogans or cultural metaphors.

To investigate this double bind and how it was reflected in the advertisements themselves, this paper focuses on 'visualization', i.e., on the palette of techniques that were specifically used to create images both literally – with the various ways in which visual elements establish meaning – and semantically – with the various procedures designed by drug marketing experts to tell stories, consolidate the properties of therapeutic agents and secure their markets.

Scientific Marketing and Strategies of Visualization in Post-War France

There are two preliminary points to make before discussing these scientific marketing strategies more concretely. The first deals with the question of semiotic analysis. A vast body of literature on signs and advertisements has emerged since Roland Barthes's and Jean Baudrillard's ground-breaking studies in the late 1950s and the 1960s.[4] More often these studies are social-scientific analyses of modern consumer societies focusing on their specific and changing cultures and on the way advertisements as signs use and reshape identities, norms and needs. Whatever its immense intrinsic interest, this literature barely touches upon the question of science and – apart from very general notions like connotation, chains of interpretation or systems of signification – is of little value for the purpose of this paper, which is to understand how advertising achieved the sort of 'boundary work' inherent to the strategies of scientific marketing. The paper will therefore address and make use of a different body of semiotic literature, the literature associated with the marketers themselves. Since the 1960s, semiotics – along with psychology, cybernetics, management theories and sociology itself – has been incorporated into the palette of disciplines from which promotion professionals borrow. As aptly summarized by Ron Beasley and Marcel Danesi, the idea has most often been to increase the impact of promotional action through the analysis of specific advertisements (or entire campaigns) understood as 'signification machines' combining signifiers to produce texts and subtexts providing specific connotations and motives to buy.[5] In direct relation to the professionalization of marketing, a critical aspect of applied semiotics has thus been the creation of general typologies of both the techniques used and the psychological or cultural tropes referred to. Although these typologies almost never discuss the specificity of drug marketing and the science issue, they are important categories of actors and provide the background for valuable analytical tools, some of which will be discussed below.

The second methodological point to be considered is the professionalization process of marketing. The history of this process has been traced to the US context and goes back to the beginning of the twentieth century, even though the massive incorporation of experts and tools into the sales divisions and routine work of large corporations happened in the 1920s. There is no equivalent knowledge for the French case, which is at the core of this chapter. The general scenario that can be tentatively used is the one proposed by the historian Marie-Emmanuelle Chessel, who argues that the professionalization and 'scientifization' of general advertising is a late phenomenon that took place after World War II, when international exchanges between Europe and the USA promoted the circulation of new tools and techniques in the fields of communication and marketing, paving the way to the constitution of a new discipline, scientific marketing, and offering new research prospects.[6] French advertising professionals thus perceived all these tools – market studies, campaign planning, integrated techniques and design – as having originated in the United States. The transfer of tools '... was favoured by trips of French nationals to the US; it was brought into France not only by advertising firms and American publishers, but also by specialized books, which, one at a time, were being translated into French'.[7] It is true that advertising studies and experts' discussions of new design and material techniques, of the respective importance of written, visual or audio media, and of legal frameworks, started in France in the late 1920s and early 1930s. A specialized journal like *Vendre*, with a readership primarily made up of publicity agents, is a good marker of this activity and of early signs of professionalization. The scale and the nature of what constituted relevant expertise for marketers, however, changed radically after the war. Surveys and statistics became good instruments that were highly promoted by specialists working at the boundary between economics and management, such as professors at the private business school, the École Supérieure des Sciences Économiques et Commerciales, and at the École des Hautes Études Commerciales, both in Paris.[8] As told by Chessel:

> The implementation of marketing tools in France is linked to the development of statistics tools in the 1940s, action by the French state, US influence, the development of a mass market, and the establishment of the European Common Market in the 1950s. The implementation is closely related both to research in product conception and to legitimation work by marketing experts, as well as to the spread of motivation studies. It should be noted how crucial awareness was of the key roles of marketing and prospecting tools, which made it easier to understand the market and to shape it.[9]

This paper will therefore build on this post-war scenario. Such an assumption is all the more reasonable as the issue at stake is *not* the existence of a given promotional tool or technique, i.e., the double-page ad in professional journals, the flyer circulated by mail, the diagnostic aid delivered by visiting drug representatives, etc., but the integration of research, information and promotion typical of advanced scientific marketing. Once positioned this way, this – in France – is clearly a post–World War II issue as it was only during the period between 1940 and 1970 that in-house, company-based pharmacological, clinical and market research escalated and became the norm, thus providing the basis for the integration of data collection and drug promotion. This integration was not only reflected in the structure and motifs used in marketing, but it was also an organizational problem focused on the relationship between two newly established divisions within the biggest firms: the marketing department and the clinical research division.[10]

This article seeks to understand the structural role played by visualization strategies – that is, both the visual techniques used in advertising documents to give a drug legitimacy, and the use of science-based images, i.e., systems of signification providing the ideal medical value of a product – in post-war drug marketing. Speaking of visualization immediately brings up references to general advertising: the massive use of slogans, bright colours and metaphoric images suggesting ideas of happiness, nature, wealth or personal accomplishment.[11] Post-war advertising for physicians began to use all of these, thus promoting a new culture of health as a permanent life concern and of cure as something that could be achieved through the consumption of drugs, never losing sight of the legitimating role of the medical sciences. The advertisements employed graphic tools, pictures, layout, text selection and other visualization methods as a means to provide – on the surface area of the advertising material – a landscape intertwining pharmaceutical, medical and legal elements in order to produce chains of signification that were not only general cultural narratives but also specific, specialized, medical stories pertaining to the reference cases every medical student has to learn, in order to generate or enlarge markets through the promotion of a very specific mode of consumption: by prescription.[12] As the editors of this volume argue in their introduction, the shift towards scientific marketing can be interpreted in the context of a very rapidly changing market featuring the diversification and growing numbers of specialties claiming their origin in research activities, as had been the case with sulphonamides and the first antibiotics. It is also grounded in a very important, albeit gradual, shift of the main targets from patients and families to prescribing physicians. The move was supported by broader changes in the healthcare system with the generalization of insurance coverage. In the French case, the universal public health insurance system, the Sécurité Sociale, included from 1945 onwards benefits for all drugs that doctors would consider prescribing as soon as the pharmaceuticals were included in the list of reimbursed therapy, something that before long became almost systematic. It should not however be forgotten that in spite of the rising importance of prescription drugs, sales of over-the-counter (OTC) specialties remained massive. OTC drugs were largely responsible for the fact that regulations and significant restrictions of promotional practices were reinforced in the 1950s and 1960s with, as we shall demonstrate, important consequences on the content of all drug advertisements. It was in this context of a massive influx of science-related words in the realm of drug promotion that strategies of visualization acquired new prominence. What kind of material can be used to analyse them? The promotional media that large firms started to use included new vehicles like films, thus giving a new meaning to the already widespread health education films massively employed by public health and hygiene movements in the inter-war period, as well as more conventional media mimicking academic literature and designed especially for physicians.[13] These could be house organs informing on many aspects of the firm's life not exclusively limited to its research activities, quasi-scientific journals made up of article reprints, new contributions from col-laborators or medical associates, special collections of articles on a specific topic sent as a dedicated volume or as a reprints package, volumes collecting the papers presented at sponsored conferences and seminars, or an incredible number of brochures focusing on one drug and its uses. Given that they both represent the bulk of post-war advertisement and most strikingly embody the Janus faces of scientific marketing, the corpus selected for this paper exclusively comprises printed advertising material for physicians, i.e., journal ads, inserts and flyers. For reasons of limited access to French industrial archives, they originate in three sources:

- the advertisements inserted in the 1960s into the journal *Concours Médical,* a widely circulated, privately owned weekly, the readership of which included most if not all French doctors, both general practitioners and specialists,[14]
- the archives of the French firm Roussel-Uclaf, because even though its material is very scattered and uneven, it includes some interesting 'series' of flyers received in succession by doctors over months or years,
- the archives of the Swiss firm Geigy, which had specific representation in France, was a major operator on the French market and circulated large quantities of promotional material, for the most part elaborated in Basel and showing little specificity in comparison with that used for French-speaking Swiss physicians (at least until the early 1970s).[15]

This diversity of sources should be kept in mind as it is related to various degrees and forms of professionalization. Although similar in size and market shares, Roussel and Geigy worked on different bases. Geigy established an internal spe-cialized department for the design and preparation of publicity, packages and promotional material as early as the 1940s. In the post-war period, this depart-ment worked increasingly with the medical department, which was in charge of all relations with physicians for both research and information.[16] In contrast, Roussel did not set up a specific department. Instead, its sales division worked with (changing) external advertising firms. As stated by Pierre Herbin, author of the most-read 1970s textbook on pharmaceutical marketing, this was common practice in France: 'Thus, specialized advertising firms [handled advertising for a number of pharmaceutical companies], and besides, an increasing number of advertising firms developed their own pharmaceutical units'.[17] Another differ-ence with Geigy was that at Roussel, until the 1970s, coordination between the sales department, the advertising firms and the medical division remained loose or, better said, left no traces in the archives. The argument will be developed in two parts. First, the paper explores the general status of visualization in French post-war drug marketing and the specific meaning it acquired in relation to the regulation of pharmaceutical publicity. Second, the paper presents and discusses a typology of visualization tools as they surface in this corpus. It will accordingly concentrate on a few examples of their combined use to construct meanings and to organize campaigns defining the use value of the drugs with the aim of expanding their (potential) market value.

Regulation of Drug Advertising and the Double-Bind of Visualization

Visualization strategies were embedded in the publicity documents that were produced, but for two reasons, they should not be approached at this level only. The first is that the rise of scientific marketing was associated with the diversification and integration of the media and promotional channels into campaigns, the organization and chronological succession of which (launch, reminder, change of medical niches, etc.) was the daily business of the new in-house professionals. One already-mentioned major consequence was the fact that no document was designed and circulated in isolation: all became part of promotional corpuses (inserts, letters, envelopes, leaflets, etc.) that could be deployed simultaneously or in succession. The temporal order of their production and mailing thus became a major topic of discussion, with professionals mobilizing applied psychology and market surveys to define the right 'dosage' (frequency of republication, time intervals between mailings, etc.) necessary to achieve memorization without saturation or negative reactions from the targeted physicians. A second and even more decisive reason for not looking at advertisements in isolation is that the strategies of marketers working in the pharmaceutical sector were deeply affected by changes in the ways of regulating drugs.[18] The post-war generalization of administrative regulation of drugs had direct consequences on marketing practices as they gradually fell under the umbrella of specific laws or legal constraints in most industrialized countries.[19] In the French case, the regulation of drug promotion not only made a distinction between publicity for the general public and publicity for doctors, it also developed increasingly specific requirements regarding the nature of the material, the information it should or should not include, and the forms of circulation. One very specific aspect of French pharmaceutical publicity regulations was the establishment of a specific 'visa' (approval) system different from the standard visa, a form of marketing authorization introduced by a decree-law enacted by the Vichy government in September 1941.

The decree-law had established a difference between *publicité technique* (or medical information) exclusively directed to health professionals, and *publicité commerciale* aimed at general (lay) consumers. Article 16 of the law thus stated that medical publicity targeted to physicians and pharmacists was free, '"free" meaning that the content of the information was not screened', as explained by Sophie Chauveau in her book on the history of French pharmacy.[20] In contrast, commercial advertising had to be legally authorized and get formal approval, called a 'visa', which only the Secretary for Health and Family could grant after the special committee in charge of reviewing commercial visa applications had examined and approved their content. Firms could however bypass the publicity visa if they 'only mention[ed] the name of the product, its composition, the name of the pharmacist maker of the drug, his university, his credits and his address'.[21]

The situation changed radically in 1963 with Decree-Law No. 63–253 dated 14 March of that year. This decree should be viewed in the context of growing criticism of the administration that had been triggered by the public scandal caused by the marketing of Stalinon, a drug used in the treatment of furunculosis that had caused hundreds of deaths although it had received unproblematic administrative approval.[22] The Stalinon affair led to a major reform of the visa, which on the one hand reinforced the pre-marketing evaluation of toxicity and production practices, and on the other came to terms with decades-long pleas from the industry to establish a proper system of patents for pharmaceuticals.[23] Although the advertisements for Stalinon were not central in the dynamics of the affair, pharmaceutical advertising was included in the reform package by the Health Ministry.

Medical publicity would also require a pre-use authorization, i.e., a visa that would be granted based on the report of a special committee evaluating the legitimacy of the claims made, conformity with the conditions of use defined in the drug visa and a proper relationship between the form and content of the material. To avoid the screening process and get a visa exemption, firms could supply the mandatory pharmacological, industrial and legal information. The list of mandatory information was extended and the number of items would grow over time to reach sixteen in 1976. In 1968, the fourteen information items required for visa exemption included:

1   Name of drug
2   Name and address of the manufacturer
3   Formula with generic name and active principle doses
4   Categorization of the speciality in accordance with the law on poisonous substances
5   Registration number referring to marketing authorization
6   Pharmacological class
7   Main therapeutic indications and potential contraindications as appearing in the marketing authorization file
8   Compulsory information imposed by the marketing authorization decision
9   Adverse effects or side effects, especially when used with other drugs or certain kinds of food
10 Information on toxic incidents and potential allergy complications

11 Habit forming or addiction risk

12 Way of monitoring patient to detect potential complications

13 Instructions for use and dosage

14 Retail price; prohibition of any coded formula; other compulsory information imposed by the law on prices; and information on relevant social legislation[24]

It is clear from looking at this list that there is little information related to clinical indications. In a follow-up to the 1941 law, most information items dealt with the product and the laboratory at which it was produced on the one hand, and the legal marketing context on the other. The latter had two sides: information on marketing authorization ('visa' and later *'autorisation de mise sur le marché*', or marketing permit), and the economic status of the drug (price, reimbursement). Although indications became a major target in scientific marketing, these were not legally defined and were left to the decision of the profession. The required scientific information had mostly to do with pharmacology and toxicology including many items (points 3, 4, 6, 8 and 13 in the list), while the question of indications was only mentioned in point 7 as having to comply with what was stated in the marketing permit.

One additional feature of the 1963 decree was that illustrated advertising would always require a visa, but again there was plenty of manoeuvring space insofar as advertisements that included only drawings or pictures useful for knowledge of the product or its form of use would not be considered as illustrated publicity: 'An advertisement is not considered as "illustrated" when the related pictures and images are helpful for a better understanding of the product involved or of its instructions for use'.[25]

This addition testifies both to the importance of images and more generally to the fact that visualization had gained ground in the promotional practices of pharmaceutical firms and its problematic status in the eyes of many doctors. It made the work of the Comité Technique des Spécialités examining visa applications highly circumstantial and a matter of internal jurisprudence. The 'illustrated' category was vague, leaving committee members to evaluate whether a drawing or a picture was useful to medical knowledge or not. The 1963 decree thus registered the core problem of scientific marketing and turned it into a regulatory issue: unifying information and promotion without giving the impression that the scientific content of ads was biased for commercial purposes but also without endangering the efficacy of the promotional message with too much excessively complex scientific content. Given this double-bind, how did visual strategies manage to integrate promotion and information?

A Typology of Visualization Techniques in the Scientific Marketing of Drugs

A general feature needs to be underscored, which is that there is no strict boundary between what may be considered medical information presented in a dry and objective way on the one hand, and marketing discourse building on metaphors, cultural images and promises on the other. The difference is there in the advertisements, partly for legal reasons, partly because the staging of science had as such acquired a marketing value, but the relations between the two are best described as a form of 'boundary work' performed through visualization strategies. For example, in the above publicity insert for Triamcinolone (Figures 6.1 and 6.2) the first page displays the image of a prescribing physician and the second, medical information. This blending is rooted in some of the general changes that may be observed during the 1930s–60s period. An analysis of the advertisements for hormones and psychotropic drugs published in *Concours Médical* thus shows how the nature of images and what is visually represented changed significantly: on the one hand, the number of photographs and the size of the advertisements increased while colour was introduced; on the other hand, although the product was already massively present before the war, after the 1950s advertisements included, at a rapidly growing pace, representations of the effects of the drug as well as of the symptoms.[26] What needs to be understood here is therefore how the drug is represented in the images, i.e., not only which medical information is represented (or not), but also how, by which means and with which techniques. Images of patients might have, for instance, been included in a 'story' referring to his/her (professional or family) life or, alternatively, to medical work, depending on which texts and other visual elements were included in the advertisement. Similarly, the effects of a drug might have been represented through images of life before and after treatment through graphs and curves alluding to clinical trials or through actual medical images (anatomical, pathological or microscopic). The combination of all these elements in the 'story' was intended to give physicians assurance on the efficacy and utility of the drug.

As a consequence of the professionalization of marketing, whether the drug marketers worked within a firm or in general advertising firms, such a *mélange* typical of drug advertising was increasingly organized according to recommendations developed in specific manuals.[27] These manuals were actually adaptations of more general marketing manuals that developed categories to describe the psychological mechanisms involved in illustration: dimension, colour, rhythm and movement for the purpose of capturing readers' attention, comprehension and memorization.[28] In the case of drugs, the recommendations are to seek to render the scientific information less technical, more easily visible and unforgettable, while the promotional text and subtext are filled with scientific references and results both in the typical publicity items (slogans, metaphors, logos, etc.) and through the use of standard forms of representation in the biomedical sciences (graphs, tables, schematized chemical reactions, etc.).

During the late 1960s and the 1970s, an atypical form of knowledge mobilized by marketing professionals was semiotics. This became an important theme of reflection and training, for instance at the Institut de Recherche Publicitaire (IREP).[29] A good, albeit later, example of the application of a semiotic approach to the understanding of drug marketing is provided by Jean-Marie Floch's work on French advertisements for psychotropic drugs.[30] Having collected several dozen advertisements in the professional press, he established that 'twelve plastic and visual categories plus three figurative categories [were] used by laboratories to code their advertisements for psychotropics'.[31] These categories were classified as binaries including clear/dark, nuanced/contrasted, coloured/black and white, small/large, simple/complex, symmetrical/asymmetrical, up/down, pictorial/graphical, figurative/abstract, etc.[32] They covered the description of the surface area of the ads and the arrangement of signifiers. As for signification, the argument was that most of the advertisements relative to psychotropics shared a common system. According to Floch, the shared structure of the ads was to oppose these categories in order to illustrate (visualize) the two states of euphoria and dysphoria (originating in the 'thymic' medical explanation of mood disorders) to create a narrative of recovery and health linking prescription of the drug with the return of euphoria taken as a beneficial state of mind. This narrative built heavily on medical knowledge. It was encoded in the visual structure of the advertisements. It was also at odds with practitioners' perception of mental health as it considered one of the phases of a pathological oscillation as normal instead of representing the idea of attenuation, dampened cycle and leverage that most physicians considered to be the main purpose of prescribing psychotropic drugs.

Borrowing from this example, a strategy of visualization can be considered as a specific package of techniques and know-how shared by groups of experts and professionals in pharmaceutical marketing and used to produce what they saw as the meanings (motives for prescription) that were needed to open or extend specific market niches. Analysis of the strategies therefore implies, in a parallel move to the semiotic approach of the relationship between signifiers and signification, both an analysis of the arrangement of elements constituting the advertising copy, and the decoding of its signification, of its subtext. Analysing the double-bind of scientific marketing however requires putting a special emphasis on the iconic message and setting aside the syntactic, prosodic and logical analyses that could also be performed, given that semiotics also teaches us that the literal message conveyed by the slogans, the scientific messages or the legal notices are visually encoded and participate in the creation of product images. As Alain

Fourcade rightly insisted, the iconic dimension of an advertisement is rooted in the 'general morphology, chromatic code, visual rhetoric elements, typographic code and photographic code' of the message.[33]

Based on the examination of the above-mentioned corpus, two sets of techniques may be distinguished that were used to combine copy and visuals, organize representations and establish the signification chain characteristic of a given drug advertisement story (Table 6.1). The first set of techniques focuses on the nature of the media and includes rather general procedures used in all industrial sectors. Its importance originates in the fact that in post-war France the materiality of printed drug publicity experienced dramatic changes with the generalization of colour and photographs and the enlargement of the surface area devoted to one product.

The second set focuses on elements of script or storytelling, for instance tropes, bearing a strong element of specificity to the pharmaceutical sector. Floch, for instance, called 'tropes' the modes of organizing narrative that would ensure a 'dynamic representation of the symptoms' and a specific understanding of the impact of the disease on the life of patients.[34] What was at stake here was more specific than the standard semiotic chain of signification as the story to be told, which could act as a motive for prescription, was a clinical combination of symptoms, diagnosis, course of treatment and outcome. Hence the idea that these particular types of stories were 'scripts' as they focused on the modalities and results of drug uses. The scripts were encoded in the visualization strategy, hence associated with recurring techniques, the number and sophistication of which grew with the investments made in drug marketing and the specialization of the personnel associated with it.

For instance, the 'emblem' technique presented similarities with the logo technique but with a major difference: an emblem did not, or did not merely, convey the image of a firm; it symbolically summarized either a pathological state or the results obtained thanks to therapy. Just like the logo, which was a 'visual representation' generating 'a 'signification system', the 'emblem' could be either figurative or abstract.[35] The emblem was immediately understandable and, according to Floch's theorization of the 'logo' notion, had the feature of 'being adaptable to multiple modes of page layouts and space settings, which [was] crucial for general communication (e.g. signature, header, etc.)'.[36] For instance, the first campaign (in 1962) for Insidon, Geigy's main tranquilizer, included an emblem such as this, which was a visualization of the effect of the drug: 'The introductory campaign uses the symbolic image of a patient liberating themselves from the glass sphere in which they are captive, illustrating both the patient's psychological state and the effect of taking the medicine'.[37] Here the patient's psychological imprisonment was symbolized by his position inside a transparent ball, which was broken down by the drug, providing liberation from his imprisonment in depression. This advertising motif had its basis in the corporate science of Insidon, according to which the effects of the drug were defined as consisting of a two-stage process, the first providing relief from anxiety and tension and the second acting more like an antidepressant, leading to mood enhancement.[38] This motif was not only used in letters, but in brochures and packages as well.

Table 6.1: Typology of visualization techniques

Techniques linked to the medium	Techniques linked to the script
Double-page ads	
Coloured photographs	Emblem
Folded leaflets	Tropes
	1. Medical work
	a) Consultation
	b) Dialogue
	c) Clinical examination
	d) Prescription
	e) Home visit
	2. Laboratory work
	3. Patient's life
	4. Public health
	5. Originating in cultural works (paintings, literary work, music, etc.)
Series of leaflets or brochures	Mathematical/statistical representations: graphs, curves, tables, etc.
Slogan and catchphrase, isolated or in special font, colour, etc.	Before/after scenario

To elaborate on these two levels and their articulation more precisely, a few of these techniques need to be discussed in more detail. One of the most important techniques was the use of a double page. If we believe the results of the GEPHAMA analysis of the *Concours Médical* advertisements, the double page was used increasingly in the 1960s. Considering the case of psychotropic drugs, previous to the war only 5 per cent of such ads covered more than one page while in the 1960s the share was nearly 25 per cent.[39] This more systematic recourse to the double-page technique was related to a decisive change in visualization strategies.

The ad used above (Figure 6.2) shows that the technique was not yet stabilized. The first page includes the indication 'please turn'. In this early version, Squibb chose to hide the exact purpose of the ad by only mentioning the therapeutic class of the product on the first page, thus using the double page as a way to play out a medical scenario leading the (not yet accustomed) reader to move from the therapeutic class to its (supposedly) best variations. One decisive feature emerged, however: all the legally required information was featured on the second page, albeit in rather small print. In the 1960s, this divide became standard and the diversification of images used on the first page was remarkable, leading pharmaceutical marketers into the general pattern of using standard signifiers from general marketing, often unrelated to medicine or any specific representation of drugs. The double-page system had the great advantage of setting a spatial divide between the delivery of medical and legal information and the construction of an image and marketing identity for the product. The technique thus addressed the physician first through visualization. The copy was limited to a minimum, usually the name or a short definition of the drug, possibly completed with a summarized indication (a symptom rather than a diagnostic category). Often the wording was also a purely metaphorical phrase, for instance *nez aux champs*, which means 'nose in the fields', in an ad for a drug against allergies. The connotation here was that one would be safe from spring allergies originating in plant pollen in the countryside, provided, as one learned with the unfolding of the visualization process, that one took the drug visualized on the second page. Once seduced, amused or intrigued, the physician could turn the page and read the second side reserved for product specifications and the technical discourse. The link between the two was often made through the slogan on the first page.

The double page thus gave the impression that marketing information and scientific information had been separated by the layout and this was probably one of the reasons why it was widely used. It was a means to give professional marketers, who had uneasy relationships with physicians and medical departments, much greater latitude when designing the first page, which was the one chiefly devoted to large colour images, elaborate graphics, etc. If the arrangement of the pages is reversed, however, the marketing value clearly appears as residing less in the actual separation than in the linking enabled by the double-page technique. Reversing the two pages destroys the effect: the technique no longer works. If the symbolic, metaphorical understanding of the drug were to come second, it would lose its edge and appear as a superimposed layer of meaning barely related to an already scientifically defined product. The association game could only work if it was part of a scenario in which the doctor turned the page and moved from his or her cultural and social identity to his or her biomedical competence. This game was often framed as an unveiling process, the first page playing on a form of mystery regarding the specific identity and targets of the drug being promoted.

From the late 1950s on, this form of articulation was reinforced by a more systematic use of colour photographs on the first page.[40] For example a 1963 double-page ad for Néomycine-Hydrocortisone (Laboratoires Diamant) presented a colour photograph of half a woman's face including mouth, ear, nostril and eyelid, each superimposed with one of the galenic presentations of the product, i.e., skin pomade, ear drops, nose drops and eye drops. The story thus built is one of convergence between medical and cosmetic advertising. The woman in the photograph has a smooth and elegant face.[41] She is obviously a young woman using make-up: she is wearing very red lipstick and thickly applied eyeliner. The viewer gets the feeling that this is an advertisement for cosmetics. This interpretation is reinforced by use of a colour code belonging to the realm of cosmetics ads: the cap of the nasal solution is coloured the same red as the model's lips.[42] But this is medical information. The focus is on the diversity of presentations of hydrocortisone/neomycin and its usefulness. The confusion between medicine and cosmetics generated by the placement of products over body parts leads to the notion that medicine not only cures but also provides aesthetic benefits. Instead of a clinical image, for instance the skin of a patient suffering from skin inflammation, the ad presents a young and healthy (woman's) face, which could seduce (mostly male) physicians. Here, in addition to its distinctive way of displaying and dividing the technical and the promotional, the double page is used according to the conventions of general marketing. It is a case of a very general strategy which connects the idea of beauty with the product. As explained by Judith Williamson, 'the assumption here [was] that because the containers [were] the same (in terms of colours) the products [had] the same qualities'.[43] It is interesting to note that in spite of its blurred boundary with cosmetics advertising, this ad does not have a visa number. Although we do not know whether the visa commission discussed the case, due to its connection with galenic forms, the woman's face was ultimately considered as part of the explanation of how the drug worked and not as an illustration.

Colour codes are very general and widespread advertising techniques. Their use in drug advertising however reveals something more specific than the standard connotations discussed in marketing manuals, for instance the association of blue with the ideas of calm, tranquillity, rest, etc.[44] The work of Geigy's *Werbungs-Abteilung* (advertising department) is a good example. On the one hand, the firm designers created a systematic colour pattern for all the firm's packages, hence a visual identity for the brand and for specific product lines. On the other hand, colour codes were used in the material sent to physicians both as elements of continuity (for instance when series of flyers related to the same product were distributed) and as signifiers of therapeutic properties. In the early 1960s, the launch of Tofranil, Geigy's first antidepressant, in France was based on a collection of brochures sent by mail. They were all designed in purple and white colours, with black-and-white photographs. While the latter showed patients assumed to be depressed (viewing life in a sad absence of colours), the general design in purple and white provided images of security against the disease (with its strong risk of suicide): the image of security is illustrated by the drawing of an anchor and the colour purple is used to code the feeling of melancholy.[45]

Other interesting uses of colour codes are found in the context of what may be called mathematical or statistical techniques, which tell stories of objectivity and exactness. In a second Tofranil series of brochures for the French market, the reader is given the results of clinical trials (open and non-controlled). The efficacy of Tofranil is first presented in the standard scientific form of a table included in a long text. What is however much more visible is a second illustration, a diagram in three colours. The latter is not a simple repetition of the former. The colour code technique has specific effects, and these provide a new script and promotional value. The diagram is centre page; much quicker to understand than the table, it encapsulates the notion that Tofranil works in most (if not all) cases. This is coded with the choice of colours as the three colours are actually two (green and red) when taking into account the fact that purple is a derivative of red. The diagram thus simply opposes improvement (red and purple) and failure (green). Moreover, since complete remissions are coloured purple, the most convincing and supposedly impressive cases are directly linked with the emblematic hue of Tofranil.

The slogan, a central item for professional advertisers, became a typical boundary technique for drug marketers. As shown above, Fourcade's typology includes the slogan in the iconic – therefore visual – dimension of advertising. Approached from the perspective of material techniques, the slogan was built through its layout, colour and position on the page. In terms of script or storytelling, the slogan was increasingly used in the 1960s as a means to reshape some of the medical information in an encapsulated way, sometimes playing on literary strings, like rhythm or repetition.[46] Given its boundary status, a great deal of the work of the visa committee focused on the exact wording of slogans, discussing at length their veracity and multiple meanings. Given that the slogan has the role of a caption to guide the visualization and the interpretation of the ad and might therefore mislead the viewers, the committee in charge of advertising authorization spent a great deal of time evaluating the interplay between the image and the formal scientific texts of the ads, discussing for instance whether the slogans would extend the indications beyond what the marketing authorization specified. This 'illegitimate' extension was, for example, the reason why in May 1979 the committee denied approval to the Organon material promoting Orgametril, a sexual hormone intended for the treatment of menopause.[47] The committee also paid great attention to the incorporation of clinical trial results in the slogans, for instance percentages showing success rates. In a 1977 report on the problems raised by slogan building, the committee thus commented: 'Slogans do not provide all the information on the context of the study; information may be imprecise and lead to a wrong interpretation. This figures-based information must be replaced by more general formulations'.[48]

To finish with this first list, there is one more technique to be mentioned, the use of which also seem to have expanded during the post-war period as it acquired important value in bringing together medical information and product imaging. It is the technique of using 'series' of brochures, leaflets and, more often, flyers. Series were typically built around a consistent set of images associated with the various indications of a given drug. More generally, the production and distribution of series worked not only as a 'reminder' like multiple mailings did; they were designed as a collection: a collection of cases or medical situations as well as a collection of similar objects with a continuity of form and/ or references (a series based on paintings, for instance) to hold them together. As Herbin observed, the fashion of series also had regulatory motives: 'Most of the time, it was by offering series that the pharmaceutical industry solicited visas ... As gifts were forbidden, series were the only gift allowed.'[49] Practitioners could thus collect series of beautiful reproductions of famous paintings placed on the front page of mailed inserts, put them in the waiting room, or give them to consulting patients or families. For example, in the late 1970s, Geigy not only sent doctors printed paintings with accompanying slides for projection; it also mailed analyses of specific musical works of composers whose lives had been plagued by depression, accompanied by a recording.[50]

The second set of techniques is more specifically related to telling a medical story, or creating a script that would provide motives for prescription. The case of the emblem has already been discussed. A second class of script-oriented techniques was the use of tropes. These can be defined as assemblages of visual motifs conveying a specific interpretation of medical use value that are repeated in all sorts of advertisements, crossing the boundaries between product lines or therapeutic classes. Given their narrative complexity, they are mainly represented in brochures, series and double pages. As summarized in Table 6.1, a majority of tropes focused on the clinical experience, starting with medical work in its various dimensions: consultation, writing a prescription and physical examination. Often the image did not work in isolation or through 'inter-textual' association with slogans and icons. Added to it were more direct references to medical practice, for instance the summary of the dialogue that was supposed to have taken place between a woman and her doctor. Such images use the trope of a human, understanding encounter, while the text provided the medical specificity of the drug, i.e., the problems of menopause and their legitimate pharmaceutical solution.

Paradoxically, although the trope of medical work was a very frequent one, it did not provide the most elaborate scenario: what was visualized was almost always either the efficacy of treatment or the benevolent but competent attitude of the physician. Medical work and its technical dimensions might have been too intricate for marketers to reflect upon in a very detailed manner. The trope of patient life, in contrast, shows how scientific marketing could operate with full case histories, with both their medical and biographical dimensions introducing family, professional and personal circumstances. As Floch aptly remarked in his analysis of psychotropic drugs:

> The communication relative to psychotropic attempts to capture not the words, but the stories and the images used by patients to describe their diseases. The stories and images they depict in the visuals of the ad help to convey the anxious and depressive moods of the patient, and by opposition ... the result of the medical treatment.[51]

Let us consider another double-page ad from Geigy's campaigns for Insidon. The motif here is that of the 'problem patient', i.e., the patient who comes again and again complaining of changing symptoms for which the physician is unable to find a clear-cut somatic cause and diagnosis. The issue is a problem in consultation: a case burdening the doctor's schedule for which the quickest solution is the use of Insidon. The perspective is that of general (social) medicine, taking the entire life of the patient into account with the notion that psychosomatic complaints are delusions but real sufferings, very often originating in problems of daily life. The imagined case report in the form of a clinical dialogue on complaints and working conditions is thus reinforced with the image of the woman at work and an iconic pseudo-ID card.

This medical problem came to play a major role in Geigy's marketing of antidepressants in the late 1960s and early 1970s. As Jean-Paul Gaudillière discusses in his chapter in this volume, building on the growing interest of psychiatrists in ambulatory care and on their debates on the relations between depressive states and somatic complaints, Geigy pushed the notion of 'larved [*larvée*], or masked depression', a disorder without the usual mental signs of depression but with psychosomatic manifestations. Changing the meaning of depression from a series of severe and relatively rare diagnoses usually handled in psychiatric hospitals to a unified illness defined on the basis of symptoms rather than etiology and found among 10 per cent of the patients seen by a regular general practitioner was a powerful strategy that would extend the consumption of antidepressants to general practice.[52] It rested on the entire palette of scientific marketing media and mobilized a number of new visuals and tropes. We shall mention one example of each.

In France, the first campaign directed at redefining depression took place in 1962–3. The new indication was summarized under the slogan 'masked [*larvée*] depression = functional disorders with no organic basis'. It was associated with an emblem in the form of a spider's web, repeated on most of the material. The spider's web played visually on several meanings. The most obvious one, echoing many images used to promote psychotropic drugs, was the idea of the patient caught in a web of delusions and the popular saying linking madness to 'having a spider on the ceiling' (*avoir une araignée au plafond*). The web here also echoed the popular imagery of the spider as an organism (wrongly) akin to insects and their larval stages. The 'larved' nature of the depression was thus both a question of its not being fully developed (it would become worse if not treated) and of its having a different shape or appearance (absence of the usual symptoms and presence of somatic complaints that could mislead the physician). The visual actually reinforces the latter as the web somewhat hides the spider, which is at the centre. Caught in a web of somatic manifestations, the patient (like the untrained general practitioner) does not see the spider/depression responsible for all these knotted intersections ... until it is too late. The material of the brochures elaborated this meaning in its own way as the cover transparency on which the web was printed could be superimposed over a drawing of the human body showing the organs that were the most frequent targets of somatic manifestations, as explained in the fifty-page medical text that followed. Mental depression thus found its way into the organic body that the physician was accustomed to examine.

Generalizing depression also built on a rare trope, that of population and medicine as a collective practice. Geigy marketers visualized depression not only as a problem of isolated biographies, but also as a rising disease, a problem of public health and populations, the roots of which were in the isolation and pressure modern urban and industrial life imposed on the individual. A brochure of 1962 promoting Tofranil thus begins with the picture of a typical urban crowd, in black and white as a clear allusion to the situation of the modern man, isolated in the midst of others. The nature of the crowd is then changed with a header/slogan saying 'depression, a world problem', which brings another identity to these individuals, that of supposedly depressed people. A new graphic technique then tells the end of the story: the photograph is associated with a transparency that can be superimposed on the crowd and shows a percentage: the average rate of success claimed by Geigy for Tofranil in the treatment of all forms of depression. If properly handled, the world problem could therefore be solved.

Tropes did not necessarily belong to the world of medicine and pharmacy. They could have more diverse social and cultural origins. This was especially the case when marketers played with references and mobilized well- (or less well-) known cultural items. As physicians were perceived as belonging to the intellectual classes, firms often played on their supposed interests in literature, painting and other forms of art. Cultural references were accordingly very often used for the construction of a series. Consider one series for Roussel's painkiller Glifanan. The figure of the martyr is used to interpret chronic pain, the main indication of Glifanan. Like the martyr, the patient affected with chronic pain suffers in an essential manner. His/her pain is not a mere incident soon to be over; it is an element of identity – for the martyr because suffering is the consequence of faith; for the patient because suffering has become chronic. There is, however, deliverance: for the martyr in the form of death; for the patient in the form of Glifanan pills.

Conclusion

To end this survey, we need to return to the basic question of scientific marketing, namely its role in building markets and, for our purposes, in reshaping prescription patterns. We have seen that as scientific marketing was professionalized, a whole palette of techniques were introduced or expanded to create new layers of meaning supplementing the mere (sometimes mandatory) inclusion of medical information in promotional material for physicians. Advertising thus accomplished two operations: one was to simplify, broaden and generalize the results of corporate-based research; the second, more related to the skills of professional marketers, was to link the use value of the drug with more encompassing professional and cultural values. In both instances, what was at stake was the establishment of a chain of signification providing motive for prescription since physicians and their consulting rooms had become the main gate-keeping mechanisms of pharmaceutical consumption. We do not know – nor did most drug marketers – what their effect was on consumption and prescription even though belief that it was significant was widely accepted and occasionally documented with correlations between the chronology of campaigns and that of changing sales. What is, however, possible to document is how various visualization strategies were combined to define use and indications, enlarging them beyond mere repetition of what was written and included in the technical summaries based on visas and marketing authorizations. It is the argument of this paper that the presumed efficacy of scientific marketing was – in the eyes of its practitioners – strongly predicated on the impact of visualization. Hence the need for a more specific understanding of the strategies employed.

Having to deal with physicians rather than patients, scientific drug marketers were caught in a (relatively) novel double-bind: they had to unify research-based information and promotion without giving the impression that the scientific content of ads was biased for commercial purposes, but also without endangering the efficacy of the promotional message with too much, excessively complex scientific content. This double-bind was not only a professional problem but also a problem in administrative regulations. The typology of visualization techniques presented in this paper is an attempt to characterize the tools involved in this boundary work. It is obviously not a final result, but a provisional listing of two sets of techniques, i.e., material- and script- oriented, intended for understanding the specific place drug marketing occupies in the history of marketing. Any typology of this sort is first an analytical and heuristic tool. In this respect, an enlargement of the corpus examined is indispensable to refine the French chronology of use, but it would also bring in new techniques, for instance tropes or emblems associated with the biomedical laboratory rather than with the clinical setting. Two additional lines of investigation are worth mentioning: the first is the question of the arrangements typical of various therapeutic classes; and the second perspective is related to the firms themselves, their marketing organization, and their personnel.

7 A BALANCING ACT: ANTIDIABETIC PRODUCTS AND DIABETES MARKETS IN GERMANY AND FRANCE

Tricia Close-Koenig and Ulrike Thoms

Introduction

When insulin was first isolated in Toronto and subsequently administered, the news was given major resonance in public and scientific bulletins alike.[1] News on both sides of the Atlantic announced a miracle with headlines like 'Brought back from death with insulin' or 'Diabetes case, given up as hopeless, saved by serum'. The Toronto lab received thousands of letters from families of diabetics, doctors, hospitals and pharmacists from all over the world.[2] The news was also closely followed by pharmaceutical firms, which collected large numbers of press clippings on the subject.[3]

Like the later case of antibiotics, insulin was a major success for the relatively young American pharmaceutical industry, leading to a shift from Europe as the major place of pharmaceutical research and production to the USA. This shift corresponds to the very same period in which marketing was advanced as a science and a practice, such that it is often assumed that marketing developed on the American front. In recent publications on the history of the pharmaceutical industry the American model is widely accepted as the blueprint for developments in other countries. Since the 1980s this model has been widely questioned and replaced, or at least complemented, with the concept of 'glocalization'. Glocalization has been adapted to numerous fields, from culture to business and sports. It points to the fact that firms adopt their products, marketing techniques and management structures to local specificities in culture and markets.[4] This is exemplified by the case of Insulin from the 1920s onwards: Eli Lilly and the University of Toronto targeted a worldwide, global market from the very start, but tried to set up an organization that paid tribute to national differences in medical systems and drug laws with national insulin committees around the world. In the case of Germany such a committee was successfully instituted to grant licences and oversee insulin production, while this policy failed in France.[5]

The enthusiastic reactions to the news point clearly to the exceptional sales potential of this long-awaited drug; it might be assumed that any advertising would have been superfluous, especially as supply did not immediately meet demand and the drug was to be sold at relatively low prices with the property rights in the hands of the University of Toronto.[6]

In general, advertisements for insulin represent an insignificant portion of the products advertised to practitioners.[7] A detailed study reveals characteristic national differences: of the 2,742 ads reviewed from the German general medical journals *Deutsches Ärzteblatt* (*DÄ*) and *Deutsches Medizinisches Wochenblatt* (*DMW*) between 1920 and 1980, there were only three for insulin and sixty-nine for other antidiabetics.[8] Interestingly, there were many more advertisements for insulin in France than in Germany for the same time period. In the French journals *Le Concours Médical* (*CM*) and *La Presse Médicale* (*PM*), there were sixty-eight ads for insulin and 482 for antidiabetics.[9] Although this was partly the artefact of a greater overall total of advertisements in the French journals, there was a significantly larger number of manufacturers advertising their insulin. Herein, we might ask how such numbers can be interpreted in terms of marketing schemes.

From an ethical point of view, the pharmaceutical market was different to other markets because the commercial interests of pharmaceutical enterprises could conflict with the well-being of patients, and so advertising in this field was regulated.[10] Consideration of how pharmaceutical firms approached marketing, communication and education with medical practitioners and patients can reveal a shifting balance of power amongst the various actors involved, which may differ in different countries. Our study examines the diabetes market and the marketing of antidiabetics and other products for diabetics through advertisements aimed at practitioners and at patients in Germany and France.

While insulin undeniably changed the lives of diabetics, it also changed pharmaceutical interest in diabetes. With insulin, diabetes changed from a fatal to a manageable chronic disease, and a permanent, life-long demand. The advent of insulin occurred in the 1920s just as pharmaceutical enterprises were reaching industrial scales. In the first part of this paper, we will present the messages conveyed in insulin advertisements in relation to the changing pharmaceutical enterprise.

Although insulin brought a radical change into the diabetes market, there were also strong continuities. Medical diabetes specialists and their diabetic patients worked in established structures, and these networks remained in place.

Doctors had long provided treatment in their specialized, often private, clinics. Companies had specialized in dietetic products and food for diabetics, and there was a market for educational literature. From the 1930s, however, a new actor entered the field: the patient association. As self-organized groups of diabetics, they took the patients' perspective. Such groups were (and still are) regarded as 'authentic' and free of commercial interests.[11] As recent studies have shown, however, they can be used as back doors to address patients directly and circumvent the German and French regulations that prohibit direct-to-consumer advertising of prescription medicine.[12] Patient associations' bulletins clearly offered the possibility of reaching the target group directly.[13] Consequently, this was an alternative media for diabetics and diabetologists to promote themselves openly, and an ideal place to address diabetics and diabetologists directly.

In the second part of the paper, we investigate the role played by advertising in French and German bulletins of diabetes associations between 1945 and 1970. This will be based on an analysis of the advertisements from the French *Journal des diabétiques* and the German *Der Diabetiker.* These advertisements offer some insight into the construction of medical and auxiliary medical markets for special products, in which the diabetic is considered a patient-consumer, and patient associations may be seen as representations of these very specific types of consumers.[14] This provides a shift from the usual history of pharmaceuticals that has largely been written as the history of pharmacy, the medical profession and regulative bodies and procedures, while the history of the use or consumption of pharmaceutical products has been left almost unwritten.[15]

Our aim is to present a comparative story of antidiabetics markets and marketing in France and Germany through a study of advertisements. For the German study, advertisements are supplemented with advertising inserts in the journals, as well as leaflets and other documents found in the Bayer and Schering company archives and the University of Toronto Archives. Although access to industry archives was limited in France to a few documents from Roussel, these were further developed with documents from the French Ministry of Health Autorisation de mise sur le marché archives and from the Agence française de sécurité sanitaire des produits de santé (Afssaps) Commission chargée du contrôle de la publicité sessions, as well as from the University of Toronto Archives.[16] By cross-analysing these various primary sources, we reflect on how the market for diabetes products developed and what marketing strategies were used to expand it. The study includes an account of the market targets themselves: diabetes specialists and diabetic patients. Our paper follows a chronological time scheme with the first part focusing on pre-1939 observations and the latter on post-1945. Whereas advertisements are but the polished tip of a longer and larger process of pharmaceutical marketing, the message or image advertisement is used here as a window on the larger goals, company images and market representations that portray what market groups were targeted – and how – in the mid-twentieth century.[17]

Advertising Insulin in Medical Journals

One of the three aforementioned German ads for Insulin, published in the *Deutsches Ärzteblatt* (*DÄ*), advertised a foreign product, 'Engl. Insulin "A. B. Brand".[18] Interestingly, German medical journals ran ads from Dr Fresenius, who proposed English Insulin, but never any ads from the producers overseen by the Insulin Committee. The large German producers refrained from advertising their insulin in the medical press so as not to destroy their self-portrayal as scientific firms. A 1930 ad for A. B. Insulin from the *DÄ* is otherwise typical of the 1930s.[19] It displays no pictures or graphics and states the brand name, producer and distributor straightforwardly. The sales argument here is linked to the achievements of A. B. Brand in terms of quality: the 'greatest purity' and the 'strongest effectiveness'.[20] By stressing a scientifically reached high-quality product, the ad aims to make a clear distinction between A. B. Brand insulin and unreliable products. It is of special importance here that German clinicians criticized German insulin as being weaker and less effective than that from Britain or America.[21]

A French ad from the same decade (pictured in Figure 7.1) is somewhat more sophisticated as it includes an illustration of the product. Its claims are, however, not unlike those of the German ad: consistency and ease of use. As it was produced in France, the producer's address is also provided.[22] The message of scientificity, however, is almost overshadowed by patriotism: this insulin was French.

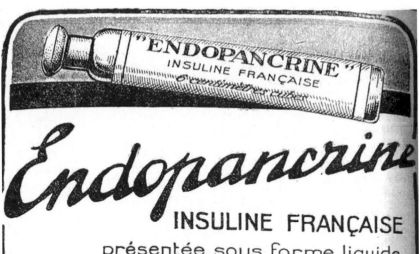

Figure 7.1: Advertisement for Endopancrine (1935); image reproduced by kind permission of Elsevier Masson.

Source: *La Presse Médicale*, 70 (1930), p. 1186.

Archival material in Germany shows that within the given historical context of pharmaceutical marketing of the 1920s and 1930s, it was not so much advertising *of* Insulin but advertising *with* Insulin that was important. Much more than in any other business, the business of pharmaceutical firms is based on innovation, scientific achievements and trust grounded on the quality, safety and reliability of drugs. It was thus of utmost importance for these firms to be amongst the early producers and suppliers of insulin. In Germany, doctors were expected to trust the large 'scientific' and reliable companies. The Insulin Committee members did so. They expected that only reputable, long-standing firms like Merck and Hoechst should be given licences. Firms sent samples to the members of the Insulin Committee, which were then tested and – if the quality was found satisfying – labelled as 'Tested by the German Insulin Committee'. This was a perceptibly important quality certificate and firms were eager to obtain it.[23]

Under these circumstances insulin was very much a prestige product that allowed the firms – if they succeeded in producing it and in acquiring the Insulin Committee quality certificate – to publicize their scientificity and modernity.[24] Although firms complained that the low sales prices for insulin left little funds to advertise it broadly, the approach concurred with pharmaceutical companies like Bayer, Schering and others, whose principal marketing schemes emphasized scientific and industrial production.

The situation in France was somewhat different: there was no French insulin committee. There was no patenting of medication, serums, vaccines and biologicals, and authorization for sale or distribution was to be granted by a scientific commission of the *Académie de médecine*.[25] Despite the fact that there was neither a patent or a national insulin committee to encourage large pharmaceutical companies to produce insulin, the insulin advertisements of existing small enterprises imparted a message similar to that of the German ads: scientificity, quality and reliability. What vouched for their quality was not an insulin committee – like for other pharmaceutical products it was the approval by the *Académie de Médecine* or by citing the use of their brand in certain hospitals or clinics. In the ad above, for example, the reliability and quality of the product Endopancrine is notably vouched for by its use in Paris hospitals. Not only did French insulin ads underscore that the insulin was developed from non-imported raw or prepared material, they also forwent the 'Insulin' label, preferring to register their own trademarks, such as Endopancrine by the Laboratoire de Thérapeutique Générale, Insulyl by Roussel or Insulosan by Choay.[26]

Insulin ads refrained from sensationalism and superlatives. Usually, they displayed little more than the product and the company and indicated the standardization and efficacy of the drug, pointing to the reputation of a respectable firm.[27] Their participation in the insulin business may not have brought instant profit but it offered an entry into the diabetes business and paved the way for later expansion with improved, as well as ancillary, products. As early as 1923, IG Farben established contacts with the the the editor of the patient journal *Diabetes*, in order to engage him in support of Hoechst Insulin. In turn the firm delivered Sionon brochures to him that he could then distribute to his readers. This may thus have been considered a worthwhile investment, despite waiving some profit, to gain social capital and secure possible future profits from the expected innovations.

One such innovation was the development of depot insulin (also known as 'retarded' or 'longer-acting' insulin) in the mid-1930s. This opened the market to competition and segmentation that used scientific progress as a marketing argument. This may be inferred from Degewop's leaflet for P.Z.-Insulin (pictured in Figure 7.2) from the late 1930s, which also exemplifies that while firms may not have advertised insulin broadly in medical journals, they used other means and ways of advertising. A search in company archives turns up numerous periodical inserts, brochures and leaflets, many of which were distributed by sales representatives during their visits to doctors and hospitals.[28] The example pictured here illustrates modern and rationalized insulin production at Degewop, one of the five German producers supervised by the Insulin Committee.[29] In fact rational and scientific production did not only help to produce high-quality insulin, it also reduced prices and increased profits. Efforts to standardize and rationalize production helped Schering to bring down the production cost of insulin by 20 per cent between 1939 and 1941.[30] As a side note, by adding protamine zinc to insulin to prolong its effects, the initial Insulin patent was no longer an issue, as manufacturers held their own patented formulas outside the Insulin Committee's jurisdiction.

Similarly, a French advertisement for Insulyl-Retard from 1940 promoted retard insulin with a graph that clearly denoted the scientificity of the product not in its production, but rather in its use with fewer daily injections.[31] The advertising argument puts forward this innovation and, again, leads the firm to be identified as scientific. There would further be other innovations in which these manufacturers would invest and, as in the advert illustrated with the Insulyl-Retard graph, not only the scientificity, but also the patients' lives, would be acknowledged.

Expanding the Diabetes Market beyond Insulin

Another of the many inserts produced by the pharmaceutical industry to provide information on insulin is particularly interesting. Dated 21 May 1930, 97,000 copies of a Bayer insert advertising insulin were printed. Like the Degewop leaflet it was illustrated, but it differed from the majority of earlier ads not so much in terms of the image, but rather in that the style resembled ads for other types of consumer products.

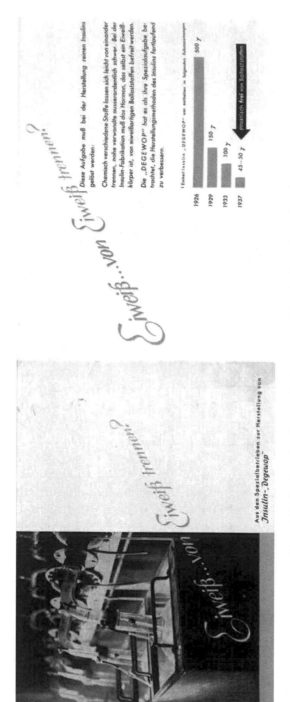

Figure 7.2: Leaflet advertisement for Degewop PZ-Insulin from the early 1940s; image reproduced by kind permission of Schering Archives, Bayer AG.

Source: Bayer Archives, Schering Archive, Bayer AG, S1/68.

It was illustrated in a rather modern graphic style with a drawing of an insulin bottle and package and a cursive font. What is remarkable is the flipside of the ad, which is an advertisement for Sionon, an artificial sweetener. The ad shows an open package of the product with a spoon in it.[32] At the foot of the package there is a brochure called '30 Desserts for Diabetics' ('30 Süss-Speisen für Diabetiker') containing practical advice on how to use the product in recipes.[33] This ad marks a decisive shift in target from doctors to patients and their everyday life. Another leaflet from 1934 is equally interesting, not so much for the design, as there are no pictures or drawings, but for the fact that it also advertises both Insulin and Sionon. Ten thousand copies of this leaflet were inserted in the general medical journal *Medizinische Welt* while another 15,000 copies were distributed to doctors, pharmacists and hospitals, most likely for further distribution to patients.[34]

Companies thus advertised widely to broaden their insulin sales, and in this aim they also extended the indications for insulin use. Bayer and Hoechst for example used the impact of insulin on appetite to offer it to tuberculosis patients and also introduced it successfully as a means to induce physiological shocks in schizophrenic and psychiatric patients.[35] Similarly, French producers advertised Endopancrine to help gain weight.[36] Some insulin products were even marketed in France without any mention of diabetes in their indications. Insulanol, for instance, an Insulyl-based ointment by Roussel, was advertised for itchiness, varicose ulcers, haemorrhoids, burns and atonic wounds.[37]

Concurrently, the success of insulin itself contributed to the growth of the market as it meant that survivors turned into lifelong customers who not only needed insulin, but also accessories for injections and blood-sugar tests such as Glykorator, Clinitest or IniematicStar.[38] The need to stick to a strict dietary regime opened the doors to producers of dietary and food substitutes.[39] Furthermore, retinopathy, neuropathy and vascular diseases were long-term complications of diabetes. Diabetics were not only prescribed insulin, but also other pharmaceutical treatments for these complications, which were prominently advertised starting in the 1950s.[40] The non-prescription products for diabetics were not however profusely advertised in medical journals. A more direct means of communication was to address the patients themselves.

Advertising Directly to Patients

Responding to the specific needs of patients was a rather effective method of advertising, as it addressed the essential target group, whose aims may have differed from those of professionals. Diabetics were faced with the challenge of a restricted diet, but this was not the only stress they were exposed to. Their special needs brought about economic as well as social stress. Initially they had to pay for their (expensive) treatment themselves, were seen as being severely ill and unable to keep proper jobs and were refused government positions. Moreover, they could not buy life insurance, and health insurance excluded diabetics. In fact they were excluded from many aspects of public and social life.[41]

Advertisements promised to fill such gaps. Consider, for example, a 1956 advertisement in the *Journal des diabétiques* that, unlike the faceless insulin ads that have been thus far mentioned, shows a happy man wearing a shirt and tie sitting at a table, a radio in the background and a smiling woman, his wife, serving him what we might imagine to be an after-work beer, a Kronenbourg Diet Beer.[42] This is a 'normal' ritual, but one that, like many everyday activities, was off-limits to diabetics and contributed to social stigmatization. This French beer advertisement promised to solve these problems: it sold hope for joy and an almost normal life. Very similar ads were published in the German pendant, *Der Diabetiker*, such as one for liqueurs by the firm Bols pledging that 'The little joys of everyday life are there for you, too'.[43]

Patient groups for diabetics were very much at the forefront of the self-support and patient empowerment movement.[44] The German Diabetes Association (Deutscher Diabetiker Bund, DDB) was established in 1931, nine years before the American Diabetes Association came to light, seven years before the French association (Association Française des Diabétiques) and three years before the British Diabetic Association. Like the British association, it was founded by diabetics, whereas the American and French associations were founded by medical doctors.[45] The bulletins of the diabetes patient groups offer an entry point into the marketing of products for and to diabetics. The price for advertisements was stipulated according to the assumed efficiency of the advertisements. For example, in 1965 the German scientific diabetes journal *Diabetologia* charged only DM 600 per page, whereas *Der Diabetiker* charged DM 1,040 per page; the price difference mirrors assumptions about the effectiveness of advertising in the journal.[46]

As of its institution in 1931, the German group published a bulletin called *Wir Zuckerkranken* (We diabetics) to establish a community of diabetics and to share information about treatment.[47] Beginning with a circulation of about 5,000, its low price did not cover expenses and the publisher discontinued it. From 1932 on, the association produced a newsletter with the participation of local doctors. It was published and sent out from Garz, where Gerhard Katsch and his diabetes clinic, Diabetikerheim Garz auf Rügen, were located.[48] After the end of war, the DDB was reorganized and the new monthly bulletin *Der Diabetiker* (The diabetic) was published from 1951, by a philanthropic journalist and benefactor of diabetics who had established a recipe service for diabetics in 1949.[49]

The DDB aimed mainly at education and at social and welfare support for diabetics with the representation of disadvantaged diabetics in legal issues and the implementation of social measures for working diabetics. Overall this programme was a mix of practical help, lobbying for diabetics and research support.[50] The number of members grew from seven founding members to over 10,000 in 1965.[51]

Membership fees, which included a subscription to the monthly bulletin *Der Diabetiker*, were kept low to make membership affordable to everyone.[52] Starting in 1953, the journal generated a surplus, largely as a result of the advertisement space it sold.[53]

The bulletin provided dietary advice and recipes, news from the association, legal, insurance and tax advice, a garden corner and a feuilleton, as well as personal reports and examples of successful diabetics. Every year, it included two complete teaching courses for newly diagnosed diabetics written by different specialists. All in all, the bulletin gave advice on how to live a satisfactory and active life with diabetes, and it may be seen as the organ of a working community of doctors and patients, and their representatives.[54] While doctors insisted that it was their task to decide on drug and diet therapy, the letters to the editor clearly show that patients refused this one-sided, patriarchal view. Above all they themselves wished to make decisions regarding their lifestyles.

A closer look at the bulletins reveals commercial interests, as *Der Diabetiker* published an increasing number of ads. Surprisingly there were ads for insulin, which, as a prescription drug, was not to be advertised to patients. These were however largely outnumbered by ads for other pharmaceuticals, the services of local pharmacists, and spas and clinics that specialized in the treatment of diabetes. The latter were run by diabetes specialists, many of whom contributed articles to the bulletin. It might be suggested that these doctors were contributing articles to the bulletin to promote their own services.

Table 7.1: Number and distribution of ads in *Der Diabetiker* and in *Journal des Diabétiques* by different categories of products

	Services		Devices		Food		Medication					Other		
	Spas and clinics	Pharmacies	Measuring devices	Injection devices	Food	Stimulants	Insulin	Oral anti-diabetics	Diabetes complications	Dietetics and Anorexigenics	Insulin producers	Other	Total
Der Diabetiker (DDB)													
1951	11	0	10	0	32	8	5	5	0	1	0	6	75
1955	36	0	2	3	60	16	1	0	4	0	0	0	124
1961	72	0	19	14	99	36	2	0	3	2	0	8	257
1965	76	0	25	14	144	27	0	0	2	2	0	7	302
1970	151	0	33	10	61	16	0	0	2	3	0	6	289
Journal des Diabétiques (AFD)													
1950	0	1	4	0	3	6	6	4	0	0	2	2	30
1955	2	3	4	2	4	9	4	0	0	0	8	1	37
1960	4	5	4	7	4	12	3	0	0	0	12	0	51
1965	4	0	6	14	10	16	4	0	0	0	13	0	67
1970	4	0	0	12	4	20	0	0	0	0	0	0	40

Source: GEPHAMA database.

It is not surprising that diet foods were the most important products advertised (see Table 7.1), while the indispensable needs of diabetics – that is, insulin and the devices used to inject it – were present in far fewer advertisements. Although the absolute number of food ads grew, their relative importance decreased because the number of advertisements for spas and clinics almost doubled between 1965 and 1970. In other words, doctors, who generally opposed drug promotion to patients, advertised their own services and intensified their advertising activities in a phase during which the overall number of ads in the diabetes association bulletin was declining.

On the other side of the Rhine, the French patient group (Association Française des Diabétiques, AFD) was founded in 1946. It was the post-war successor to the Association amicale des diabétiques formed in 1938, and its aim was to improve the fate of diabetics.[55] The membership of the association, as well as the executive committee, were made up of diabetics and their friends and families, albeit an honorary or scientific committee was composed of medical professors and doctors. Like the DDB, the AFD also aimed to provide education as well as social and welfare support to diabetics, to support scientific research, and to implement social measures for working diabetics.[56] Members of the AFD paid annual fees, which went to scientific research, summer camps and social missions, as well as the publication of the bulletin. In addition to the bulletin, from the 1950s on, members received a diabetes handbook.[57] Membership fees were supplemented with investment funds (*fonds placés*), subsidies (*subventions*) and advertising revenue.[58]

The *Journal des Diabétiques* was a quarterly limited to sixteen pages, or thirty-two pages after 1952.[59] Its articles were mainly written by diabetes specialists and offered information on rights, treatment, scientific results, and international news and statistics. The chairman, an attorney, was particularly involved in fighting for the rights of diabetics and communicating news on the struggle through the bulletin, and clarifying questions of improved ration cards, social security coverage and employment, notably as a civil servant. It also provided a review of products and treatment.[60] These articles were supplemented with columns providing dietary advice, recipes and food charts, recapping frequently asked questions of the most general order but also repeatedly warning against charlatans, as well as offering a space for diabetics to place their classified ads.

Advertisements filled 15 to 28 percent of each bulletin.[61] The *Journal* editors acknowledged the ads to be contributions with a note calling the readers' attention to the advertisements by stating, 'This bulletin can continue to be published thanks to support from our advertisements. They help us ... Think of them ...'[62] Alternatively, in issues in which this notice did not appear, a note indicated how to contribute to the AFD, with one suggestion being to advertise in the journal. Statements that sought to draw readers' attention to the advertisements was not unique to the French bulletin, with a similar note appearing the 1931 German bulletin: 'Diabetics take notice of the advertisement section. Its information is no less important than the editorial section'.[63]

Some French advertisers were not just looking to promote their products. In the 1950s, pharmaceutical laboratories such as Choay sought, rather, recognition for their contribution to the cause of diabetes. Their advertising space, for example, stated: 'Choay laboratory is pleased to be able to contribute to the publication of this bulletin'.[64] In the 1960s, the 'patronage' aspect became more uniform with a list of the pharmaceutical laboratories that had made contributions provided below the table of contents on the first page of the bulletin. Not all of those listed had purchased advertising space in the bulletin, and those that had simply stated the name of the laboratory and its location, leaving much of the advertising space empty; they did not even state what they manufactured, but they were all insulin producers.[65] This was an alternative means of seeking credibility in the public mind, and more importantly in that of patients or consumers. Their role extended beyond producers of insulin and drugs to the role of benefactors sympathetic to diabetes. In return, diabetics were to have empathy for the pharmaceutical company and, it can be assumed, to choose or request their products. This scheme allowed pharmaceutical firms to relay the message that they were looking out for diabetics. The strategy is comparable to pharmaceutical industry's financing the publication of educational literature, with the AFD acting as intermediary, assuring targeted and authoritative distribution.[66]

Aside from the far smaller number of advertisements appearing in the *Journal*, largely due to this being a smaller bulletin, another distinct difference from the German ads was that there were no ads for hospitals, and only one for a clinic (see Table 7.1). In addition, nothing was advertised for diabetes complications, though there were occasional ads for pharmacies. Syringes, injectors, sterilisers and other instruments and accessories represented a significant and rising share of the ads. More importantly, in terms of the advertising space they occupied, food products were marketed to supplement diabetic diets. These and stimulants – sugar, chocolate and even cough lozenge alternatives and substitutions – made up the greatest part of the advertisements. These categories all involved appealing to the daily needs and pleasures of diabetics, providing them with a sense of normality.

Conclusion

In this study of the early insulin market, we are struck by the imagery and language of industrial production, of product reliability and of scientific progress in the insulin ads. Effectively, the 1920s and 1930s mark the rise of pharmaceutical production on an industrial scale, a markedly different process from the back room of a pharmacy. Insulin was promoted as exemplary of the industrial and scientific strength of pharmaceutical industries. Moreover it served as an example of the altruism of the researchers who made their patent available freely, for the benefit of humankind. However, this is not to say that there was no marketing at play. Notably the later depot insulins of the 1930s were marketed through common channels, i.e., to key opinion leaders and through leaflets and not primarily through medical journal advertisements.

But these were not the only mechanisms central to this paper, which presents how a whole palette of diabetes products were developed, building on the scientific renown of insulin. In contrast to the widely accepted narrative that dates the history of patient associations to the 1970s, we have shown that consumer marketing through patient associations' bulletins since the 1930s was another channel for communication from pharmaceutical companies and physicians to diabetics. In this channel, the scientific achievement of insulin production forms the basis on which a second layer of marketing was founded, which accepted scientificity as a matter of course, but used arguments of life style, comfort and personal well-being. That is, it built upon the mechanisms and elements of scientific marketing, but took it to another level, herein answering to the associations' goals of patient empowerment and well-being by ensuring they took responsibility for their own therapeutic regime, while opening up new approaches to educate patients and define a target group.

Diabetes is a disease of equilibrium: a proper balance of diet, insulin and exercise is needed to keep sugar levels stable and normal.[67] Measurement, quantification and equilibrium characterize the general line of diabetes treatment.[68] Balance and equilibrium were also recurrent terms in both ads and patient education. For example, a 1955/1960 Novo zinc insulin advertisement heralded 'diabétiques équilibrés'.[69] Nevertheless, there were major imbalances. One of these is the fact that doctors presented themselves as benefactors respecting the moral economy of science and the Hippocratic Oath, thus refusing to advertise for drugs, although they did advertise their services in the German patient association bulletin. Second, there was another imbalance, or at least tension, between physicians' concern for the future and patients' interest in the present. Doctors advised keeping blood-sugar level at a stable, low level in order to prevent long-term consequences or complications. Far-sighted diabetologists were therefore interested in having patients inject insulin regularly and follow a strict diet. Patients, on the other hand, were just as concerned with living well, every day.[70] The difference in their interests was recognized in marketing schemes, and this imbalance was reflected in the products advertised in the medical versus patient periodicals.

The diabetic market is interesting and relevant as insulin has remained, over the past nine decades, the only means of living with Type I diabetes mellitus. This means that diabetics are literally insulin-dependent for the whole of their lives.

This unites them as a highly special group of patients who share not only the need for a drug essential for them to live, but also a similar social situation. Along with their medical needs, their needs for a 'normal' life style, with the rights and comforts of other citizens, unite them as a special consumers' group, with diabetic patient associations acting much like consumer associations. All too often, their desires differ from their needs, demands and interdictions. This was exactly the situation out of which a market grew that was by no means limited to insulin and other drugs, and included instruments, diet foods and drinks, specific services such as spas, journals for scientific and mainstream information, scientific books, advice literature and, more recently, upscale lifestyle magazines. With the number of diabetics on the rise, this market is bound to expand further.[71]

In the case of Germany, the Toronto insulin policy paradoxically contributed to, instead of inhibited, the mercantilization of diabetes. The strong position of the committee in the scientific networks solidified existing market structures and, in particular, the strong position of large pharmaceutical companies, which the committee deemed scientific, experienced and trustworthy. The companies were well aware of the value of the Insulin Committee's label and used the insulin business to reinforce their image as trustworthy, scientific and innovative firms with a strong foothold in the diabetes field. By following this path Hoechst would become *the* diabetes company after World War II, when most other firms had abandoned production of insulin due to the difficulties of the time. This led to its holding a nearly monopolistic position in the field of oral antidiabetics, for which it charged very high prices, eventually attracting the attention of the Federal Cartel Agency to their pricing of Euglucon.[72]

The same imbalance of forces was not at stake in France. While German firms further increased imbalances by forming monopolies through patents and by adding the production of instruments, artificial sweeteners and diet foods to their portfolio, this was not the case in France, most probably because smaller producers dominated the field. In other words, ironically, regulation of the insulin business, which was meant to ward off commercial forces, was fully instrumentalized by an already powerful industry that promoted itself to doctors and thus sought, and still seeks, to make use of existing imbalances for its own purposes. This shows that globally the same forces and developments were at stake in different countries, while a closer look reveals local differences. Depending on different medical systems and cultures it took different forms. Consumer marketing opened up a channel, aside from usual advertising to medical practitioners and through pamphlet distribution, which became more and more important for increasingly informed and self-conscious patients. In fact, this could result in conflicts with the ideal of scientific marketing and the insistence on scientificity, as it addressed non-scientific issues such as well-being and life style.

8 VARIATION IN DRUGS AND WOMEN: STANDARDIZATION AS A TOOL FOR SCIENTIFIC MARKETING OF ORAL CONTRACEPTIVES IN FRANCE AND WEST GERMANY (1961–2006)

Lisa Malich

First introduced in the USA in 1960, oral contraception was not ordinary medication as it focused on preventing pregnancy, a condition that was not regarded as a disease. This is why Lara Marks calls it one of the first 'designer' or 'lifestyle' drugs.[1] Women and doctors accepted the pill faster than its manufacturers expected them to, and it soon came into wide commercial success. Two years after the company Searle launched the first pill, Enovid, on the US market it had increased its sales by 27 per cent, reaching a record high. Within ten years after its introduction, several international firms from countries such as the USA, France, Germany and the Netherlands were producing oral contraceptives.

From the start, however, the pill also triggered many concerns regarding its safety. Debates on an increased risk of thrombosis and cancer led to more extensive research designs, new epidemiological approaches, and an increased focus on the standardization of drugs. Accordingly, a central goal in the marketing of oral contraception was to communicate its safety and its nature as a standardized drug. This paper discusses the ways in which standardization was represented in scientific marketing of the pill in two Western European countries: France and Germany.

Today Western Europe is the region with the highest incidence of pill use worldwide. France and Germany are part of the group of the few countries where more than 40 per cent of women rely on this form of contraception.[2] Nevertheless, most studies on the pill concentrate only on the USA and Great Britain.[3] The few investigations on Germany or France only take a view of one of the two countries in isolation, its sales figures and its cultural context. For West Germany,

many studies focus only on the early period to 1980.[4] There are also only a small number of surveys of the French situation, and most of them focus primarily on the percentage of users and on legal issues.[5] To fill this gap, my article will compare France and West Germany covering the period from the 1960s to 2003. I will target not only the specific conditions in each country and the national therapeutic cultures, but also transnational trajectories and common changes in culture, gender and drug marketing.[6] After all, the pill was always involved in international developments: events like the ban on contraception in the encyclical written by Pope Paul VI in 1968 and the Nelson hearings in the 1970s, which discussed long-standing concerns about drug safety, had worldwide effects.[7] Moreover, many pill manufacturers operated in international markets.

Most existing studies on the pill have neglected marketing materials. Only some of them have mentioned the first important advertisements, especially those for Searle's Enovid in the USA or those for Schering's Anovlar in the Federal Republic of Germany (FRG).[8] My analysis will therefore draw from flyers, marketing materials and advertisements for the contraceptive pill in gynaecological and obstetric journals. Medical journals were chosen because both countries prohibit direct-to-consumer advertising of drugs. Advertising is a useful source because it reveals how companies tried to represent their products, what the dominant notions of the pill user were and how the design, images and marketing strategies changed over time. Overall, promotion is a to-and-fro proposition: it both seeks to influence opinions and ways of thinking and is influenced in return by opinions and ways of thinking. This is especially true for scientific marketing, which uses methods like polls or market research and tests advertising efficacy. This approach has gained in importance for pharmaceutical advertising since the 1950s. Ads thus function both as mirrors and as agents of social transformation. Looking at the pill from Donna Haraway's point of view as a material-semiotic configuration tells us that advertising, a semiotic activity, is also always connected to materiality.[9]

My investigation and analysis of German and French advertising for the contraceptive pill from 1961 to 2003 is developed in two steps. First I will describe general national differences in how the pill was marketed in the two countries. Thereafter, I will analyse references to standardization and how they were employed as tools for scientific marketing. I will argue that two different uses of standardization can be found: first, and most obviously, the pill is framed as a standardized drug, and second, the pill user is also standardized. In both cases, standardization is represented as emphasizing both the safety and the uniqueness of the advertised product. Since representations of the pill are closely linked to images of its female users, I will also take into account changing notions of gender and sexuality, and the agency of patients.

Material

The main source of my analysis is print advertising in medical journals. I examined six French and two West German gynaecological journals.[10] There is a larger selection of French journals because the country offers a greater variety of relatively important gynaecological magazines, many of which have changed their names or were only published for a short time. In the FRG, the situation is more homogenous, with only a few key journals dominating the field. Additionally, German and French 1960s and 1970s information brochures, advertisements and flyers designed for physicians by Schering AG, the manufacturer of the first European pill, were analysed in order to include earlier advertising.[11]

Source analysis included examination of not only slogans, advertising copy and lists of indications, but also of graphic design, visual elements and images, providing an additional visual-history approach to the investigation.[12]

Early National Differences: French Multipurpose Drugs versus German Contraceptives

Comparing the source material for national patterns in marketing, advertising style and presentation of the drug reveals major differences only in the initial period, from the 1960s to the late 1970s.

The early differences in advertising reflect important legal and political differences regarding contraception in France and in the FRG. Whereas contraception remained prohibited in France for several more years, it was legalized in West Germany in 1961, the same year the first German or European pill, Anovlar, was launched by Schering. In the conservative climate of the era, the pill – or the 'green bomb', as it was sometimes called – was seen as a method to regulate marital reproduction.[13] It was to be prescribed only to married women who already had children. According to Eva-Maria Silies's study, these restrictions were characteristic of the first phase (1961–66) of pill use in the Federal Republic of Germany (FRG).[14] At the time, contraception and sexuality were hardly ever addressed as topics, discussion of the pill was framed in moral terms and only a small number of women used it. Moreover, the media were already reporting potential side effects of the drug such as depression, and a higher risk of cancer and thrombosis. These fears were increased by the thalidomide tragedy in 1961–62, which ultimately led to the alteration of drug regulations.[15] The pill nevertheless slowly gained in popularity, and the first public debates began appearing on whether oral contraception ought to be prescribed to every woman who wanted it, including young and unmarried women, marking a rapid increase in the use of oral contraception in the second phase (1967–72). In 1969, for instance, about 16 per cent of all women between the ages of 15 and 45 were taking the drug.[16] This development came with social changes such as a liberalized view on sexuality and the rise of women's and student movements. Use of the pill in the third phase (1973–9) remained stable at almost 30 per cent and did not increase much for a while. Feminist perspectives on the pill also began to change: while the women's movement had fought for oral contraception in the early years, now it regarded the pill as an instrument of male-dominated medicine intended to control female reproduction. Many older women stopped taking the drug, but the drop in use was offset by increasing numbers of young users.

Some of these developments are reflected in the advertisements of the first two decades in the FRG, notably illustrating the three phases identified by Silies, although sometimes with a few years' time lag.[17] In contrast to France, German marketing materials highlight contraception as the main effect of the drug. During the early years, however, from 1961 to 1968, this was done in a very restrained and often implicit way, focusing strongly on family and marriage. At that time, the texts mentioned the physician's task to be mostly 'marriage counselling' or 'counselling of young mothers' and support to 'family planning' or 'responsible parenthood'.[18] Otherwise, they stated that the pill could offer a break between pregnancies. The advertisements seemed to downplay the idea that the product could prevent any pregnancy at all. This focus is mirrored in the images used. In accordance with conservative views and prescription policies, early marketing materials picture married women, often mothers. One advertisement for Anovlar, for instance, contains an image of a couple whose marital status is explicitly indicated by their wedding rings. Another for the same pill from the early 1960s shows a woman with her two children at the doctor's office. Sitting down and literally looking up to the physician, she is saying: 'Two children in such a short time were just more than I could take'. Her subordinate position, the children and her simple, rather poor and conventional clothing emphasize that she is a helpless patient and a mother with moral integrity. The picture takes the perspective of the male physician and the slogan is addressed to him: 'Anovlar 21 supports you in the counselling of young mothers'. This, and the triangular composition of the picture, puts him in a superior position, helping a woman in social and economic distress with his professional knowledge.

From 1968 onwards, West German print advertising and marketing materials openly mentioned 'contraception' more often in their slogans and copy, as well as in the lists of indications.[19] Starting in the 1970s, the lists mention contraception either solely or as the first indication amongst others such as dysmenorrhea or ovulation pain. From 1975 on, contraception became the only indication in most cases. The imagery was also diversified and included more neutral themes not depicting women exclusively as wives and mothers.

Legalization and distribution took longer in France. Six years later than in West Germany, in December 1967, contraception in general and the pill in particular were legalized by the so-called '*loi Neuwirth*'. The law was nonetheless implemented very slowly by the French administration, so prescription of hormonal drugs for contraceptive purposes still remained relatively illegal for a few years. Although hormonal drugs with contraceptive effects were found on the French market beginning in 1961, they could only be prescribed for indications such as sterility or dysmenorrhea. In 1973, the first hormonal medications obtained the French marketing authorization (*autorisation de mise sur le marché*) as contraceptive drugs. In 1974, the law legalizing contraception was extended and facilitated access to the pill for a broader range of women.[20] According to Sophie Chauveau, this delay in implementation can be attributed to moral concerns but also to increased safety standards in drug regulations after the thalidomide tragedy.[21]

The debate on the law had many effects. It divided the field of gynaecology, which in France was more heterogeneous than in Germany and consisted of four distinct groups (*compétences*).[22] The first and strongest group, a combination of obstetricians and gynaecologists, rejected the approval of the drug. The group was largely dominated by its male membership and a surgical orientation. In contrast, the smaller group of medical gynaecologists, which comprised many female physicians and had an endocrinological concentration, was in favour of the law. The French women's movement had a longer struggle and a stronger fight to lead for access to the pill.[23] Many women thus regarded oral contraception as a sign of female empowerment. Unlike in other Western countries, the feminist medicalization critique of the 1970s did not, in France, target hormonal medication.[24]

The legal situation affected the sales figures, which were much lower than in the FRG. Thus in France, prevalence of the pill cannot be divided into three phases like in West Germany. There were rather two phases, approximately related to the two stages of approval. In the first phase, to 1970, fewer than 5 per cent of women between fifteen and forty-nine years of age used the drug.[25] In the second phase, starting in 1971, the share grew strongly and continuously. By 1974, 17 per cent of the women in this age group were taking the pill. By 1988, ten years later than in West Germany, the rate had risen to more than 30 per cent.[26] Prevalence in France was thus lower and grew more slowly than in Germany, but the increase was spread over a longer period of time, more continuously and with no stagnation periods.

Given the French administrative regulations and law of the time, it is not surprising to find that the most striking feature in early French advertising for the pill was its subtlety. Regarding the purpose of the drug mentioned in slogans, advertising copy or lists of indications, the French sources are even more discreet than the – already quite discreet – German ones. Early marketing of the pill could not explicitly address contraception at all. To be consistent with other products, the (subtle) focus had to be put on the unique quality of the drug. The most common way to achieve inconspicuousness was to concentrate on different reasons to prescribe the drug. In simple advertisements, often containing neither pictures nor lengthy copy, only issues like dysmenorrhea, amenorrhea, problems caused by ovulation, endometriosis and sterility were mentioned as possible indications.[27] Advertisements for drugs that could be used as oral contraception did not then differ significantly from advertisements for other hormonal drugs at that time, and early French marketing material required the physician's expertise and knowledge of the brand name to identify the drug as oral contraception. Such was the case, for instance, of the 1963 advertisement for Enidrel, the first French pill manufactured by Byla.[28] It listed many indications that were also typical of a number of non-contraceptive medications used to treat so-called 'female maladies' and also had a very neutral, unobtrusive design.[29] Another common type of marketing strategy was to not mention any purposes or indications at all and just rely on the brand name. The advertisement for the oral contraceptive Planovin(e) by Novo Industrie is a good example and also illustrates national differences (Figures 8.1 and 8.2). Appearing in 1968 in Germany and in France, the picture in both countries showed a stone statue of a woman holding an infant.[30] In the image, the whiteness of the statue stood out on a dark background and the figure of the baby dominated the composition. The materiality of stone, the contrast of black and white, and the cool colours evoked associations of purity, transcendence and spirituality but avoided the notion of sexuality and corporeality. By focusing on the abstract idea of a child, contraception was addressed but transferred into the positive realm of planned reproduction. The visual language and adherence to conservative ideals were thus very similar in both countries, but while the German advertisement included a text describing the contraceptive qualities of the drug, the French one contained only the name of the drug and its company and provided no further information.

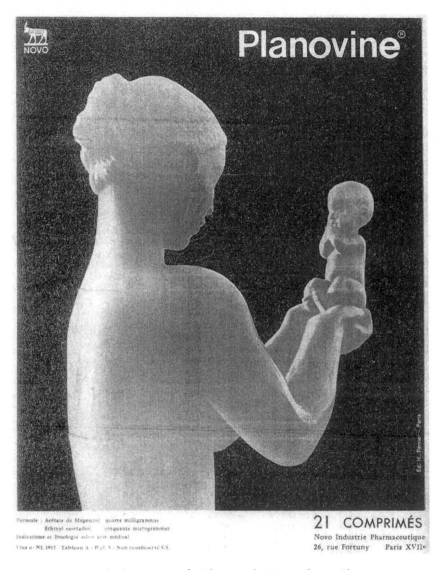

Figure 8.1: French advertisement for Planovine by Novo Industrie Pharmaceutique
Paris; image reproduced by kind permission of Novo Nordisk.

Source: *Gynécologie pratique*, 19 (1968), p. xviii.

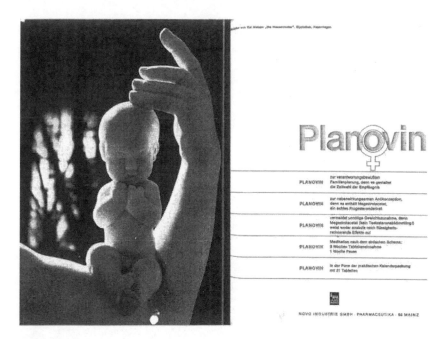

Figure 8.2: West German advertisement for Planovin by Novo Industrie GmbH Pharmazeutika Mainz; image reproduced by kind permission of Novo Nordisk.

Source: *Der Gynäkologe*, 1 (1968).

Nonetheless, many advertisements also attempted to stress the specificity of their products with an additional hint at the contraceptive qualities of certain hormonal drugs. For instance, several advertisements for pills such as Lyndiol by the Laboratoires Endopancrine[31] or Anovlar by Schering included a sentence like *'mise au repos de l'ovaire'* ('putting the ovaries to rest'), which explained that the medication would halt the function of the ovaries during its use.[32] Often highlighted by its size and colour, the sentence helped to identify the product as oral contraception by stating a medical effect that had contraceptive consequences without addressing contraception explicitly.[33] Only after 1974, the year when the law was extended, was contraception mentioned in the list of indications, but the older indications such as dysmenorrhea and ovulation problems still remained, and it took five years longer in France than in Germany for contraception to become the sole indication of the pill in most advertising. Problems with ovulation were still mentioned as reasons to prescribe the drug in France until the early 1980s. The same medication appeared in French marketing for a relatively long time as a multi-functional drug aimed at several purposes connected to 'female maladies' when it had been defined solely as a contraceptive in the FRG years earlier. So although the ingredients were similar, one could speak of the marketing for two different drugs in the first fifteen to twenty years: a multi-functional medication in one country and a contraceptive in the other.

It seems quite clear that the initial differences in marketing style stemmed from a profound discrepancy between national forms of drug regulation, primarily and most importantly between administrative regulations.[34] In the French context, the laws of 1967 and 1974 and the accompanying public debate had a major impact on the marketing and advertising of the drug. Notwithstanding, the legal situation in France does not completely explain the relatively late appearance, in the early 1980s, of contraception as the sole indication of the pill. It could be hypothesized that, due to how the drug had been depicted during its period of introduction, a cultural and medical notion of the pill as multi-functional drug had been established and had remained valid even after 1974. Many women and physicians probably perceived it not primarily as contraception, but as medication against menstrual problems. Additionally, economic factors and industrial regulations were also at play in this process because listing many indications also increased the number of prescriptions written, hence the sales of the drug. Consequently, France featured a specific national 'therapeutic culture' in the prescription of the pill until the early 1980s.[35]

There was another minor disparity between the French and German images. Like in the above-mentioned advertising for Anovlar by Schering, in West Germany the female user was often shown in combination with a male physician. In contrast, no physicians were pictured in the French advertisements. This was probably because in France gynaecology was more diverse and fragmented, and the country had a higher percentage of female doctors. The figure of the male paternalistic physician did not offer a general model with which to identify, as was the case in Germany.

Despite these differences, there were already many similarities between the two countries in the first two decades following the launch of the pill. Notably, the way advertisements portrayed the pill user changed over time in similar patterns. In the first years, notions of the woman as wife and mother and as a patient in need of medical advice were central. The late 1960s brought in a larger variety of images, including close-ups of the smiling faces of beautiful women wearing make-up and fashionable clothes. Moreover, most advertising from the 1970s on displayed young women, reflecting the fact that at the same time, an increasing number of users were unmarried and began to take the pill at an earlier age.[36] For example the French ad for Organon's Ovanon explained: 'For the young woman. She wants to feel good, she wants to be sure' ('Pour la femme jeune. Elle veut être bien, elle veut être sûre').[37] The picture showed a confident woman looking straight into the camera and holding her briefcase – this pill user did not give the impression of a mother, but rather of a university student or a businesswoman focusing on her own life.

As the following chapters will show, there was another resemblance. West German and French advertising represented standardization in the same way. In the first two decades, both specifically highlighted the quality of the pill as a standardized drug. Despite differences in legal systems and in national therapeutic cultures, changing attitudes towards gender and sexuality, as well as concerns regarding drug safety, influenced the marketing in the two countries in a comparable manner.

The introductory period was followed by one of similarity in the depiction of contraceptive drugs. From the mid-1970s on, French and German materials coincided more and more, and after the mid-1980s, hardly any national differences in style, content, size, appearance or indications could be found. The marketing strategy and rhetoric changed in similar patterns in both countries. This demonstrates the growing interconnectedness of post-war developments in different Western European countries, and that France and West Germany participated in them in equal measure.

Standardization: Reducing Variability and Producing Variety in Drugs and Women

In advertising and marketing, references to standardization can be an advantage due to its positive connotations such as safety, reliability and quality. This is related to the function of standardization as a 'technology of trust', ensuring and facilitating communication amongst groups of scientists, physicians and pharmacologists.[38] Standardization can, however, conflict with another marketing characteristic: the tendency to focus on the individuality, innovativeness and uniqueness of the product. The analysed material partly reflects this tension, especially in its emphasis on certain aspects of drug standardization and its disregard of others. In most of the advertising, however, the conflict between standardization and individualization cannot be detected. Instead they seem to be quite pragmatically combined. One reason might be that in the imaginary world of an advertisement the main principle is not necessarily logical coherence but coherent appearance – marketing, if scientific or not, primarily needs to look good and to sound good.[39]

Standardization not only focuses on drugs, it is also instrumental at many different levels in the construction of patients.[40] This was also true in marketing. Overall, two different uses of standardization are of importance in the source material: first and most obviously, the pill is framed as a standardized drug, and second, the consumer of oral contraception is standardized and categorized. The first use played a central role in the two decades following the introduction of oral contraception, when health concerns were the focus of public debates.[41] The latter became more important in the 1980s and 1990s as a consequence of the saturation of the market, the search for new user groups, as well as the growth of consumer culture.

Representations of a Standardized Pill

If standardization is defined as a way of reducing variability, the standardizing of drugs can be characterized by three goals: (1) to create qualitatively identical goods with known properties; (2) to control clinical uses; and (3) to standardize the pharmacological effects.[42] In the early marketing of both countries, aspects of these different dimensions were employed to establish the notion of hormonal contraceptives as standardized products. The three goals did not, however, assume the same importance, and their modes of presentation changed over time.

The first goal, the creation of identical goods, only played a minor role in the marketing of the pill. The standardization requirement was met simply by specifying in the advertisements the chemical ingredients of the drug as well as the daily and monthly dose. The reasons for this marginal position are twofold: on the one hand, the goal of identical goods dates back to the first standardization techniques of the 'chemical approach' associated with the Industrial Revolution at the end of the nineteenth century.[43] This kind of information has been ubiquitous in the pharmaceutical field since the beginning of the twentieth century. On the other hand, many contraceptive pills are made of similar or related compounds and active ingredients. Therefore a conflict between standardization and product individuality might actually be a causal factor for the relative reluctance in this case. It was not a good idea to focus on chemical compounds and the known properties when emphasizing the uniqueness of a particular pill.

The second goal, control of clinical uses, received more attention, at least in the early years and at least in one respect. Of the many clinical uses in existence, one practical aspect was particularly stressed: advertisements and flyers often emphasized the easy-to-use packaging system of the drug, which included a list of the days of the week, alerting the patient to remember when to start and stop taking her medication. This was a major topic throughout the 1960s and early 1970s in German as well as in French samples, which was addressed in the texts but also underscored through pictures of the pill packages and application systems. An example is the French ad for Ovariostat by Organon.[44] Here, the front view of the package and the plain, graphical design gave the impression of clarity and simplicity. Also the copy stated the 'facilité d'emploi' (ease of use) and provided information on the user-friendly and functional system, something that was characteristic of many advertisements.[45] The packaging of the pill was thus presented as the perfect tool for standardizing the use of oral contraception. As a consequence, only the female customer emerged as the source of variability and error in use of the pill, connected to old ideas of femininity as irrational and disorderly. In contrast, other possible sources, like the physician or a possible interaction with other drugs, were omitted. Although the packaging systems seemed to be quite similar, they were advertised as specific features of a certain pill and as innovative medical devices. Thus, in this regard and in the early years, standardization and individualization did not seem to conflict, and were instead combined: within the conceptual framework of an advertisement, the standardizing potential of its package made a pill unique. Starting in the mid-1970s, however, this no longer seemed a noteworthy and distinct characteristic. The easy-to-use packaging system including the weekdays had become common and had been established as the standard for almost all contraceptive pills. This process occurred at the expense of individualization, so emphasis on the packaging vanished and made way for different representations of standardization.

The third goal, on pharmacological effects, was what was most frequently displayed in marketing materials, underscoring the control and safety of the product. Here the standardization and the individuality of the product seemed to be consistent because the standardization of the pill was presented as one of its unique qualities. This goal was mainly depicted in three different ways: recording of effects, emphasis on the great number of satisfied consumers and reference to scientific elements. These three strategies of representing the standardization of drug effects will now be discussed.

The first and most obvious way was to list drug information in the advertisements, which gradually included more and more effects and side effects. A second way was achieved by emphasizing the great number and wide range of women who took the pill, highlighting the universality of its effects. This was particularly frequent in the early marketing of the 1960s. An illustrative example is the 1968 French advertising flyer for the pill Anovlar 21 by Schering.[46] It shows photographs of women's faces presented in an apparently global context: one woman in a sari seemed to represent India, and other women wore clothing that called to mind various African, Asian or Western countries. The slogan said: 'In the whole world, more than two-and-a-half million women are treated each day with Anovlar' ('Dans le monde entier, plus de 2 millions 1/2 de femmes sont traitées chaque jour par l'Anovlar'). This presentation implied that regardless of cultural background and living conditions, the effects of the drug were universal, safe and satisfactory. The variety of consumers was used as evidence to reveal the homogenous effects of the drug. The number of women mentioned and the reference to a universal finding thus seemed to represent certainty about the drug that might otherwise be expected from a clinical trial.

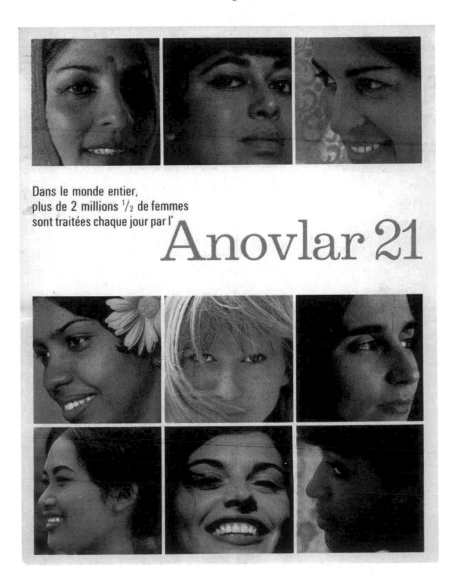

Figure 8.3: French advertisement for Anovlar 21 by Schering; image reproduced by kind permission of Schering Archives, Bayer AG.

Source: Schering Archives, 1968.

This leads us to the third strategy, i.e., referencing scientific knowledge and standardized research designs. This strategy often concentrated on desired effects and on side effects. Nevertheless, only specific side effects like weight gain, nausea or breast sensitivity were addressed.[47] In contrast, the media and a number of scientists began speculating in the 1960s about much greater health hazards such as a potential risk of cancer or blood clotting.[48] The ads rarely mentioned these objections. While a few advertisements at least highlighted the limited risk of thrombosis due to a specific drug,[49] concerns about carcinogenic effects were never explicitly brought up.

This third way of representing standardization was particularly indebted to methods of scientific marketing that had been developed after World War I and which had been expanded upon since the 1950s. One of its characteristics was the use of seemingly scientific elements such as graphs, curves, tables or pictures of smear samples.[50] Sometimes these images were used to illustrate content, for example to demonstrate that specific side effects decreased or that an intended effect increased, but they also functioned as part of a decorative artwork in the background of the ad, conveying the sense of scientific control and credibility.[51] An example of this strategy is a German advertisement for Lyndiol by Organon.[52] It recommended the pill for first prescription and emphasized its safety. It contained photographs of different young women partly faded out by a purple curve in a diagram showing the concentration of plasma in the drug after eight hours. While the women's pictures represented the random variability of patients, the graph illustrated the controlled and standardized effects of the pill.

Connected to the use of scientific elements was another strategy: the explicit reference to individual studies. This remained very common from the 1960s to the 1990s, in particular with regard to side effects. In some advertisements, these references were quite detailed, with mention, for instance, of even the exact sample size of the quoted study,[53] or a description of the results of many different studies, each for one specific side effect.[54] A last way of establishing the notion of scientifically proven and standardized effects in marketing was the publication of studies by drug companies in journals similar to those of academic institutions but published by the maker. An example of this is the 1972 study by Schering on the properties of the oral contraceptive Microlut, which was aimed at physicians and scientists and published in the company's series *Medizinische Mitteilungen Schering*.

Conceptualization of the pill as a standardized drug thus took many shapes. Of the three standardizing goals, the first was neglected, while control of drug uses remained important until the 1970s. Overall, the third dimension of standardizing effects was the most dominant and was portrayed in a number of ways. It could notably be found in marketing materials from the 1960s to the 1980s. The similarity of West German and French marketing implies that despite important legal differences, both markets were shaped by a number of forces in common. Discussions about the health risks of the pill and new professional and administrative regulations following the thalidomide tragedy played a major role in this regard.

The drug standardization dimension seems to have become less important in marketing since the late 1980s. Moreover, almost simultaneously with the representation of the pill as standardized, another process had started: standardization of its user.

Standardizing Women

Beginning already in the 1970s and increasing in the late 1980s, a different use of standardization can be observed, one aimed not at the pill, but at women who take the pill. Several classification schemes, typologies and standards were established, reducing the variability of female consumers. In doing so, however, this very variability was decreased and at the same time emphasized. The classification schemes produced a controlled and well-regulated variation of women.

This occurred in a period of transformation, not only in gender-related notions but also in the fields of medicine and pharmacology. To start with, the feminist movement grew stronger in the 1970s; it fought against restricting women to motherhood, and in favour of equal rights and liberated sexuality. Feminists also criticized the medicalization and objectification of female bodies and opened women's health centres. In addition, patient groups emerged that also challenged the paternalistic power of physicians. The relationship between doctor and patient thus became less authoritarian, more information-oriented and more cooperative. Gradually, passive patients turned into active consumers who chose medical services according to their individual demands.[55] This development was partly influenced by the transformation of pharmacy into a profound capitalistic industry with a strong market orientation. Additionally a growing number of 'lifestyle' drugs were introduced in the 1980s and gained wide commercial success. Focused not primarily on illness but on conditions like impotence, hair loss and weight loss, these drugs promised a better quality of life and the accomplishment of social norms. Subjective choice and consumer rights became more important, as well as issues like life satisfaction, informed consent and optimization.

At the same time, the material side of the pill as 'material-semiotic configuration' also changed. In the 1970s there was already a wide variety of products on the market. Compared to the first pills, they often contained a lower dose of hormones and had less severe side effects. Pills that were based just on progesterone and were free of oestrogens, as well as sequential pills, had been on the market since the 1960s and proliferated in the 1970s. Drugs with reduced progesterone were also developed in the late 1970s. There was more diversity and competition, but the market was also being saturated. In 1973 for instance, between twenty-five and thirty different kinds of oral contraceptives were on offer in many Western countries.[56]

By the 1970s, the pill had become popular in West Germany and in France. Growing numbers of younger and unmarried women were using it, and moral concerns had begun to wane. Twenty years after the drug had emerged, its prevalence entered a period of strong growth. In France, an extended second phase followed the first phase of prohibition, with long and continuous growth of user numbers. In 1978, around 28 per cent of women between twenty and forty-four years old were taking the pill and ten years later, this figure had practically reached 34 per cent.[57] By 1994 it had risen to approximately 40 per cent. Prevalence of the pill remained higher in West Germany than in France. The numbers in the two countries cannot, however, be compared directly because statistics were based on different methods and on samples with changing age ranges. In 1985, approximately 38 per cent of German women fifteen to forty-five years old were taking the drug. After the country's reunification with East Germany, in 1992, almost 51 per cent of the same age group were taking the pill.[58] Thus, despite growing competition and market saturation, pill prevalence continued to rise in both countries through to the early 1990s.

In this context, standardization in advertising focused increasingly on the pill user. Initially, the strategy was closely connected standardizing the effects of the drug. As discussed above, emphasis on drug standardization highlighted the universal effects of the drug on all female bodies. It underscored the supposed homogeneity of women, particularly in 1960s advertising, like in the Schering example. A few years later, the variety of women and their bodily differences came to the fore, and focusing on this variety was used as a marketing strategy. Special subgroups of women were set in order to reduce and to regulate this variability, which at another level, also helped to find new consumer groups and to deal with the increasing competition and saturation of the market. 'Frauen sind verschieden' ('women are different'), the marketing slogan for two pills by the manufacturer Glaxo, illustrates this process.[59]

When the categorization of women came about in the 1970s, it included primarily physiological characteristics. Subgroups were determined such as 'very young women', 'progestogen-sensitive women', 'older women' and 'women with special cycle problems'. Initially, these subgroups were intended to be matched with a specific pill type that suited them: Ediwal was explicitly advertised as a solution to menstrual problems,[60] Diane as one for acne,[61] and pills like Exlutona or Ovanon were targeted to young women.[62] The standardization and categorization of women thus corresponded to the standardization of specific drug effects. A variation of women was produced in correspondence with pills that matched their individual constitutions.

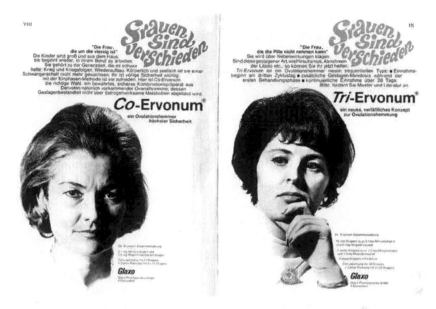

Figure 8.4. West German advertisement for Co-Ervonum and Tri-Ervonum by Glaxo; image reproduced by kind permission of Schering Archives, Bayer AG.

Source: *GF*, 29 (1969), pp. viii–ix.

A good example is the Glaxo advertisement in Figure 8.4. It presents two pills, Tri-Ervonum and Co-Ervonum. Supporting its general claim that women were different, the ad classified various types of patients. While the first drug was advertised for 'the woman who cannot take the pill and who will complain about side effects', the latter was aimed at 'the woman around 40 who could not cope with another pregnancy'. The types were illustrated with portraits and with longer descriptions of the personal conditions of characteristic users. A photograph in black and white depicted each woman looking into the camera with a serious face. This method of representation was reminiscent of medical cases and conveyed the notion of an objective classification of differences. At the same time, the texts and images personalized the different drug types and gave each pill an individual face.

Although physiological features played the major role in Glaxo's advertisements, they also mentioned social and psychological aspects. The description stressed, for instance, that the older woman belonged to the war generation, had raised several children and had had a hard life. This anticipated a development that had its full effect in the mid-1980s and early 1990s. The image of the individual woman as consumer of the pill became increasingly important. Her personal and psychological situation, her wishes, feelings and thoughts were, more and more, addressed in marketing materials. Emphasis on women's personalities at this time can be linked to an emphasis on women as consumers with individual wishes and demands. It also reflects a gradual change in the doctor–patient relationship, evolving from a paternalistic configuration to a more cooperative and service-oriented one, and the general turn to the increasing use of social sciences for marketing, which resulted in the establishment of consumer types.[63]

Moreover, many advertisements addressed sexuality much more explicitly and without constraining it to marriage and reproduction. An example is the German advertisement of the pill Diane. In 1979 it recommended, in relative neutrality, prescription of this drug for women with severe acne and argued primarily in favour of its therapeutic effects for this condition.[64] Here, acne appeared primarily as a physical condition. In 1994, however, an advertisement for this drug stated in the slogan that this pill was 'more than therapy against acne' because it also 'interacted with self-confidence'.[65] This was followed by a thorough and emphatic explanation of how negatively severe skin problems affected a woman's emotional and mental well-being.[66] This was illustrated by a colour photograph showing a beautiful, young, scarcely dressed woman. Lying down with her eyes closed, she appeared to be enjoying the kiss the man behind was giving her. The focus here was on the consumer's personal situation, her psychological needs and her right to have a good quality of life, including a fulfilled sex life. A specific type of user was connected to a specific pill.

Personification could also be found in French advertising for the pill Cilest,[67] though it employed a different way of standardizing women and combining pills and users. The ad introduced three women: Nicole, Brigitte and Patricia. Not only were they individualized with names, there were also photographs and reports on their personal situation, particularly on their wishes and needs. Each woman came to represent a standard. Nicole, for example, had just had a baby and wanted to continue with the pill while Brigitte wanted to change the type of pill she was using because of side effects. The proclaimed variability of women was first reduced to different categories and then satisfied with only one solution: Cilest.

The conceptualization of different sorts of women connected with elements of psychologization, and an emphasis on emotions, culminated in a typology of the psyches of teenage girls in a 1989 advertisement by Schering.[68] Illustrated with a picture and exemplified with a longer description, the advertisement presented different types of girls, for example 'Type 2: She wants what other people want' or 'Type 3: She really knows everything better'.[69] The images depicted a woman looking into the camera, again reminiscent of photography of medical cases. The same model 'played' each different woman in varying postures and wearing different clothes to suit the individual types. The advertisement stated that this typology was based on a scientific study sponsored by Schering. The emphasis in the scientific study was in fact placed more on the differences in the women taking the pill rather than on the effects of the pill itself. As a result of this classification – and therefore standardization – of women, the advertising that followed recommended prescribing the pill Femovan for each of these types. As with Nicole, Brigitte and Patricia, different categories of women were not matched with specific pill effects. In contrast to the older advertisements by Glaxo, this time the same pill was suitable for all. Psychological individuality was not only emphasized and categorized, it was also homogenized: now one pill was set as a standard for all women. The individualization and de-individualization of women were produced at the same time. This made it possible to fabricate the variation of women – but not of drugs.

The tension between standardization and the uniqueness of a product was thus resolved into a specific solution. The advertising rhetoric gave the impression of a very close fit between a category of woman and an individual pill, but it was always the same pill. The uniqueness of the pill was represented by the uniqueness of the women taking it, and simultaneously, standardization of the pill was represented by the fact that it was effective for all these different kinds of women.

Overall, while framing the pill as a standardized drug was central in the 1960s and 1970s, standardizing and categorizing the oral contraception consumer became more important in the 1980s and 1990s. The standardized woman took on two shapes: in one, she was a specific user type matching a specific pill, and in the other she was one of many different user types for whom the same one pill was recommended. Parallel to this process, the notion of the user changed. Instead of a passive patient, the ads portrayed an active consumer. Individual needs and personal situations now mattered in marketing. This process was influenced by increasing market saturation, the search for new consumer groups, more service-oriented medicine and the general growth of corporate capitalism.

Focus on the consumer's quality of life eventually became dominant in advertising. In the 1980s, the material aimed increasingly at issues such as lifestyle, leisure and happiness. This is the most noticeable trend today, while representations of standardization are less significant. Starting in the late 1990s, advertising only occasionally referred to different user types, classifications or the control and safety of a drug. Instead, there were many pictures of young women extravagantly and stylishly dressed up,[70] or of tanned and smiling people at the beach.[71]

At that time, pill prevalence remained more or less stagnant in both countries. In 1994, nearly 40 per cent of French women between twenty and forty-four years old took the pill, and in 2000 almost 46 per cent.[72] In 2004/5, the prevalence of users between fifteen and forty-nine years old stood at around 40 per cent.[73] Consequently, for the period going from when the pill was introduced to 2009, three phases can be distinguished in France: a first phase of little usage until 1970, a second phase of constant increase until the mid-1990s, and finally a third phase to the present, with a usage rate of about 40 per cent. In Germany, pill prevalence has always remained higher than in France. In 1992, almost 51 per cent of German women between fifteen and forty-five years old used the drug.[74] In 1998, prevalence of users aged between twenty and forty-four years old even reached 58 per cent.[75] In 2011, Germany was one of the countries with the highest prevalence of oral contraception, with more than half of women between eighteen and forty-nine years old taking it.[76] Two more phases have therefore to be added to the three phases of the first twenty years identified by Silies.[77] The third phase with a constant level at 30 per cent in the 1970s was followed by a fourth phase with a new increase in the 1980s and a fifth phase since the 1990s with prevalence remaining at around 50 per cent. So from the introduction of the pill until today this process can be divided into three distinct phases for France and into five phases for Germany, where with stagnation at a high level, marketing seemed to rely on establishing a brand name and concentrating on consumer satisfaction and wellbeing. A good and final example is the advertisement for the pill Leios by Wyeth.[78] There were different versions, showing for instance a woman with a snorkel and diving goggles or a woman at the hairdresser's. One image depicted a woman lying stretched out on the floor, smiling with obvious satisfaction.[79] She was surrounded by numerous shopping bags and the slogan of the advertisement was 'Was Frau will' ('what woman wants'). The bird's eye view revealed a world full of consumption opportunities; a world of which the pill was now a part.

Conclusion

Two different aspects of French and German advertising were discussed in this paper, starting first with national differences in the decades following the introduction of the pill. In Germany, the pill was marked early on as a contraceptive, whereas in France the pill was advertised for a long time as a multipurpose drug. Due to the legal situation, French advertising had to strike a balance between stressing the homogeneity of the pill with other products and subtly indicating its contraceptive properties.

Second, the paper examined representations of standardization as tools for scientific marketing. Despite the legal differences, they were similar in both countries. Two different uses of standardization were found. First, the pill was framed as a standardized drug. This played a central role in the two decades after the introduction of oral contraception, when health concerns were the focus of public debates. Here, advertisements presented standardization of a pill as one of its unique features. They notably emphasized the control of clinical uses and the standardization of pharmacological effects. Second, women taking the pill became increasingly standardized in the 1980s and 1990s. Ads mirrored this standardization but at the same time increasingly addressed the variation of consumers, whose medical, psychological and social needs were now put centre place. This development was accompanied by increasingly saturated markets and the development of consumer culture and lifestyle drugs.

In both countries, the notion of the female pill user changed according to similar patterns. While she primarily appeared as wife and mother and as a patient in need of medical advice in the early years, she was later often portrayed in a sexualized way and as a consumer with individual needs and wishes.

These similarities demonstrate not only the growing connection between developments in different Western European countries, but also that France and West Germany participated in equal measure in many post-war developments. Despite different legal and social situations, specific therapeutic cultures and diverging pill prevalence, common forces shaped the marketing in both countries. In the first two decades, these forces were new professional and administrative regulations following concerns about drug-related health hazards, as well as the women's movement and a critique of medicalization. In the next decade, increasing competition due to market saturation, the development of different types of oral contraception, more liberal gender roles and the growth of lifestyle drugs played a major role. This was accompanied by a focus on consumer satisfaction and branding in the late 1990s. The case of oral contraception might provide a broader framework for understanding different methods of scientific marketing: in general, reference to biomedical research seems to be more relevant when a new product is controversially introduced and publicly contested. In contrast, knowledge according to the findings of social and communication sciences seems to become central when stagnating sales numbers plea for the diversification of the market as to expand it further on its margins.

Overall, the pill emerged as a dynamic historical configuration, in which material and semiotic elements were deeply entangled. Depending on the context, the pill was a multipurpose drug, a safe medication, a contraceptive, a solution to individualized problems or a lifestyle drug. These configurations were the results of different power relations between multiple actors: between state administrations, regulatory agencies, feminist groups, patient organizations, practising physicians and scientific research. Nevertheless, the dominant actors were large capitalistic firms with vast financial resources and widespread definitory power through marketing.

9 MARKETING LOOPS: CLINICAL RESEARCH, CONSUMPTION OF ANTIDEPRESSANTS AND THE REORGANIZATION OF PROMOTION AT GEIGY IN THE 1960s AND 1970s

Jean-Paul Gaudillière

In the context of this volume the notion of scientific marketing has two different meanings. First, it points to the transformation of marketing into a form of science, i.e., a practice informed by the input of sciences ranging from economics and psychology to the sociology of medical practice. In other words, it is a way to underscore the rise of market research within the world of pharmacy. Second, scientific marketing highlights the systematic mobilization of biomedical sciences, primarily clinical research, for marketing purposes. This chapter addresses the emergence of this second dimension of the construction of drug markets, how it was diversified and how it was integrated into the organization of major drug companies after World War II.

The historiography of post–World War II clinical research has been best epitomized in the work of H. Marks, I. Löwy or A. Cambrosio and P. Keating, which provide a good understanding of how statistical evaluation in the form of controlled clinical trials emerged in medicine, how the tools of would-be evidence-based medicine were transformed into regulatory instruments by the US Food and Drug Administration (FDA), and how this endorsement was unevenly imparted to various fields of medicine, with cancer as the one specialty in which clinical research became such standard practice that trials became a distinctive feature of the care routine.[1] This historiography however has to a large extent left out the firms themselves as well as the issue of the links between the trial culture routine work in medical general practice and the mass consumption of drugs.

Looking at the practices of scientific marketing is a way to fill this gap, at least from the perspective of the transformation of pharmacy into a fully-fledged capitalistic industry. To qualify such a broad statement, a brief reminder will be useful of a few patterns running parallel with the transition from 'propaganda' to 'scientific marketing'. What the work of historians like S. Chauveau, V. Quirke, J. Greene, D. Tobbell, D. Carpenter and many others in the past fifteen years teaches us is that post-war reorganization of the Western world of drug making can be characterized by five main features:

- the changing scale of a market increasingly supported by new forms of benefits provided by health insurance, national or private, and thus turned into aggregated, collective spending;
- mergers or the disappearance of vast numbers of small family-run firms that had originated in pharmacies established by graduated professionals;
- the introduction into the market of whole new classes of drugs, opening the door to chemotherapy in areas that had either not at all been working with therapeutic substances (cancer) or not doing very successfully with them (tuberculosis);
- the rising importance of administrative rather than professional or industrial regulations, with, as a consequence, a significant drop in the number of specialties sold on the market in all major industrial countries; and
- the generalization of chemical-biological-clinical screening as the dominant path to drug invention, which in the eyes of most firms gave them the possibility of finding radically new active substances rather than copying, modifying and combining those included in the pharmacopoeia, therefore legitimizing massive investments in internal research infrastructures.[2]

What is less often stressed in the literature is that within thirty years this combination had radically altered the construction of drug markets and placed the search for 'innovations' centre stage. The idea here is not – as suggested by the misleading expression 'innovation society' – that research and development were becoming the determinant factor in investment choices or in the generation of economic value. The perspective is rather that the advent of pharmaceutical capitalism changed the relationship of market operations with the making of both the use value and the exchange value of drugs.[3] The core of the argument is that large post-war pharmaceutical companies, rather than anticipating development and growth on the basis of competition through prices and short-term management by taking sales data as the major if not the sole indicators, increasingly relied on monopolistic practices rooted in patent protection, competition for entire therapeutic classes and long-term planning of launches and marketing. For the purpose of this chapter, two major shifts were decisive: (a) the transformation of substance-based patents into a normal state of affairs allowing not only the control of production channels but the control of all the uses that could be envisioned for a given compound; and (b) the advent of scientific marketing as a way of shaping prescription practices and generating new medical uses.[4] In both cases, control of medical use value – both anticipated and realized – took precedence over questions of production processes and production costs, at least at the level of strategic planning and upstream market construction.

Psychotropic drugs are an ideal example for exploring how scientific marketing became a decisive part of this reorganization process. The first reason that psychochemicals are such a good case to study is the unique role such drugs played in the so-called therapeutic revolution. Even though some drugs were actually used in asylums and hospitals before the 1950s and 1960s, for instance insulin in shock therapies or barbiturates for sedation or deep sleep therapy, pharmaceuticals did not at that time appear as major tools in the psychiatrist's arsenal. This situation was radically changed with the introduction of neuroleptics and antidepressants.[5] Moreover, while general practitioners had a long tradition of using sedatives, sleeping pills, roborants and barbiturates in routine cases of nervous weakness, neurasthenia or psychosomatic symptoms, the scale of such practices changed dramatically after World War II with massive prescription of amphetamines and tranquilizers.[6] We therefore have every reason to believe that there was a complex relationship between psychotropic drugs – their invention, production and marketing – and the deep post-war transformation of clinical practices in psychiatry and more generally in mental health.

The second motive for looking at psychotropic drugs more closely is the existing historiography. The role of pharmaceutical companies in reshaping medical practices is far from being uncharted in this area. For tranquilizers and antidepressants in particular, D. Healy has articulated a powerful narrative in the case of mood disorders and depression.[7] In very crude phrasing, he argues that market and industrial interests have transformed depression from being both a symptom (a depressive state) and a narrow psychopathological category designating instances of severe mood disorder taken care of in psychiatric hospitals (classified as endogenous depression, psychogenic depression, involution depression, etc.) into a very broad and unified diagnosis calling for the prescription of antidepressants. Healy's claim of the central role of marketing practices and firms' shaping of clinical research covers two waves: the introduction of monoamine oxidase inhibitors (IMAOs) and tricyclic antidepressants in the 1960s and the introduction of serotonin recapture inhibitors (SSRIs) in the 1980s, with a strong emphasis on the latter, as this coincides with the generalization of DSM–III symptomatic criteria for the diagnosis of depression.

This scenario of an industrial and market-based redefinition of a disease category is far from impossible. What it is lacking, however, is a serious investigation: into industrial practices; into what the antidepressant-manufacturing companies actually did to change knowledge and 'create' medical use value and a new market; and into the ways in which psychiatrists and general practitioners reacted to and collaborated with these firms. The aim of this chapter is to address this issue through the lens of 'scientific marketing'. This implies shifting the focus of analysis from the profession, academic papers and debates on the classification and the aetiology of psychiatric disorders – now relatively well documented – to the industry itself and its research, management and marketing practices.

As we experienced in the course of the GEPHAMA project, the Swiss Basel-based firm Geigy, which merged with Ciba in 1971, provides a good case for such investigation. In the immediate post-war period Geigy was a relatively small firm with a strong reputation in the sales of chemicals – DDT was prominently listed in its catalogue – rather than pharmaceuticals.[8] Between the mid-1950s and the merger with Ciba, however, the firm's portfolio became increasingly linked to human medicine, and thanks to the discovery of tricyclics, Geigy became, in the 1960s, a world leader in the emerging antidepressants market.

The core hypothesis in this chapter is that during the three decades that separate the 1959 market launch of Tofranil (brand name of imipramine), which was Geigy's first psychochemical, and the quasi-termination of this line of research in the context of a new merger in 1996 between Ciba-Geigy and Sandoz, scientific marketing at Geigy took on two configurations associated, respectively, with different ways of conducting clinical research and different ways of organizing the promotion of drugs to physicians. To analyse this transition, the chapter is divided in two parts. The first focuses on the early 1960s and takes Tofranil as an example of how Geigy operated to build the antidepressants market. The second section deals with the late 1960s to early 1970s reorganization of the company within the context of its merger with Ciba and the trajectory of another antidepressant, Ludiomil, which originated in Ciba's research but became the new company's flagship psychochemical.[9]

Geigy, Tofranil and Scientific Marketing, Version One

Geigy established a special *Werbungsabteilung* (advertising department) in the late 1940s and early 1950s.[10] In the first ten years of its existence, the department gradually specialized in the manufacturing of packages and all sorts of graphic material used by the medical and sales departments (the former focusing on the firms' relationship with physicians, the latter on its relationship with pharmacists) but did not deal with questions of what was considered medical information – be it the advertising copy in medical journals or the flyers and brochures elaborated for them. Such questions and decisions remained the province of the medical department with its special *Wissenschaftliche* (scientific) *Information* section. The publicity section was thus made up of designers, drawers, packagers, movie-makers, etc ... Their work produced a unified 'Geigy' style of products, making a decisive contribution to the image of 'modernity' the firm intended to put forward.

This separation was however challenged by the expansion and professionalization of the medical representative system, which gradually emerged as a core 'segment' in the management of relationships with physicians. In the late 1950s and early 1960s, this workforce, which had not been central to the chemical model of market construction, expanded at a rapid pace.[11] Training of representatives was formalized, combining teaching of sales techniques with biomedical knowledge.[12] Its coordinators – a majority of whom were medically trained – were, for instance, from the mid-1960s onward, sent for a few weeks or months to collaborating laboratories and clinics to update their understanding and knowledge of rapidly changing medical practices.[13]

Tofranil was Geigy's first antidepressant. It originated in an attempt to find analogues of chlorpromazine, the first neuroleptic. It was designed as a compound that would help Geigy to enter the new market of hospital psychiatry. Following the research conducted by the psychiatrist R. Kuhn, who would become a long-standing associate of Geigy, Tofranil proved a weak antipsychotic but a promising treatment for hospitalized patients affected with severe depression.[14] In Kuhn's early results, severe endogenous depression occupied the first rank as putative indication.

How did Geigy's scientific marketing work in the case of Tofranil? What choices of medical targets were selected once imipramine (the name of the chemical) was redefined an antidepressant? France, Switzerland and Germany were the countries in which the 1958–62 launch campaigns were implemented, but these were all organized in Basel, targeting hospital psychiatrists and using similar if not identical brochures, flyers and letters to physicians.[15]

The campaign not only combined materials of different formats and clinical meanings (with a strong emphasis on clinical biographies and case summaries on the one hand and statements of supposedly high-profile psychiatrists on the other hand); it also played heavily on the repetition effect with regular mailing of printed materials. A good example is provided by the series of letters accompanying reprints of medical articles produced by Geigy's medical partners that were sent to Swiss clinicians in the course of 1961 and 1962. Thirteen different mailing campaigns were done with eight different articles, the topics of which included the side effects of Tofranil, depression in ambulatory psychiatry or general practice, and the usefulness of Tofranil in ageing.

The medical knowledge mobilized in this combination of materials all originated in a core group of Swiss clinical collaborators including not only Kuhn but major Swiss psychiatrists like P. Kielholz in Basel or J. Angst in Zurich. These psychiatrists provided the firm with a set of 'basic' references (articles and exemplary cases), all gathered in open research. Geigy did not commission specific inquiries into its clinical partners. Neither did it define ways of selecting patients or administration protocols. Rather, it provided pharmacological information and dosage recommendations, leaving the heads of psychiatric services to decide which diagnoses (and putative indications) were worth pursuing.[16] The exchange system was such that the firm traded supply of new promising molecules against reports of clinical cases combining summaries and a very simple form of aggregation per diagnosis with semi-quantitative evaluations of the outcomes (improved, partially improved or unchanged) and a list of problematic secondary manifestations.[17]

In terms of clinical targets, Geigy's medical department heads juxtaposed a list of (neurasthenia-like) symptoms and existing classifications (both Kuhn's and Kielholz's schemes were used) to advocate the general use of Tofranil (it improved almost all forms of depression) *and* at the same time a specific hierarchy amongst the various diagnoses, keeping endogenous depression as the most appropriate indication, as Kuhn and others had initially recommended. The campaign also followed clinical routine in advocating use of Tofranil in combination with two existing treatments – shock therapy and psychotherapy – arguing in favour of supplementing other forms of care with chemotherapy. Tofranil was thus presented as a way to lessen the burden of suffering, opening on to the possibility of conversation and interaction with the physician. In the case of electroconvulsive therapy, the argument was that Tofranil reduced the number and violence of the shocks needed for lasting improvement.[18]

Finally, Geigy tried to break away from the strong divide between hospital and ambulatory care, and between psychiatry and general practice – although in a low-key manner. The first argument, which echoed the psychiatric literature directly, was that the new antidepressant improved the situation of severely depressed patients in such a dramatic way that they could soon leave the hospitals. Ambulatory care would then become a second step in the treatment, after hospitalization, ensuring its real success. In the case of France, this perspective met with strong resonance as psychiatrists were already engaged in a search for new forms of care centred on outpatient services and a controlled return to life in the city as an alternative to long-term institutionalization.[19] The second perspective linking Tofranil and general practice is evidenced in the series of letters sent to Swiss general practitioners building on the accepted notion that old age could trigger depressive states which were initially mild but could evolve into severe involutional depression. These could be handled in general practice on the basis of long-term quasi-preventive treatment, using a specially designed low dosage form (10mg) of Tofranil.

The last feature in the trajectory of Tofranil that needs mentioning is the relation it bears to the then-booming tranquilizers market. What kind of strategy was in play? It is quite clear that Geigy soon sought out the tranquilizer market and that its leaders had been very much impressed by the rapid success of Roche's Valium in particular. Insidon was Geigy's most serious attempt to occupy this market segment. Insidon was envisioned as a hybrid molecule – a combined tranquilizer and antidepressant. The profiling of Insidon thus differed from that of Tofranil, as Geigy promoted it in parallel with the latter but for general practice only. The focus was what the medical literature called 'problem patients', namely those accounting for a significant segment of a general practitioner's clientele who would come again and again with shifting and unclear functional problems, problems deemed 'psychosomatic'. Nonetheless – as we have shown elsewhere – commercial success did not follow.[20] Insidon remained the problematic child of Geigy's management: it never reached the US market (the FDA denied it a marketing permit, presumably on the grounds that its clinical targets were too broad and too vague) while sales in Europe remained quite marginal compared with other tranquilizers in the same range as those of the much more selective Tofranil.

Table 9.1: Sales of Tofranil and Insidon in France and Germany (in millions of Swiss francs)

Year	Tofranil, France	Tofranil, Germany	Insidon, France	Insidon, Germany
1959	3.2	0.9	—	—
1960	5.13	1.95	—	—
1961	5.3	2.33	—	—
1962	?	?	?	?
1963	5.2	2.0	5.0	?
1964	4.8	1.81	4.62	1.86
1965	6.7	1.86	4.8	3.65

Source: Data computed on the basis of PP1 A. Produktion Pharma Geigy Pharmaka. Jahresbericht 1947–1959/1962–1966 and PP 130–1 – PHARMA – Jahresberichte der Pharmazeutischen Abteilung, 1960–1968, GAB.

1966: Reorganizing and Standardizing Clinical Research

At Geigy, the second half of the 1960s was dominated by a process of internal reorganization focused on the question of clinical research. By 1966, management had launched a major reshuffling of the medical department, the main objective of which was to introduce formalized and statistics-based clinical trials. The origins of this move are partly to be traced back to the changing role of the FDA and the difficult experience Geigy had already had with the US agency regarding its new requirements for toxicity assessment and controlled efficacy trials (the Insidon case remained somewhat of a traumatic experience). Other motivations were more internal, originating in both the changing scale of clinical collaborations (already visible in the Tofranil campaigns) and in a slowly emerging management culture that was following the same general patterns in the pharmaceutical sector promoting strategic planning and standardized criteria for decision making.

The organizational scheme proposed in 1966 thus consisted in separating the medical department into one unit focusing on preclinical studies as well as small-scale, more or less open, investigations, and a second unit (Medizin II) in charge of what the FDA had started to label Phase II and Phase III trials.[21] The aim was to terminate the perceived chaos of trials authorized and supported by each doctor in the department and produce an integrated organization that would allow an overall management of screening, from the early stages of selecting chemicals to market launch decisions. The trials were thus redefined as the basic planning units. They had to be approved by the heads of the department and based on explicit questions and protocols that could deliver information associated with each stage in the formal decision making tree that had been developed by the new department heads. To foster coherence of action, a central catalogue was produced of all trials, listing titles, targets and answers to a series of standard questions (regarding effects, tolerability, side effects, dosage, metabolism, associations and relations to other therapeutic interventions).

Intended for gradual implementation in the late 1960s, the scheme was also designed as a critical tool to advance international collaboration, enabling the circulation of data between Geigy's national representations or subsidiaries (starting with those in the United Kingdom and in the United States) so as to ease the registration processes. The reorganization was also viewed as an element of convergence with Ciba as talks about a merger progressed rapidly after 1969.

Relationships with clinicians then took a different turn. Although Medizin I kept the network of open trials alive, maintaining the possibility for elite psychiatrists like Kuhn or Kielholz to work with very new compounds in whatever way they liked, Medizin II took over the development of standardized protocols for multicentre collaborative studies.[22] In the case of psychotropic drugs, however, such protocols faced many problems: the absence of accepted biological markers or endpoints for mental disorders, the heterogeneity of local practices and the multiplicity of classification schemes. Beyond just writing up agreements with physicians regarding the choice of patients, the nature of control groups, the dosage of drugs and their administration patterns, Geigy's management therefore increasingly emphasized the need for homogeneous forms of evaluation and reporting. The perspective was to move into a state of affairs such that trial data should be coded to permit computer-based statistical analyses. It was within this configuration that in-house physicians started to advocate the use of psychometric scales based on semi-quantitative rating of symptoms, behaviour and psychic manifestations like the nomenclature of psychiatric diagnostic criteria developed by Heidelberg's clinicians, which provided the background for Geigy's electronic processing of data.[23] In the case of depression this meant importing Hamilton's recently developed rating scale, the features of which were incorporated into the design of trials, at least those planned to involve multiple investigators and centres, and contributed to focusing attention on the measurement of symptoms rather than on the assessment of the origins and aetiology of disorders.[24]

Although most of the changes of the late 1960s focused on clinical research, the reorganization did not leave marketing untouched. The main institutional innovation was an expansion of the market research section. Its tasks were very broadly defined including the entire spectrum of medical, economic and sociological questions centred on the monitoring and analysis of prescription patterns. The targets of marketing research would thus include:

- the pharmaceutical products themselves (chemistry, pharmacology, clinical use, presentation, packaging and prices);
- the treatments (means of medical education, practices, sources of authority, and temporal and geographical differences);
- the diseases (incidence, seriousness, course, therapeutic options, economic and social impact, geographical differences, climate, and ethnology and civilization)
- the social and economic factors (influence of the global economic context and of general social changes on drug consumption and influence of the insurance system and of regulations);
- the physicians (relationship to patients, authority, training, on-going education, sources of information, specialization, age, professional and social status, nature and size of their clientele, and attitudes to pharmaceutical firms and their products);
- the patients (their influence on prescription, their medical knowledge, general opinion on medical questions, acceptance of treatments and compliance);
- the firms (market shares, product lines, new market introductions, withdrawals, prestige and cartel policies);
- the propaganda (market structure and dynamics); and
- the sales.[25]

Before this encompassing programme of medicine and prescription studies took on any practical meaning, Geigy had resorted to purchasing information generated outside the firm by specialized agencies. In spite of the cost, which was deemed very high, management had decided to subscribe to the monthly information on pharmaceutical sales in Germany that Intercontinental Marketing Services (IMS), a US-based private consulting agency, had started to produce and sell. Given its importance, the psychotropic drug market was also estimated to be worth making specific marketing and research investments. Following the Insidon debacle in the United States, Basel joined with Geigy-Ardsley, its US subsidiary, to commission a specific survey of the entire American market for psychochemicals.[26]

The first outcome of these initiatives was an internal reassessment of the relationship between tranquilizers and antidepressants. Management then endorsed the idea that to surpass the success of Tofranil and ensure future growth, the objective was to lessen the divide between the tranquilizer and antidepressant niches. Given the strength of Roche products and the failure of direct competition with profiled tranquilizers like Insidon, such blurring would best be achieved through the invention of an antidepressant targeting the mild mental complaints encountered in general practice:

> a) From a commercial perspective, the interesting preparations are those used in a great number of mild cases (like Librium). Viewed from the market, the difference between tranquilizers and antidepressants plays no role, contrary to what we have been inclined to think internally ... b) For the time being, tranquilizers (starting with Librium and its analogues) are the most widely used specialties for handling the most frequent, mild mental and psychosomatic disorders ... There is a very large potential market for an efficient, non-toxic and popular antidepressant (a sort of 'first efficient tonic'); c) in contrast, the market for psychopharmaceuticals against psychosis has already reached its ceiling.[27]

Ciba-Geigy and Scientific Marketing, Version Two

A proper analysis remains to be done of the organizational changes that the merger between Geigy and Ciba brought about in the late 1960s and early 1970s. In the context of this chapter, suffice it to point out two features regarding the blending of clinical research and marketing. This blending was not circumstantial. It should be viewed as a direct consequence of the simultaneous expansion of scientific marketing and the internalization of the organization of clinical trials. The former resulted in new, market-driven demands for specific research while the latter provided new opportunities to control, transfer and mobilize data. Circulation between clinical research and marketing thus started to operate at two levels: that of daily promotion and campaign running with the selection of clinical data and its shaping and transformation into promotional material; and that of long-term planning, selection of market segments and specific requests for new trials and/or product development.

The first series of changes fostering this blending of clinical research and promotion was a new mode of production and circulation of information, which originated in the fact that the product lines of the two firms were not merged but juxtaposed. Ciba's medical representatives remained in charge of Ciba products already on the market while Geigy's medical representatives kept promoting those from the Geigy line.[28] New products would be distributed according to their origins in the research infrastructure. Coordination was therefore deemed essential and specialized committees were set up at several levels to insure minimum commonality of decision.

At the top level, weekly meetings of a 'working group for medical-pharmaceutical information' (*Arbeitsgruppe pharmazeutische-medizinische Information*) gathered the heads of both the clinical and marketing departments to discuss products already on the market as well as the future of those in the clinical trial pipeline. The memos of these meetings were circulated at all upper levels of management. These documents summarized major decisions regarding the surveillance of sales, the production of publicity material (the major tools of which were printed brochures and books on the one hand, and films on the other), the organization of campaigns and the outcome of prioritized trials.

Medical marketing information was actually given such priority that an entire 'product management information' section was set up to coordinate the follow-up of trials and the preparation of product-oriented material for medical representatives. The section was placed under the authority of a physician and a pharmacist. It was responsible for writing the bulletin and the information sheets for the sales force. Paralleled with intensified product-based training sessions, the role of these new tools was evidently to provide standard arguments and data to be used during the visits paid to physicians, but it was also to foster convergence of the two networks of representatives.

A second significant change was the reinforced planning of research activities. A good marker of this tendency is the yearly organization of research conferences gathering the upper management of the marketing, biology *and* clinical research departments from Ciba-Geigy-Basel on the one hand and their counterparts in the firm's US subsidiaries. These yearly meetings were general assessments of research perspectives with position papers reviewing all areas and products lines, i.e., central nervous system psychochemicals, and cardiovascular, metabolism, chemotherapy (antibacterial, anti-virus and cancer), anti-inflammatory and anti-allergic drugs. To facilitate discussion, specific sheets were prepared summarizing the status of all compounds that had been granted some clinical value, i.e., that were already on the market, in clinical trials, or on the verge of crossing the frontier from preclinical to clinical studies.

Biological research took on unprecedented importance in these evaluations. The stabilization of an in-house screening system for psychotropic drugs based on a battery of animal tests was mobilized in two different ways. As Lucie Gerber shows in this volume, the first was to reinforce an approach of putative clinical value focusing on symptoms like fatigue, sleeplessness, anxiety or vegetative manifestations rather than disease categories, mobilizing analogues of these target symptoms in animal tests. The second, as exemplified in the summary sheet on C49802 – a promising compound from the Ciba pipeline – was the search for biochemical endpoints, in this case the combination of assays for the inhibition of noradrenalin and serotonin reuptake.[29]

Products sheets and position papers only provided the in-house research background for planning purposes. Market studies, starting with sales data and documentation on competing firms' positions, were the second line of documentation on which 'strategic' coordination and long-term investments were to be decided. General outcomes of the research conferences were therefore on the one hand short-term actions regarding the fate of products under development (for instance, which trials would be included in a new drug marketing application submitted to the FDA) and general investigation priorities.

The 1973 conference for instance estimated that, in the central nervous area, antidepressants remained a high priority both in the United States and in Europe while tranquilizers, despite their massive importance in global sales, should rank second.[30] Ranking and planning was thus shifted in the direction of product classes and lines viewed as providing similar market opportunities. The 1975 conference estimated that the antidepressants niche could still grow and that the above-mentioned C49802 should be prepared as a follower of Ludiomil, the new antidepressant Ciba-Geigy had just introduced in the market, with 1982 as a possible date of registration.[31] A couple of years later, tranquilizers had further regressed to third-rank priority in Europe, replaced by research on drugs targeting the mental conditions related to ageing.

The Research and Marketing Blend in Practice: Ludiomil as a Broad Antidepressant

How did the reorganized scientific marketing work in practice? The launch of Ludiomil is well documented in the Ciba-Geigy archives and provides a good example of the strong interplay between clinical research and promotion.

Ludiomil originated in Ciba research. Its preclinical trajectory was comparable to that of Tofranil since it had also been synthesized as an analogue of chlorpromazine. Its transformation into an antidepressant was however a product of the merger between Ciba and Geigy since: (a) its antidepressant properties were consolidated within the Geigy animal screening system; (b) C34276 (then not yet Ludiomil) was passed on to Geigy's core set of Swiss psychiatrists in 1970; and (c) in 1971, when its marketing was decided, Switzerland was chosen as the first target country given that Geigy had solid experience in negotiating with Swiss registration authorities.

As discussed in the protocols of the working group for medical-pharmaceutical information, the 1972 Swiss launch was a three-phase process mimicking the clinical research pipeline organization, with psychiatrists targeted in the first phase and general practitioners in the second.[32]. In practice, there were actually three steps. The first was a general 'orientation' during which all Swiss doctors were made aware of the existence of Ludiomil by means of a letter describing its properties as making a difference with other antidepressants (Tofranil and its follower Anafranil), namely owing to its broad spectrum of action (Ludiomil showed action on both mood and anxiety) and its reduced adverse effects. The letter was accompanied with a Ludiomil leaflet and a sample.

During the second phase, all Swiss psychiatrists and neurologists as well as a selected group of general practitioners listed for their interest in psychiatry (1,800 physicians in all) received a visit from a medical representative mentioning Ludiomil and presenting brief material on its spectrum of action. This was followed by a 'personal' rather than mimeographed letter that did not present conventional advertising material but a research volume, i.e., the proceedings of a special symposium on 'Depressive States – Diagnosis, Evaluation and Treatment' that Ciba-Geigy had organized the previous year in St Moritz, gathering not only its core network of psychiatrist collaborators but specialists from France, Spain, the UK and the US. The volume juxtaposed papers on the classification, rating and general treatment of depression with papers on the pharmacology and early trials of Ludiomil.[33] Mailing of the volume was followed within less than six months by three letters containing specific flyers on the trials. Finally, psychiatrists received six supplementary 'reminder' information sheets.

The last phase, in the direction of 8,000 general practitioners, was no less oriented towards clinical research. They not only received conventional flyers – ten in less than six months – but also the volume on the symposium (40,000 copies of the book were distributed, including the later English translation) and one brochure, the title of which was 'Man's Psychopathological Manifestations'. In addition, six inserts were placed in Swiss general medical journals.

Emphasis was thus placed on research data and on mobilizing 'opinion leaders', i.e., not only psychiatrists but also general practitioners with some reputation in the treatment of patients with mental disorders. The flyers did not summarize a specific case or picture indications and advantages, as had been the case with Tofranil. Instead, each element of the Ludiomil series presented the results of a clinical trial.

The third flyer that was circulated, for instance, did not simply put physicians' records in a new format; it presented aggregated data directly produced by the Ciba-Geigy medical department and its information management system. The flyer summarized a paper that the medical personnel had presented at the St Moritz symposium based on the statistical treatment of the first 238 case report sheets that the firm had received from thirteen trials (still on-going at the time of presentation), including three in Brazil, two in Switzerland, two in Germany, one in France, one in Austria, one in Spain, one in the UK, one in Italy and one in the Netherlands.[34] These trials had been designed to respond to marketing rather than regulatory concerns as they were all comparative assays with control groups treated with either Tofranil or amitriptyline (marketed by Merck Sharp & Dohme under the name Elavil), the latter considered as the direct competitor of Ludiomil. The paper itself included two types of data: a qualitative comparison of the three groups in terms of effects on a series of 'target symptoms' belonging to the core set of depression (sleeplessness, inhibition, agitation, depressive mood, feeling of oppression and reduced work ability); a quantitative rating of the action of Ludiomil on the sixteen items of the Hamilton scale. Only the table summarizing the latter was included in the flyer. This table actually became such an icon of Ludiomil marketing that it was reproduced in dozens of mailed documents all through the 1970s.

This intimate joint management of clinical trials and promotion did not rely on the work of specialists. In contrast to what had been done with Tofranil, the clinical research on Ludiomil mobilized, very early on, general practitioners belonging to the 'interested' group of general practitioners Ciba-Geigy had selected on the basis of the previous Insidon campaigns. This early involvement of general practitioners in clinical research was a major innovation as it did not represent a form of Phase IV trial, but rather blurred the separations between phases, bringing into the pre-marketing phase the question of routine use and final prescribers. With this new practice, the clinical research department acknowledged the specificities of general practice both as a commercial segment and as an autonomous form of medical practice. On the one hand, these trials were a sort of 'seeding' operation that blurred the distinction between the circulation of molecules for research and the distribution of samples. On the other hand, because Ciba-Geigy considered hospital psychiatry to be a closed world in terms both of patient selection and of evaluation criteria, the inclusion of general practitioners was deemed essential to gather information on 'real practice' conditions. At stake was psychiatrists' fascination with the design of local classification schemes and the search for etiological rather than symptomatic categories.

Such marketing of clinical trials may be viewed as selective dissemination of simplified research results, leaving the impression that the clinical use value of Ludiomil was chiefly established in discussions between psychiatrist opinion leaders and Ciba-Geigy's clinical-research managers while the market value of Ludiomil emerged in a second step out of the intricate combination of promotion and actual prescription (documented both in the trials including general practitioners and in the monthly follow-up of Ludiomil sales). As illustrated in the information material prepared for the representatives, the role of general practice research was however more than just application and follow-up. The memo circulated in April 1973 for instance included a detailed description of one of the two Swiss clinical trials. The memo was aimed at training the representatives and was designed as in-house information rather than for external use.[35] The trial had already included 1,400 patients and compared Ludiomil with Pfizer's doxepin (trade name Sinequan) according to two different protocols. The first group of physicians (seventeen psychiatrists and seventy-five non-psychiatrists), called 'within doctors', conducted a non-blind but randomized assay of Doxepin and two dosages of Ludiomil. The second group (thirty-six psychiatrists, 114 non-psychiatrists), called 'in between doctors', conducted an open trial of one preparation only, which could be any of the three. Efficacy results were requested in the form of a simplified semi-quantitative rating taking five symptoms into consideration: depressive mood, inhibition, anxiety, agitation and sleep disorders. More detailed information regarding adverse reactions had however been demanded by marketing.

Market-Based Knowledge: Promoting 'Larved' Depression

Scientific marketing, version two, was therefore much more than just publicizing selected clinical results originating in the controlled work of Ciba-Geigy's medical partners. It also meant the active shaping of prescription patterns based on the production of market-based and market-oriented knowledge. This had already been evidenced with the shift from etiological to symptomatic categories that had accompanied the marketing of Insidon.

Where the trajectory of Ludiomil is considered, the point is however best illustrated with another shifting of targets, this time to the promotion of disease categories in addition to the marketing of products with their cortege of specific indications. This move stemmed from the new organizational structure blending clinical research and marketing in two different ways. The first was the previously mentioned rise of long-term planning in the organization and increased reasoning in terms of therapeutic classes, which resulted in Ciba-Geigy's repositioning antidepressants in general practice in addition to psychiatry and hospital care. In the eyes of management, promoting an antidepressant that could occupy the tranquilizer segment did not only mean stressing new properties marking a difference with Tofranil and first-generation antidepressants – for instance milder side-effects or quicker therapeutic action – it also implied changing the meaning of 'antidepressant' to address an enlarged series of symptoms including such symptoms as anxiety or sleeplessness, which were not necessarily included in the clinical tableau of severe (endogenous) depression. The second connection resides in the loops between clinical research and marketing made possible by the new organization. Such loops worked both ways. Clinical research and its results obviously shaped marketing practices as it constrained the range and content of advertising. The in-house government of trials however opened the possibility of another loop through which marketing demands would be turned into new research, documentation and information/promotion material. This is precisely what was at stake with Ciba-Geigy's reinvention of 'larved' or 'masked' depression.

The category was not entirely new. Larved depression was occasionally mentioned by psychiatrists in the early 1960s and the category had actually surfaced in the early Tofranil campaign. Before its merger with Ciba, however, Geigy had mentioned it only in the context of the French market. The choice may be interpreted on the basis of sales results (Table 9.1), namely as an attempt to capitalize on the relative success of Tofranil amongst French physicians. In comparison, German sales amounted to only one-third of French sales, and were almost exclusively associated with hospital prescription and severe depression.

The meaning the medical department attributed to 'larved depression' was clearly shown in the first brochure that it circulated starting in 1963 under the title 'Dépression larvée – Troubles fonctionnels sans support organique' (Larved depression – Functional disorders with no organic basis).[36] Larved depression was presented here as a disorder typical of patients presenting various, often shifting, organic complains for which no clear diagnosis could be stabilized. Such patients also fell under the 'psychosomatic' label. Geigy linked such situations with depression through the argument that these patients were suffering from 'larved depression': depression with somatic projections or somatic manifestations. Tofranil could help doctors and patients face these problematic conditions. The clinical cases used in the brochure to illustrate the existence of 'larved depression' had all been selected from the psychiatric literature on Tofranil. Interestingly enough, even though the authors insisted on the somatic component of these cases, the patients had all been diagnosed and presented differently, i.e., as suffering from anorexia, endogenous depression, organic depression or hypochondria.

The brochure, as well as the few flyers, sent to French physicians strongly suggest that the aim of this sub-campaign was less to isolate a new category than to link Tofranil with a specific realm of practice: that of psychosomatic medicine.[37] Building on general practitioners' interest in sorting out 'true' organic disorders, the material on larved depression did not offer a new classification of depression but provided physicians with a minimal entry point for suspecting a depressive *state*, listing core bodily symptoms unrelated to the conventional depressive complex, i.e., fatigue, weakness, exhaustion, pains and loss of weight. The idea of a psychopathological specificity seemed far from the considerations of Geigy's medical experts. As the firm's literature explained, given the complexity of the manifestations of larved depression, the issue was not to establish a proper diagnosis but to achieve a pre-selection of patients for whom a prescription might be suited and to then take the success of the Tofranil treatment as confirmation of the condition. In contrast to other brochures, which insisted on the selective efficacy of Tofranil on mood and on the thymic system as an explanation of its specific value in depression, here Tofranil was granted *double* efficacy: both on mental and *somatic* symptoms.

This attempt was however short lived. Larved depression soon disappeared from the marketing of Geigy's antidepressants. When Anafranil, heir to Tofranil, was launched in 1967, the 'larved' category did not surface.[38] Another element is the atypical structure of the French antidepressants market (on this, more below). Extension of the market outside core psychiatry was pursued in another way, namely through the idea of the preventive action of antidepressants. Anafranil in small dosage could help general practitioners control the early manifestations of depression and therefore avoid the evolution of the disease into a severe disorder for which hospitalization would become necessary.[39] Larved depression was also absent from the material produced during the first phases of the Ludiomil launch. There was for instance one single paper discussing it included in the 1972 St Moritz symposium and in the Ludiomil book that came out of it.[40]

Rather than reflecting a professional change, the return and massive use of larved depression in the early 1970s should be viewed as a marketing choice, a choice grounded in the new set of practices associated with scientific marketing, version two. For example, in July 1974, in the context of preparing a new Ludiomil campaign in Germany, the medical representative information material bringing in larved depression as an indication stated quite clearly:

> Previous key-point in the praxis: 'psychovegetative disorders' indication
>
> New key-point in the praxis: 'larved depression' indication
>
> Rationale: The 'larved depression' indication is a more adequate description of Ludiomil as a general-practice-oriented antidepressant than the 'psychovegetative disorders' tranquilizer label
>
> Argument: When promoting Ludiomil in physicians' practice we repeatedly stumble on the competition of tranquilizers. ... The results conveyed by our cartel partner in Germany suggest that the choice made during the first marketing phase, which was to profile Ludiomil as a small-dosage psychochemical with as main indication 'psychovegetative disorders' actually allowed entry on the market but one cannot speak of a breakthrough in any sense of the term. Making this equivalence between Ludiomil and tranquilizers ... be it at the profile level or at the indications level – is not the right way. The practitioner must be convinced through our explanation campaigns that an antidepressant (like Ludiomil) is not an alternative to a tranquilizer and that, in parallel, tranquilizers are not an alternative for the treatment of depressed patients, including patients with larved depression.[41]

This new profiling of Ludiomil as an antidepressant with anxiolytic properties especially designed for the treatment of mild/larved depression in general practice had actually started in 1973 with the organization of a second symposium at St Moritz, the entire purpose of which was to discuss the category.[42] As discussed elsewhere, resurrecting larved depression was to some extent a reaction to the mounting visibility and discussion of depression in general practice; a change supported both by psychiatrists' epidemiological considerations and by some general practitioners' specific interest in mental health issues.[43] In the latter case, the psychosomatic boundary was linked to the value and specificity of general practice in its ability to consider the patient as a whole rather than as a collection of specialized organs or systems.

Ciba-Geigy's endorsement of larved depression was, however, not just a reaction, but a proactive move. The firm actively shaped the category. Ciba-Geigy's interactions with what would later be called 'key opinion leaders', its organization of research and its production of medical literature gave the term a specific *diagnostic* value associated with *prescription standards*. Larved or masked depression thus signified a new step, this time unequivocally rooted in scientific marketing, in the direction of a new form of depression, i.e., a unified and widespread disease to be treated in general practice with antidepressants.

This stabilization of larved depression as a diagnostic category and indication may be illustrated with the proceedings of Ciba-Geigy's 1973 symposium and how they were used. Organized by Kielholz and the clinical research department, the meeting presented highly contrasted understandings and definitions. The participants mostly discussed the putative etiology of larved/masked depression, its relations to hypochondria and vitalization, its role in what were considered mere facts, i.e., the rising incidence of depressive disorders in general practice and their manifestation through a combination of mental and somatic symptoms. Angst was the most eloquent advocate of the importance of larved depression, arguing that the core classification of depression had been worked out with hospital patients who were no longer representative of the target population.[44] Moreover, the conventional definition originating in the tableau of endogenous depression with its cortege of guilt and suicidal tendencies might be an artefact linked to Western Christian culture, while somatic expression might be the general rule. Viewed from this cross-cultural standpoint, Angst's conclusion was that practice did not only need to recognize the importance of somatic symptoms but also, and more radically, to 'move conventional depression to the periphery', giving up terms like 'somatization' and accepting that what was called 'masked' or 'larved' depression might well be the core element of depressive states.

During the symposium, Ciba-Geigy medical experts presented the results of an inquiry the firm had conducted with the Swiss psychiatrist W. Poldinger amongst psychiatry specialists in order to document their views on 'masked or larved depression'. A majority of them (5,000 questionnaires had been sent in Switzerland, Germany and Austria, and 1,162 had been sent back completed) explained that they rarely used the term, that it was understood as signalling cases in which somatic symptoms dominated and anxiety appeared more strongly than depressed mood. Such cases were taken as peculiar forms of endogenous depression.

In spite of their heterogeneous views on etiology, nosology and treatment, all participants endorsed the term and agreed that the problem was of great importance in routine mental health. Accordingly, during the final discussion, it became clear that the complexity of the relationship of the 'mask', i.e., the somatic manifestations, with the various types of depression should not preclude using a category that cut through the existing classifications. Kielholz then summarized the general feeling in one of his comments: 'You would therefore give up the qualification 'endogenous' or 'psychogenic' and use the concept of larved depression for all depressive states in which the somatic symptoms come to the fore? I can say that I completely agree with this meaning'.[45] Although uneven, the collective endorsement of larved/masked depression thus provided Ciba-Geigy with a St Moritz-based propaganda volume in all points analogous to that edited by Kielholz in 1972. This volume became an integral part of the Ludiomil campaigns and was widely circulated in Germany, Switzerland and Austria (more than 18,000 copies in all).[46]

Ciba-Geigy's management then decided to organize another symposium as a complement to the 1973 event. In 1974, the third St Moritz meeting gathered an almost identical group of specialists to discuss depression in general practice, thus addressing both diagnosis and therapeutic responses. The clinical and marketing departments' own contributions again focused on the category, this time taken in the broader context of mental health in daily practice with a survey that the firm had conducted in Austria, France, Germany and Switzerland. W. Pöldinger's presentation of the survey results strongly emphasized their convergence, which merely confirmed the larved-depression model, documenting the treatment pattern Ciba-Geigy expected. An impressive number of physicians ascribed mental health problems to their patients: up to 40 per cent claimed that more than half of the visiting population suffered such troubles. Moreover, 5 to 10 per cent of general practice patients were allegedly affected with 'larved depression'. Finally, 80 to 90 per cent of the respondents were convinced that these numbers were growing.[47] General practitioners generally handled depressed patients themselves. They treated them with prescriptions combining antidepressants and other psychotropic drugs, amongst which tranquilizers were claimed to be those most often used. Treatment was not usually prolonged until full disappearance of the symptoms. The one single strong discrepancy with the model was the significance of etiology, which was mentioned as important and taken into account by two out of three general practitioners. This went largely unnoticed.

It should be added that the inquiry also revealed strong national differences (especially regarding the situation in France) but these were only superficially addressed. What were deemed important were the commonalities that could be used in the education of general practitioners. At the end, Kielholz provided a summary indicating that Ciba-Geigy's marketing soon turned into a series of flyers recapping the salient points of the symposium. Circulated amongst both German- and French-speaking practitioners, the flyers included titles such as 'Frequency and Rise in Psychiatric Disorders in Daily Practice', 'Treatment of Depression in Switzerland from a Statistical Viewpoint', 'Length and Termination of Depression Treatment', 'Choice and Use of Psychotropic Drugs' and 'Diagnosis and Differentiation of Depressive Disorders'.[48]

The second dimension of Ciba-Geigy's construction of larved depression was its specific linkage with Ludiomil. In March 1975 the Ludiomil 'product information for marketing' thus explained:

> The time is ripe to replace this pseudo-therapy of depressive states through targeted actions. Since it is much easier to link the new perspectives offered by larved depression with a new rather than old product, we shall focus the treatment of this indication with Ludiomil.[49]

New marketing operations were to include both general education of physicians on the category and specific marketing of antidepressants:

> General measures: Competent specialists in psychiatry (St Moritz symposium) are determined to put in their authority. They are ready to engage in – and take charge of – the continued education of their colleagues in the field of depression (diagnosis and therapy). This perspective may be supported with the organization of educational workshops, regional meetings for physicians, closer contacts between psychiatrists and general practitioners, with the writing of 'post-graduate' material, with a stronger participation of general practitioners in psychiatry conferences, with the conduct of surveys like that presented in St Moritz. ...
>
> Marketing concept: In the end, the issue is to convince the physician that the prescription of tranquilizers in case of depressive disorder is actually a medical failure. Beyond that, we need to offer the physician help in diagnosis, which can take the form of three questions he should ask his patient and if the replies are positive should bring in the suspicion that a case of larved depression may be at hand.[50]

The material created for the late 1970s campaigns thus focused on diagnosis proper with numerous series of Ludiomil flyers insisting on the masked dimension of depression. The series, entitled 'Derrière la façade', 'Dass man daran denkt' and 'La dépression larvée dans la pratique courante', all included product information and diagnostic aids focusing on a short list of elementary questions for the patient: 'Are you sleeping well? Are you still able to enjoy yourself, to find pleasure in the little things in life? Are you still interested in things? Are you still enterprising?'[51]

The feedback of this renewed campaign into in-house research was not massive but nonetheless worth noticing. Demands for new clinical trials of Ludiomil coming from the marketing department included studies of Ludiomil efficacy in the treatment of larved depression and psychosomatic symptoms in depressive states, a comparison with the efficacy of tranquilizers and, again, trials of overall efficacy in general practice.[52] By the late 1970s, however, only three trials specifically targeting larved/masked depression had been conducted, all of them in Germany. As the 1977 research conference explained: 'Little interest was expressed by different countries for masked depression. Germany was very active in the indication "psychovegetative syndrome" and the ND 7 trial of Ludiomil compared with Limbatril was completed for 899 patients'. It added that Ludiomil did not show any difference in efficacy.[53].

This brings up the question of the final status of masked/larved depression. It is difficult to evaluate the commercial impact of all these activities. If only use of the category is considered, then it remained limited to the German-speaking area. The marketing material developed for France barely used it, thus confirming the early emphasis Ciba-Geigy officials had placed on the favourable ground provided by the German category of psychovegetative disorders as well as the less pressing need for such a category in the French context, where antidepressants had penetrated general practice more easily.[54]

More quantitative evaluation is provided by the IMS Health data on the pharmaceutics market in West Germany, confirming that in the late 1970s consumption of antidepressants began to grow at a faster pace – even though it remained much weaker – than that of tranquilizers.[55] Moreover, Ludiomil soon became the second most prescribed antidepressant in the country while the sales of Tofranil remained stable, presumably associated with severe endogenous depression and hospital consumption.

Considering, however, the general significance of larved/masked depression for the construction of the antidepressant market, i.e., its value as way of redefining depression for general practice and transforming antidepressants into acceptable treatment for a vast population of patients complaining of organic as well as mental problems, then the situation looks different. Larved depression was part of a more general process that did not only take place in German-speaking countries. In France as well, Geigy's scientific marketing paved the way for symptom-based, unified and general practice–oriented depression, even if in the former case its vehicle was less Ludiomil than Anafranil.

Conclusion

What is then to be drawn from these two trajectories? Building on them, the two phases that characterize pharmaceutical marketing at Geigy and Ciba-Geigy may be compared by using a grid linking organization, products, targets and tools.

Table 9.2: The two modalities of scientific marketing at Ciba-Geigy

	Scientific marketing 1 (1960–70)	Scientific marketing 2 (1971–96)
Organization	Publicity + pharmaceutical + medical departments	Marketing + clinical research departments
Main psychochemicals	Tofranil, Pertofran, Insidon Antidepressant + tranquilizers	Anafranil, Ludiomil Antidepressants
Targets	Sales, surveillance of competing products Indications defined for each molecule/brand	Information management and planning Market research and surveillance of prescription Planning of product classes On-going education of doctors
Tools	Open clinical trials Printed material (integrated advertising) Trained medical representatives	Coordination committees + marketing information sheets Phased standard trials Promotional campaigns on products and medical categories Key opinion leaders

Beyond the obvious role played by science-based promotion in building the market for first-generation antidepressants and what may therefore be viewed as an industrial making of the new depression, this grid gives some support to the idea that the birth of scientific marketing was a decades-long process, possibly initiated before World War II, coming into its full shape in the 1970s. The most salient feature in this respect is neither the existence of a more or less diversified body of announcements and company literature mobilizing research results and targeting prescribing physicians, nor the existence of a specifically trained sales force paying regular visits to practitioners. It is rather the blending of research and marketing activities, which started in many firms in the 1960s when they, like Geigy, began to reorganize and expand their activities in clinical research, taking control of trial organization and spreading the norm of standardized and controlled experimentation. This development took place partly in response to regulatory incentives first implemented in the United States but more fundamentally in the context of a rapidly growing market. This in turn made possible a unique juncture with equally booming marketing activities, which provided the core infrastructure of scientific marketing, version two.

This blending of clinical research and marketing should not be underestimated. It bears methodological, historiographical and normative meanings.

First, it underlies the intimate relationship between the creation of use value and that of exchange value in the making of economic goods. This relationship is not specific to the construction of drug markets, but in this sector it took distinctive and highly integrated forms well exemplified in the double meaning of scientific marketing mentioned in the introduction to this chapter.

Second, the blending of clinical research and marketing reveals a major factor in the generalization of the screening model in drug innovation. Screening as a general model for drug innovation does not only mean the specific combination of chemical synthesis and pharmacological testing in animal models that emerged during the 1930s in companies like Bayer, which built its pharmaceutical expertise on a chemistry-based research infrastructure. Screening also includes later steps in the research-and-development (R&D) pipeline that were stabilized in the post-war period, i.e., phase-based clinical trials and scientific marketing campaigns. The inclusion of the latter in firms' general planning through the linear organization of in-house R&D attested in the case of Ciba-Geigy might well be a major explanation for the post-war generalization of screening, a process that otherwise remains mysterious given the multiple and local routes leading to the invention of new drugs.

Third, this close integration of clinical research and marketing in pharmaceutical companies has had major consequences on the ways in which we assess the value of drugs and control their circulation. The dominant way of regulating drugs in the second half of the twentieth century is often considered to be state-based administrative regulation, which replaced the professional order of pharmacy.[56] The generalization of screening has however created a situation such that industrial entrepreneurs are the providers of most, if not all, clinical data on which administrative regulations are supposed to be developed. The intimate connections this production of medical data has had, and maintains, with scientific marketing testify powerfully to the industrial and market-based nature of contemporary drug regulation. In a more normative perspective, the birth of scientific marketing points to the historical roots, and the contingency, of what is an often-criticized situation of the almost inevitable conflict of interests currently seeming to plague the world of pharmacy.

10 MARKETING LOOPS: THE DEVELOPMENT OF PSYCHOPHARMACOLOGICAL SCREENING AT GEIGY IN THE 1960s AND 1970s

Lucie Gerber

It takes a great many guinea pigs, laid end to end, to show us the mechanisms of human comedy and tragedy.[1]

In the 1950s a range of new psychotropic drugs gradually gained entrance into clinical practice, profoundly renewing the existing psychiatric armamentarium.[2] Chlorpromazine hit the French market in 1952 under the trade name Largatil. On its adoption by the psychiatric milieu, the drug became the first chemotherapy considered 'specific' for the treatment of psychoses, carving out the therapeutic class of neuroleptics.[3] Soon after, in 1955, Miltown (meprobamate) hit the American market. The drug rapidly gathered very favourable reception for the treatment of anxiety disorders and it is considered today as having originated the therapeutic class of mild tranquilizers.[4] In 1957, the American psychiatrist N.S. Kline and his colleagues communicated on the energizing properties of iproniazid (Marsilid), a compound initially tested for the treatment of tuberculosis, on patients suffering from mild depressive symptoms.[5] Iproniazid came to be known as the first antidepressant of the monoamine oxidase inhibitor type (MAOI). At the same time, in 1957–8, the Swiss pharmaceutical firm Geigy introduced Tofranil (imipramine) to the European markets. Tofranil came to be known as the first and leading tricyclic antidepressant.

As often recounted, Tofranil was not initially developed as an antidepressant. Spurred on by the structural analogy of iminodibenzyl derivatives with chlorpromazine, Geigy had first targeted the treatment of schizophrenia. The objectification of imipramine's antidepressive properties, as well as its association with the treatment of severe hospital-based endogenous depressions, had essentially been the work of a handful of Swiss psychiatrists, most importantly R. Kuhn, who collaborated with the company. From Geigy's perspective, the advent of tricyclic antidepressants constituted a test case to change the scale and nature of both the production and mode of promotion of psychopharmaceuticals. On the one hand, Geigy deployed intensive marketing activities to build and secure the new market segment of antidepressants. On the other hand, it invested significant time and resources to turn this 'good fortune' into a rationalized drug research system. To internalize the early stages of drug discovery, as well as to scale up and systemize the production of psychopharmaceuticals, Geigy relied on the establishment of a new preclinical experimental facility including an animal assay system. In this respect, from the late 1950s on, the firm's pharmacologists attempted to elaborate new animal models that could reliably represent part of the clinical features of psychiatric disorders and/or be predictive of the behavioural and neurophysiological responses induced in patients by psychopharmaceutical drugs.[6]

These combined efforts need to be read against the post-war consolidation of a pipeline-based way of developing new therapeutic compounds, i.e., an integrated, intensive and large-scale drug development system, ranging from systematic chemical synthesis to marketing.[7] This 'assembly line' model of innovation, as it was called by N. Rasmussen, is based on the generalization, after World War II, of a chemical-pharmaceutical 'system of practices' – called 'screening' – to organize the conception and production of drugs.[8] This mode of invention through screening establishes an ad hoc, systematic collaboration between the organic chemistry department and the pharmacology laboratory. The chemists support the drug research efforts by fabricating battalions of new substances. These molecules are then transferred to the biological department. There, pharmacologists routinely run the series of analogues through standardized and graded assay systems, trying to objectify their toxicity, specify their activity and predict putative therapeutic properties and efficacy. As soon as possible, the few promising compounds are isolated from the many deceptive ones and sent over to the development stage. Along the pathways of adoption of novel production praxis, the pipeline-based model of innovation is also rooted in changing management and marketing practices. In the post-war period, medium- to long-term drug-development planning matured as the firms worked more actively on the diversification of products within a given therapeutic class and increasingly targeted medical market niches. These new market-building practices were intimately connected to the changing scale and nature of marketing activities.[9] During this period, marketing adopted new types of promotion practices, massively using technical arguments and in-house research data, both clinical and laboratory-based. Moreover, marketing was diversified and transformed into a research-like activity by adopting tools from social and economic sciences such as statistics and detailed surveys of prescription patterns.[10]

In this paper, I examine Geigy's post-war alignment with a screening strategy in the field of psychopharmaceutical drugs by focusing on the development of in-house animal modelling practices. Building on historical studies on biomedical animal modelling practices and the contemporary history of depression, I document and analyse Geigy's psychopharmacological animal activities from their official adoption in the late 1950s with the institution of a specialized experimental unit to the consolidation of a preclinical assay system in the early 1970s.[11]

By discussing the production and selection of new animal models and their integration into a standard screening battery, I will argue that the investments made by Geigy's pharmacologists cannot be understood by focusing exclusively on the interactions between the clinic and the laboratory. In the context of a company producing market goods, the translation of clinical knowledge at the experimental level was not only considered from the perspective of experimental feasibility; it was also judged in terms of market issues, especially through the use, from the mid-1960s on, of sophisticated market surveys and strategic planning. At Geigy, this strong entrenchment between experimental and economic rationales resulted in a shift of the reference point of the modelling process. Throughout the 1960s, the targets of the modelling process gradually shifted from psychiatric disorders as such to psychopharmaceuticals and from antidepressants to boundary work between the different classes of psychopharmaceuticals available on the market.

Transforming 'Good Fortune' into an Internalized and Systematic Drug-Selection Facility

In the close aftermath of the market introduction of Tofranil, the decisive role played by psychiatrists in the advent of the drug as an antidepressant shaped Geigy's approach to developing new psychopharmaceuticals. In the late 1950s and early 1960s, the firm gave the clinic centre stage, organizing the maintenance of a tight and small formalized system of exchanges with professionals. Clinicians were granted great latitude in conducting the clinical trials; neither the selection of patient groups nor the choice of evaluation criteria were imposed on them by the company. Furthermore, in the late 1950s and early 1960s, there was not a strong hierarchy between the experimental and the clinical stages of the drug development process. It was not unusual, for instance, to expect the first clinical outcomes to deepen chemical and pharmacological investigations, or even to occasionally synthesize and test a novel compound at the request of a clinician.

To some extent, persistence of the clinic at the heart of the innovation process was related to Geigy's rudimentary experience in the field of psychopharmaceutical drugs, as epitomized most clearly in the company's limited preclinical experimental infrastructure. In the 1950s, Geigy's animal testing facility in the field of psychotropic drugs was very modest. The psychiatrist A. Broadhurst, then an employee of the British branch of the company, took part in the early pharmacological testing of iminodibenzyl derivatives in Basel and recalled that '[a] part from fairly gross behavioural observations, such as the presence of sedation in treated animals, no specialized behavioural studies were carried out. Very few techniques of this type were in use, or even known, at that time'.[12] Given the unavailability of adequate preclinical testing techniques, the company had to rely as early as possible on clinical investigations for the assessment of candidate drugs.[13]

From the mid-1950s on, when Geigy definitely committed to the development of new psychopharmaceuticals, the firm's lagging experimental facility came under close scrutiny. In 1955, for instance, the chemist F. Häfliger raised a cautionary note on the company's preclinical infrastructure. In his view, it prevented the drug development programme from scaling up:

> The absence of pharmacological tests prevents any systematic investigation of the field. If the pace of the clinical assays cannot be scaled up, commercialization of a new product should not be expected in the near future. The iminodibenzyl derivatives tested so far seem to present the desired properties. However, since thirty new preparations stemming from this group are in the process of being prepared, a selection through one or more tests on animals is unavoidable.[14]

In the late 1950s, Geigy's managers decided to address this pressing issue. They split up the existing pharmacology laboratory to set up a new research unit in addition to the place for research on toxicity and pharmacodynamics. Headed by the pharmacologist W. Theobald, this laboratory was to be dedicated solely to preclinical psychopharmacology. In order to sustain and rationalize the firm's drug discovery efforts, Theobald's laboratory was in charge of producing, almost from scratch, a series of animal models, experimental techniques and protocols.

Inventing the Pharmacology of Tricyclic Antidepressants

For Geigy's pharmacologists, the production of a novel animal test system was complicated by the very fact that the objects to be modelled were mental disorders and their treatment.[15] Psychiatric afflictions are hard to predict; their causes are hardly known and their manifestations are confused and heterogeneous, with each patient displaying specific configurations of symptoms. Furthermore, they are generally held to be multifactorial disorders, involving genetic predispositions, biological dysregulation, socio-environmental factors, psychological configurations and social practices. Moreover, diagnosis of mental disorders is traditionally made through the identification of disturbances operating at the symbolic, intellect or affect level. These faculties are either reputedly absent in animals, or at best hard to objectify. All in all, the traditional dilemmas of biomedical modelling – the distance between the animal and the human, the heterogeneity of clinical situations and the controlled and artificial laboratory setting – were somehow exacerbated in this enterprise.[16]

The pharmacologists' task was further complicated by the absence, in the late 1950s and early 1960s, of any established biological criteria to correlate the experimental results and the clinical data directly.[17] The pharmacologist A.

Delini-Stula, who joined Theobald's team at Geigy in the late 1960s, recalled that at this period neurobiochemical knowledge and tools were not decisive in organizing the preclinical evaluation of psychotropic drugs, for '[t]he anatomy of neurotransmitter systems of the brain, as well as the neurobiochemical processes and the receptor structures, which constitute today's target for the development of psychopharmaceuticals, had yet to be discovered'.[18] Throughout the 1960s, the firm's pharmacologists addressed this difficulty mainly by turning to the manipulation and control of the behaviour of laboratory animals, since behaviour could be seen as both a target of intervention and an entity mediating between the laboratory and the clinic.

Transforming the behaviour of laboratory organisms into preclinical pharmacological tools was difficult. First, the overt behaviour of an organism is an extremely random phenomenon, the intrinsic variability of which somehow had to be minimized and controlled to allow the production of a stable pharmacological tool displaying comparable results throughout the successive trials.[19] Second, animals were so to speak too 'normal'; no non-human species spontaneously presented behaviour that could be identified as analogous to a depressive syndrome. Consequently industrial pharmacologists faced the challenge of generating and selecting a repertoire of artificial behavioural patterns in laboratory animals – altered functions or aberrant behavioural motives – which could somehow be representative of a depressive state and enable the prediction of an antidepressant potential in humans.

At Geigy, as I interpret it, producing and selecting behavioural patterns for predictive screening operations were initially addressed by modelling processes that considered existing reference drugs as therapeutic rather than chemical entities, using their properties once they had been appropriated and interpreted by clinicians.[20] In this sense, Tofranil represented the initial benchmark to build the battery of tests and organize the screening. Its clinical effects rather than the disorder, depression, constituted the starting point and leading thread for the assembly of a novel screening battery. By constantly referring to the clinic, pharmacologists retroactively established a range of animal models and assays that could be predictive of some selected positive and negative properties of the drug.[21] As illustrated by the history of the pharmacology of Tofranil, however, there was no spontaneous fit between the pharmacological instruments, the drugs under study and the clinical phenomena.

Imipramine: An Ambiguous Compound

The task of creating new experimental models predictive of an antidepressant effect in the clinic turned out to be deeply challenging. In the late 1950s, the available infrahuman laboratory tests used for centrally acting drugs turned out to be of limited help to codify the activity and therapeutic properties of Tofranil. Using these tests, it was for instance difficult to clearly differentiate the pharmacological actions of Tofranil from those of structurally related drugs like traditional neuroleptics and anti-allergic compounds.[22] Even though psychiatrists had attributed particular therapeutic effects and indications to imipramine, for some pharmacologists the testing facilities could not establish more than a quantitative, rather than qualitative, difference between the pharmacological effects of imipramine and chlorpromazine.[23] Furthermore, at the behavioural level, imipramine seemed to have few acute effects. The administration of non-toxic doses induced, apart from a slight sedative effect, no significant changes in the locomotor activity of experimental animals. In the late 1950s, for example, Geigy's pharmacologists ran the treated animals through a battery of behavioural tests used to measure the effect of the drug on fine motor skills.[24] There were no significant effects until high doses were administered, already leading to toxic effects, which seriously restricted the usefulness of these tests. During the early 1960s, through scientific engineering and experimental tinkering, the industrial pharmacologist tried to align the drug and the scientific apparatus to make this 'unexpressive' compound a workable entity.

To manipulate and control the behaviour of their laboratory animals and perhaps to circumvent the absence of acute effects of imipramine on the overt behaviour of laboratory organisms, Geigy's pharmacologists turned mainly to a pharmacogenic modelling strategy.[25] They used known chemical substances to generate impaired behavioural patterns that could represent either selected behavioural symptoms of depression or pharmacological effects presumed to be implicated in the action of Tofranil. In the early 1960s, this translated very concretely into the adoption of two main lines of investigation. The first was 'antagonism to experimentally induced depression of the central nervous system' and the second was 'enhancement of central adrenergic activity'.[26] The latter strategy, which I will not develop further in this paper, relied on the finding that imipramine increased certain effects of adrenergic substances. In the late 1950s, pharmacological investigations found that imipramine potentiated the peripheral effects of endogenous monoamines (noradrenaline) that were administered exogenously to laboratory animals, which led to the formulation of the hypothesis that imipramine exerted its antidepressant action by sensitizing the central adrenergic functions.[27] It was later shown that imipramine also increased the effects of synthetic stimulating drugs, like amphetamine; this potentiation was then hypothesized to be related to a central action. Based on these results and assumptions, new preclinical tests were soon developed.[28] The potentiating and prolonging effects of imipramine on the signs of sympathetic hyperfunction and, most importantly, on the behavioural excitation induced by adrenergic substances became tools in the 1960s to predict potential antidepressant properties.[29]

Prediction through Behavioural Analogy: The Reserpine Model of Depression

During the 1960s, the most stable animal model that was elaborated in the retrospective quest for pharmacological tests predictive of antidepressant properties was the reserpine model of depression. Reserpine was an indole alkaloid that had been isolated in 1952 by the pharmaceutical firm Ciba from the dried Indian root *Rauwolfia serpentina*. Reserpine, introduced on the market under the trade name Serpasil in 1954, had a very strong and prolonged sedative effect, a property that stimulated its use as an antihypertensive and as an antipsychotic drug. Work with reserpine to produce animal models of depression was based on two grounds. First, in the mid-1950s, reports began to appear documenting that reserpine precipitated mental depression in an alarming proportion of patients receiving the treatment to control their high blood pressure.[30] Second, reserpine and similar centrally depressing agents, like tetrabenazine or Ro 4–1284, induced a characteristic behavioural syndrome in laboratory animals – mostly rodents – made up of 'a decrease in or a loss of locomotion and exploratory activity ... a hunch-backed posture [and] cataleptic immobility'.[31] To some degree, these signs of behavioural depression, of akinesia and 'stupor', were equated with the depressive states witnessed in humans, and drove pharmacologists in the late 1950s and early 1960s to use reserpine to produce new animal models in order to uncover potential antidepressant drugs.

In the late 1950s and early 1960s several papers, stemming from various laboratories, were published documenting the antagonism of various reserpine effects by imipramine.[32] For instance, in 1959, in the first published review of the general pharmacology of Tofranil, Geigy's pharmacologists used various substances that had a depressant effect on the central nervous system, including reserpine, to conduct drug interaction studies with imipramine.[33] For example, rats received subcutaneous injections of a dose of 2mg/kg of reserpine, which induced a drastic reduction of spontaneous motility. If injected four hours later in doses of 50mg/kg, Tofranil completely inhibited the sedative effects of the alkaloid for one hour. In another experimental protocol, called the '*Lidspalten* (palpebral) *test*', strong doses of imipramine significantly enlarged the constricted pupil (miosis) as well as curtailed the abnormal drooping of the upper lid (palpebral ptosis) induced by reserpine.[34] Geigy's pharmacologists concluded their 1959 paper by suggesting that a positive pharmacological dynamic component, in terms of drive, might be deduced from the antagonism of reserpine effects by imipramine.[35] Nonetheless, very cautiously, they did not stretch the analogy between their experimental results and the clinical phenomena too far. They did not presume that the centrally depressing effect of the alkaloid and the related functional disturbances induced in the animals, both behavioural and autonomic, bore any relation to the underlying pathogenic mechanisms and clinical signs of depression. At this stage, it seemed that the reserpine syndrome antagonism was essentially a convenient pharmacological protocol to transform imipramine into a 'workable' drug, not yet a real model of depression. This overlap came into full bloom in 1961–2 thanks to transatlantic data and experience sharing between Geigy and the clinical pharmacology laboratory of the National Heart Institute in Bethesda (Maryland, USA), which was run by the biochemist B. Brodie. It was during this information sharing period that the firm developed its second commercial antidepressant, Pertofran.[36]

Desipramine, the future Pertofran, had been identified in 1959 by Geigy's chemists as a natural metabolite of Tofranil – the only one amongst the six that had been found for which the synthesis had not raised major difficulties.[37] The full endorsement of the development of desipramine as a commercial compound was catalysed by the results obtained in 1961 by Brodie's team at the National Heart Institute, which, having been at the forefront of the development of cerebral neurochemistry from the 1950s on, was then trying to elucidate the action mechanisms of imipramine. The team had measured the rate of imipramine found in the brains of laboratory animals after chronic treatment with the antidepressant. As they saw it, the data collected suggested that the antidepressant effect of Tofranil was conditioned by the accumulation of desipramine in the brain.[38] For Geigy's heads of research, this surprising news, which could not be confirmed in successive experiments, came with an even more stunning statement.[39] The transcription of a telephone conversation in July 1961 between Brodie and the firm's leading chemist, Häfliger, reads: '[Brodie] has a test [in animal experimentation] that enables a specific evaluation of the antidepressant effect. With it, he can rapidly distinguish substances with antidepressant properties from substances having effects of the monoamine-oxidase inhibitor or of the amphetamine type.'[40] A handwritten note added in the margin of the transcription 'Kaum zu glauben' (hard to believe) testifies that Geigy was surprised by Brodie's claim.

Brodie's test was a reserpine antagonism test that consisted of chronic pre-treatment of rats with imipramine before injecting a dose of reserpine or Ro 4–1284, inducing a behavioural syndrome similar to that induced by reserpine, but with the advantage of being infinitely more rapid.[41] Chronic pre-treatment with Tofranil blocked the appearance of the characteristic reserpine-like syndrome. In this test, desipramine not only antagonized but allegedly 'reversed' the sedation and induced a prolonged hyperactive behavioural pattern:

> This pattern consists of 'compulsive' exploratory behaviour characterized by ceaseless, steady circling around the perimeter of the cage. Placed on a high platform the animals almost invariably try to leap down ... The animals appear to be stimulated by an inner drive to which they respond even when life-threatening situations, such as a fall off a high board, arise.[42]

To Brodie and his team, their test reported for the first time the 'removal' of the reserpine-like syndrome that allowed the putative antidepressant potency of new compounds to be tested in laboratory animals.[43]

During this same period, the first reports of the initial clinical trials conducted in three Swiss psychiatric clinics seemed to confirm Brodie's experimental results. In the clinical trials, desipramine shared a common range of indications with imipramine and depressive syndromes responded well to the compound. Most importantly, the clinical reports revealed that desipramine acted more rapidly than imipramine and that its psychomotor-activating effects seemed to dominate the clinical picture of the patients under treatment, thus paralleling the experimental findings made with laboratory animals.[44] In 1962, Pertofran was introduced into the market by Geigy. From the perspective of animal experimentation, the market introduction of a new antidepressant contributed to giving strength and objectivity to the 'validity' of the reserpine-like syndrome as a model of depression; the experimental principle of the reserpine antagonism soon became the standard industrial test to screen for new antidepressants. This can be interpreted as resulting from a complex and iterative looping effect between the clinic, the laboratory and the market. The experimental procedure had initially been used in reference to the clinical reports documenting the depressant effects of reserpine in patients receiving the alkaloid as an antihypertensive. The empirical validation of the ability of the model to predict antidepressant effects, further sealed by the market introduction of a new antidepressant compound, strengthened the cohesion of this association even more, though indirectly. With the reserpine model and its variations, in 1961 Geigy's pharmacologists could praise their progress; they had ultimately found a way through the pharmacological haze of tricyclic antidepressants and reached a semblance of differential characterization predictive of an antidepressant effect.[45]

As epitomized by the reserpine model of depression, the construction of a predictive pharmacology of tricyclic antidepressants proceeded from a significant manipulation of clinical data. In my interpretation, however, the construction of an equivalence system between the laboratory and the clinic entailed a shift in the understanding of depression and its treatment. In the retrospective quest for new preclinical models, Geigy's pharmacologists did not so much try to produce models of depression as to produce animal tests in which the positive and negative clinical features of Tofranil would be expressed and could be assessed. Putting aside the mental dimensions of depression, industrial pharmacologists focused instead on a limited and selected set of secondary manifestations: loss of vitality and psychomotor impairment. In addition, focus on the clinically validated drug as well as the pharmacogenic methodology contributed to turning the behavioural parameter into the sign of an internal pharmacodynamic parameter, entirely reducible to the couple drug effects. Even more than the individual tests, it was their inclusion in the screening battery that most clearly reveals how clinical knowledge was tensioned by the construction of a screening model for drug development.

Modelling the Prescription Market

To back up Geigy's therapeutic innovation programme, the industrial pharmacologists gradually integrated the new experimental tests into a general preclinical screening strategy. I believe that the construction of this screening system partially depended on the evolution of Geigy's market targets, which, throughout the 1960s, became less focused on distinct diagnostic entities than on cross-cutting symptomatic targets: anxiety, low mood, psychomotor inhibition and agitation. As a consequence, viewed from the perspective of the firm's drug innovation programme, the clinical frontier between antidepressants, neuroleptics and mild tranquilizers became increasingly thin. This process originated mainly in market-oriented research. It reflected Geigy managers' interpretations of the constraints and opportunities of the general psychopharmaceutical market segment based on sales data and, from the mid-1960s on, on detailed surveys of prescriptions patterns. This was converted by Geigy's pharmacologists into specific research and development practices. In my understanding, as the decade unfolded, they operated a gradual and experimental dismembering of psychiatric entities into cross-cutting 'target symptoms'. On this basis, they progressively constructed a 'cross-class' screening methodology; a drug selection system operationalizing the flexible boundaries of antidepressants, neuroleptics and mild tranquilizers.

Here I will argue that the weakened differentiation between psychotropic drug classes can be traced back to complex interactions between the laboratory, the clinic and the market. On the experimental scene, this process might first be traced back to the early 1960s, when the medical handling of antidepressant drugs contributed to the emergence of symptom-oriented approaches to diagnosis and treatment. This symptomatic breakdown of depressive syndromes and treatments originating in medical concerns but also corresponding to as many market niches, progressively gained ground in Geigy's drug innovation programme. As the decade unfolded, the rising influence of scientific marketing exacerbated this symptomatic approach to drug development. At the end of the 1960s, building on market-oriented surveys, Geigy's management formulated new drug innovation goals to gain larger market shares and reach the general practice segment. Reflecting on these commercial pressures, industrial pharmacologists adapted the organization of the screening system to match the firm's shifting market priorities.

In this section, emphasis will be on the modelling dynamics, and the experimental tools and concepts that enabled the construction of a 'cross-class', symptom-oriented, screening system. My main argument is that this preclinical methodology enabled the alignment of laboratory work with marketing practices and sales volume issues. In my opinion, however, it also increased the disconnection between drug development practices and the psychiatric rationale, as it pushed the attachment of therapeutic targets to distinct diagnostic entities even further into the background.

A Focus on Secondary Symptoms

During the early 1960s, Geigy devoted significant efforts to building the antidepressant market. The launch of the Tofranil campaign had mainly targeted hospital psychiatry, thereby reinforcing the professionals' view that imipramine was associated with the treatment of severely impaired depressive patients. While endogenous depressions of the melancholic type were thought to be particularly responsive to Tofranil, these conditions still represented only a very small portion of psychiatric diagnosis.[46] As analysed by Jean-Paul Gaudillière in this volume, during the launching campaign, the primary vector used to extend the range of indications for Tofranil had been to advocate parallel use of existing etiological nosologies and a symptomatic grid.

On the one hand, the firm's advertisement used existing classifications like, for example, that of P. Kielholz, a long-standing collaborator with the firm, who listed five different forms of depression organized along a somatogenic-psychogenic axis. In this respect, the clinical efficacy of Tofranil was said to decline, qualitatively and quantitatively, the more one departed from the vital core of endogenous depressions.[47] On the other hand, the commercial brochures encouraged the professional not to place undue reliance on the etiologic classifications, which were said to be potentially arbitrary. The advice given to professionals was to reverse the burden of proof, i.e., to judge the effects of Tofranil empirically on its main 'target symptoms'.[48] In the commercial brochures, beyond the primary symptoms of depression – despair, guilt and hopelessness – these 'target symptoms' included secondary symptoms like indecision, anxiety, psychomotor inhibition, etc.[49] As illustrated in an advertisement used during the launch campaign for Tofranil, which ran from 1958 to 1962, the marketing department also incorporated the somatic aspects that may accompany depression. The brochure lists various physical symptoms that should awaken physicians' suspicion of a potential case of depression:

> The lack of appetite typically leads to weight loss. Constipation and abdominal pain are frequent symptoms. A feeling of constriction in the chest, often accompanied by heart beats or dyspnea is also to be found. Decreased libido and even impotence are also rather common signs. For women, menstrual disorders appear. Patients sometimes complain about dysuria or pollakiuria (urinary frequency).[50]

This promotional strategy, using symptoms as marketing units, was first and foremost an attempt to foster the use of Tofranil beyond the most severe types of affective syndromes, and, more marginally, to reach general practitioners.[51] In this sense, the campaign to launch Tofranil met with mixed success. On the one hand, there was no spontaneous or massive adoption of Tofranil by general practitioners. Geigy's management attributed the lack of success of Tofranil in general practice to its slow action as well as to its important side effects, including neurovegetative disorders, feelings of dryness, tachycardia and cold sweats. Geigy's management thought that general practitioners found treatment with Tofranil difficult to handle and very demanding in terms of monitoring.[52] On the other hand, there was growth in its use and a parallel rise in the ambulatory treatment of depressed patients.[53] By the early 1960s, Tofranil had become a reference compound for the treatment of endogenous depressions. It was amply copied by other pharmaceutical companies, which brought about a growing commercial offer of tricyclic antidepressants.[54] As will be argued below, the increasing range of antidepressant agents indirectly strengthened Geigy's focus on symptomatic targets when defining priorities for drug development.

While they all belong to the same generic class of drugs, as it was outlined by A. Ehrenberg, tricyclic antidepressants 'do not act with the same efficacy on each of the affective syndromes'.[55] For instance, psychiatrists learned from experience that when the secondary symptoms of agitation and anxiety dominated the clinical picture, patients often did not react very well to Tofranil. For if the treatment had already exerted its beneficial effects on psychomotor activity before the onset of its antidepressant action, or if it had exacerbated feelings of anxiety and agitation, the patients could commit suicide if there was a sudden increase in their depressed mood. As a consequence, clinicians were reluctant to use imipramine with depressive patients affected by agitation and anxiety. They rather opted for electroshock treatment or, alternatively, combined Tofranil with a sedative and/or neuroleptic agent in the early stages of the treatment. With the growing offer of antidepressant chemotherapies, however, psychiatrists could also select other compounds to treat patients affected with agitation or anxiety. Amitriptyline, a tricyclic antidepressant first sold by Merck under the trade name Elavil, had precisely invested in the economic niche of agitated depressions. This compound possessed, along with an antidepressant property similar to that of Tofranil, a strong sedative effect, so it became the main challenger to Tofranil in the psychiatric hospital market.[56]

In the 1960s, the advantages and limitations of the new generation of antidepressants contributed to polarizing the clinical view on therapeutic regimens along a stimulation–sedation line. A spectrum of therapeutic targets mirrored the symptomatic breakdown of the clinical action of antidepressants. In the 1960s, a trend emerged of establishing a cross-etiological distinction between depressions of the inhibited-apathetic type and depressions of the agitated-anxious type. In 1963, the Swiss psychiatrist Kielholz formalized this understanding of antidepressant regimens (Figure 10.1).[57]

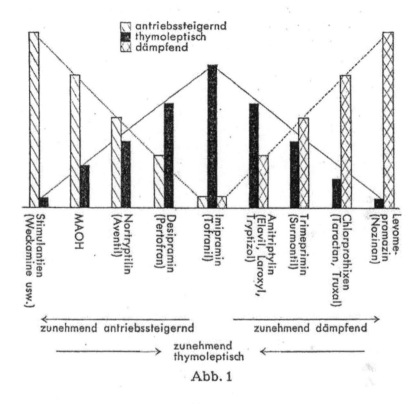

Abb. 1

Figure 10.1: A schematic representation of the spectra of action of antidepressants; image reproduced by kind permission of Georg Thieme Verlag.

Source: P. Kielholz et al., 'Therapie der Depressionen und der depressiven Krankheitszustände', *Deutsche Medizinische Wochenschrift*, 88:34, pp. 1617–24, on p. 1618; copyright © 2014 Georg Thieme Verlag KG. The graph provides a schematic representation of the differential activities of the main antidepressive drugs available on the market in the early 1960s. The dark columns represent the mood-normalizing property of antidepressive drugs, while the striped and the hatched columns respectively stand for their stimulating and sedative effects. The right arrow under the graph indicates a growing sedative activity, while the left arrow shows a growing stimulating activity. The two converging arrows below the graph indicate a growing mood normalizing activity.

Accordingly, antidepressants expressed, with a varying degree of strength, the following three effects: the antidepressant effect itself – i.e., mood normalization, a sedative effect – which could be useful to dissipate agitation and anxiety, and a stimulating effect – employed to control psycho-motor inhibition. In the figure reproduced above, these three properties are featured as following: the dark columns represent the antidepressant effect, striped columns the stimulating effect and those with a hatched motif the sedative effect. Polarization operates from left to right along a stimulation-sedation line. While nosological attributions were still considered important, Kielholz's advice was to identify the most prominent symptoms and to match these target symptoms with the profile of undesirable effects of the antidepressants and the kind of medical care (hospital-based or ambulatory).

The clinicians' focus on secondary target symptoms was in turn adopted by Geigy's management when defining drug innovation goals in the antidepressant field, and to some extent was further translated at the experimental level when conducting preclinical work.[58] In the 1960s, Geigy's pharmacologists began to look for drugs qualitatively similar to Tofranil but that would possess, beyond the core antidepressive effect, 'stronger sedative effects (similar to amitriptyline)'.[59] This innovation goal can be interpreted as reflecting a fragmentation of the clinical entity of depression into a set of distinct therapeutic targets (low mood, agitation). Drawing and assembling several tests from the entire range of available experimental models could in turn be used to meet these targets.[60] Animal models predictive of an antidepressant effect were thus used in combination with pharmacological tests predictive of a sedative effect, traditionally associated with the class of neuroleptic drugs. For instance, between 1961 and 1965, the most widely used experimental procedure at Geigy had been the narcosis potentiation test, a standard test to identify chlorpromazine-like compounds.[61] In rats and mice, neuroleptics potentiate (prolong) the sleep-inducing effects of various hypnotic drugs.[62] To predict neuroleptic potential, industrial pharmacologists measured the duration of experimental sleep. The narcosis potentiation property was not specific to neuroleptics, since it could also be found in numerous antidepressant drugs.[63] In the 1960s, to find sedative antidepressants, Geigy's pharmacologists associated this standard procedure to assess neuroleptic effects with the preclinical battery to predict antidepressant potential.[64] In my interpretation, reflecting on on-going medical and related commercial issues, the firm's pharmacologists gradually adopted a symptomatic logic. This led to the construction of what I have called a 'cross-class' screening logic, i.e., analogical reasoning between, on the one hand, the standard effects of tricyclic antidepressants, and on the other hand, isolated pharmacological effects traditionally associated with neuroleptics. This process was exacerbated in the late 1960s with the formalization of the standard screening battery.

Boundary Work between Therapeutic Classes

At the experimental level, the clinical frontier between antidepressants and neuroleptics became increasingly thin owing to a focus on shared segments of their symptomatic action. From the industry's perspective, however, the real issue from the middle of the 1960s on was the overlap between antidepressants and mild tranquilizers. I will now demonstrate that this process was not prompted so much by psychiatrists' handling of antidepressant drugs, but originated instead in the growing impact of scientific marketing on the planning of industrial research. More broadly, it can be interpreted as an effect of the firm's internal restructuring.

As analysed by Jean-Paul Gaudillière in this volume, in the second half of the 1960s, Geigy initiated a thorough internal reorganization process. Starting in 1966, the firm reshuffled its divisional structure, introduced network techniques and strategic planning, formalized clinical trials, and expanded its system of scientific marketing. One major aim was to tighten up articulation between the different working units and thereby achieve overall management of the screening process, ranging from the definition of medium- and long-term innovation goals, through the selection and development of products, to market-launch decisions.[65]

The research department was thus reorganized. As vividly emphasized in 1967 by W. G. Stoll, head of research at Geigy, research was meant to become more integrated: 'The setting up and conduct of industrial research, as well as its inclusion in the business process, depend on the innovation goals set by the company ... Research in the industry *cannot and must not lead a life of its own*'.[66] In this perspective, a decisive feature of Geigy's reorganization was the consolidation of its scientific marketing system. By the mid-1960s, the formerly named 'propaganda' activities, initially affiliated to the sales department, had been renamed 'marketing' activities and were integrated into the pharmacological research department.[67] More than just new terminology, this change was related to the shifting dimensions and tasks of scientific marketing. Beyond the considerable use of in-house research for physician-targeted promotion, marketing increasingly relied on the production of market-oriented knowledge, especially through the organization of prescription surveys. As a consequence of these changes, Geigy's management lent increasing credence to the marketing department to give a ruling on the firm's innovation priorities. This stood out most clearly when, starting in 1967 as part of the reorganization plan, the company commissioned a fundamental review of the research targets in the psychopharmaceutical field.[68] The task, delegated to the joint supervision of the marketing and the research departments, consisted in auditing on-going research goals, formulating new innovation targets and selection criteria, and rationalizing the allocation of human and experimental resources accordingly. In the words of

Geigy's managers, this review aimed at 'on the one hand, achieving a better align-ment of research activities on the wishes of marketing, and on the other hand, improving the marketing department's understanding of the opportunities and problems of the research department'.[69]

As support material to coordinate the meetings between the research and the marketing departments, the firm ordered a series of market surveys. These thorough market reviews, crossing sales data with prescription patterns accord-ing to diagnostic indications, were performed by J. Pollack and A. Fuchs from Geigy's American and Swiss marketing departments, respectively.[70] The most obvious point to emerge from this data was that 'tranquilizers [were] clearly the superior products in terms of sales performance'.[71] The figures were indeed edi-fying. In the United States, by far the largest market, tranquilizers (both major and minor) accounted for the biggest share of total sales of all psychotherapeu-tic drugs. In 1967, they accounted for an estimated USD 262.5 million or a 71.6 per cent share of the total market in this field. The same year, minor tranquilizers alone, massively prescribed by general practitioners, the leading trademarks of which were Librium and Valium (Roche), accounted for an esti-mated USD 170.5 million or a 65 per cent share of total tranquilizer sales. This amounted to 10.2 per cent of the total American prescription market share.[72] By contrast, the market for antidepressants, though a growing segment, '[fell] far short of the heights reached by tranquilizers with a volume only 15 per cent of that achieved by tranquilizers'.[73] Invited as they were to pay more attention to the actual state of the market, Geigy's managers expressed the belief that the general practitioner's market now exceeded the psychiatric segment in terms of chances for commercial growth.[74] The review process culminated in reshuffling the order of priorities for future drug development. Mild tranquilizers were upgraded to the rank of priority target: 'From a commercial perspective, the development of a 'psychosomaticum', i.e. .a compound possessing therapeutic qualities similar to Librium, would by far have the most outstanding chances of success'.[75] Neurolep-tic drugs held on to their second rank in the firm's innovation programme, while the pride of the company, standard tricyclic antidepressants, slipped from first to third rank. The second major outcome of the market reviews performed in 1967 and 1968 was a reconsideration of the relationship between tranquilizers and antidepressants. Analysing the market information, not just sales volumes but patterns of use and drug performances by indications, Geigy's heads concluded that 'in the milder psychiatric/psychosomatic cases, as predominantly encoun-tered in general practice, indications for mild tranquilizers and antidepressants can hardly be differentiated'.[76] In this perspective, Geigy's management cham-pioned the view that a major source of economic growth would be to develop a 'mild antidepressant', a 'combination of tranquilizer and antidepressant' or other drugs of various chemical and pharmacological origins that could 'find their place in the large and heterogeneous field of the little specific pharmacotherapy of mild psychic conditions'.[77] Looking at psycho-pharmacotherapy through a market lens, the firm established general drug selection criteria hovering between the antidepressant and the mild tranquilizer niches. How these 'cross-class' innovation goals were materialized at the experimental level will now be accounted for by analysing the standard screening battery, which was formalized at Geigy in the late 1960s.[78]

It was then that the pharmacologist C. Morpurgo incorporated the series of tests crafted over the decade into a predefined evaluation scheme that enabled a rapid and staggered assessment of the candidate drugs.[79] In my interpretation, the cornerstones of this assay system were the standard drug profiles Geigy's pharmacologists had gradually constructed for each of the three drug classes (Figures 10.2, 10.3 and 10.4). In this context, a drug profile generally represents the summary of a drug's pharmacological effects as measured in a range of animal (or pharmacological) tests. Drug profiles are first and foremost tools to keep track of a considerable amount of data and to manage the multiplicity of preclinical tests – one must remember that no assay was considered specific enough to stand on its own. At Geigy, the early stage of the construction of drug profiles had consisted in assembling a range of animal tests, constructed and stabilized with reference to clinically validated drugs like Tofranil, chlorpromazine and Librium, each representative of one of the three classes of drugs (antidepressants, neuroleptics and mild tranquilizers). For example, routine evaluations to screen for mild tranquilizers included experimental tests to assess three main pharmacological properties: anticonvulsive, muscle relaxant and 'taming' effects.[80] The former was assessed in chemically induced convulsion antagonism tests: the strychnine and the Cardiazol antagonism tests. The muscle relaxant properties were, amongst others, evaluated in the so-called traction test that enables the measurement of motor coordination and muscle tone. This experimental procedure consisted in 'suspending a mouse by its forepaws to a horizontally stretched wire'.[81] When placed in this position, the laboratory animal would normally rapidly grasp the wire with its hind feet. The experimenters recorded the latency or failure of the treated laboratory animal to execute this behavioural task. The 'taming' effects in turn could be measured through a series of behavioural tests in which the laboratory animals were put into a state of 'affective types of aggressiveness' induced by stressful situations like social deprivation or the presentation of noxious stimuli.[82] At Geigy, the routine test to predict a 'taming' effect was the 'Fight reaction' test, which uses mice.[83] In this test, two mice are placed in a small experimental box, the floor of which is electrified. This stimulus generally elicits belligerent outbursts with the two laboratory animals assaulting each other. This shock-induced fighting can be inhibited by the action of psychotropic drugs.[84]

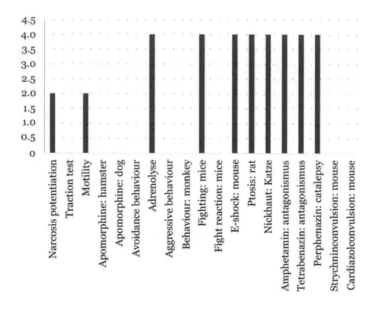

Figure 10.2: A schematic overview of the drug profile for antidepressants.

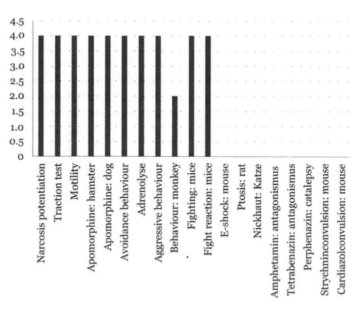

Figure 10.3: A schematic overview of the drug profile for neuroleptics.

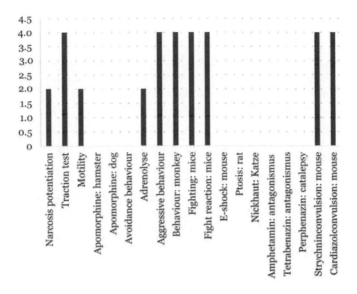

Figure 10.4: A schematic overview of the drug profile for tranquilizers.

The first step of the screening consisted of a matrix of seven testing routines. All the new chemical compounds were systematically screened through these seven protocols to make a first selection as well as a preliminary affiliation to one of the three therapeutic classes. My interpretation of the firm's archives is that each class had an emblematic test allowing a temporary classification of the new molecules. In this sense, the reserpine model distinguished the antidepressants, the narcosis potentiation test was representative of the neuroleptics and the tests for antagonism to chemical convulsions were used to characterize the mild tranquilizers. The second step of the screening consisted of a more detailed pharmacological evaluation organized according to drug classes. The candidate compounds were profiled for systematic comparison with the profiles of standard and clinically validated drugs. The profiles allowed the experimenters to 'reason by analogy'.[85] They could rapidly and directly compare the spectra of candidate compounds to one another, and against standard spectra of clinically validated compounds of the corresponding therapeutic class. This testing system also allowed a more detailed comparison of the activity of a given drug with prototypal profiles in other classes of compounds. As such, the schematic overview of standard drug profiles reproduced above shows that isolated pharmacological effects, while usually associated with one therapeutic class, might be observed in the three drug classes. For instance, the narcosis potentiation test used to predict for sedative effects, as well as the 'Fight Reaction' test commonly linked to anxiolytic properties, were present in the three profiles.[86] At the end of the screening, the pharmacologists would thus have a more or less complete picture of the activity of the candidate compound.

In 1969, Theobald and Schindler stressed in a presentation of Geigy's pre-clinical drug research efforts: 'The selection of new clinical preparations cannot be exclusively grounded on the effects of known compounds. Deviations from the activity of existing commercial drugs heighten the chances to find radically new and more effective preparations'.[87] Accordingly, the drug profile constructed was more than a standard activity spectrum. The screening strategy allowed an analogical assessment between on the one hand the pharmacological activity of the compound and that of standard products in each therapeutic class, and on the other hand the presence of isolated effects that were absent from or only weakly present in the prototype drugs but might be valued in a specific range of indications.[88] Enabling a modular reorganization of preclinical work, I believe that this type of profiling facilitated the back-and-forth movement between pre-scription, research and marketing.

Proof that this preclinical screening strategy became operational, at least for selecting candidate drugs, can be literally read in the new terminology used in Ciba-Geigy's annual research conferences in the early 1970s. In 1971, for instance, Basel's pharmacological laboratory communicated on an unusual drug, a 'pyrrolodibenzazepine derivate, [which] represent[ed], chemically and pharmacologically, a new type of psychoactive drug (*"bisleptic"*) with a spectrum of activity different from all known compounds. It possess[ed] properties that [were] specific both for antidepressant and neuroleptic drugs'.[89] Similarly, 'bipo-lar' drugs, another ad hoc term describing compounds having a bipolar spectrum of action – displaying both anxiolytic and antidepressant patterns in the behav-ioural screen – gained ground in Ciba-Geigy's internal literature in the 1970s.[90]

Conclusion

In the decade following the market introduction of Tofranil, Geigy's preclini-cal psychopharmacological activities gradually stabilized. In the late 1960s, the initial cautiousness sparked by the formidable challenge of producing animal models for psychiatric disorders had given way to a measure of confidence. In 1969, Theobald's team considered that ' [their] available testing techniques for the development of psychopharmaceuticals should continue to provide a good grounding to select, with a relatively good prognosis, candidate drugs compara-ble in terms of clinical effects to commercial drugs'.[91] Judging from this quote, the firm's primary incentive to build a specialized experimental facility proved to provide reasonable success. On the eve of the 1970s, the 'good fortune' of Tofranil had been transformed into a drug selection system internal to the firm. While none of the new psychopharmaceuticals commercialized by the firm in the 1960s stemmed directly from the screening, Geigy nevertheless had developed a full-blown screening programme in the field of psychotropic drugs, i.e., an integrated, streamlined and large-scale therapeutic innovation programme.

In this paper I have tried to show that within an industrial market-driven context, the construction of an equivalency system between the laboratory and the clinic had not only been appreciated at the level of experimental feasibility. It had also been conditioned by marketing practices, taking the form of market studies, cost and benefit analyses and medium- to long-term planning of innovation goals. At Geigy, the subsequent development of psychopharmacological screening took place during a broader and thorough internal reorganization process. At the end of the decade, this resulted in the maturation of an extended scientific marketing system, as well as in the emergence of a managerial culture promoting general management of the screening stretching from chemical synthesis to market launch. A major outcome of this restructuring was the tighter integration of research and development (R&D) activities with market building operations. At Geigy, the entanglement of economic and marketing rationales stood out most clearly in: (1) the adoption of symptoms as the basic working units when defining therapeutic targets; and (2) the weakened differentiation between drug classes. These interrelated processes can be read as resulting from complex feedback effects between the market, the clinic and the laboratory.

First of all, the fragmentation of the signs of mental disorders into a restricted set of functional units that was easier to handle was tied to the very modelling process. At Geigy, the challenge of creating new pharmacological tests was addressed by organizing the modelling process around clinically validated drugs. The firm's pharmacologists tried to produce animal models that could be predictive of the positive and negative properties attributed to Tofranil by clinicians. In this respect, the therapeutic drug, not the psychiatric disorder, constituted the reference point for modelling operations. While building on clinical knowledge and data, this modelling dynamic nevertheless tended to introduce a shift in the conceptualization of depression and its treatment. At least at the experimental level, the mental dimensions of depressions were either obliterated or translated into secondary symptoms, namely psychomotor inhibition and loss of energy.

Throughout the 1960s, the dismemberment of psychiatric conditions into 'target symptoms' was exacerbated by feedback effects between the medical uses of the drugs and marketing operations. As attested by the Tofranil launch campaign, the 'behaviour symptom' unit also became a marketing entity. Geigy attempted to shift the standards of intervention and redefine the boundary of depression by advocating a mixed use of etiological classifications and symptomatic diagnosis. At the same time, the company also recorded medical practices, failures of products and market opportunities, and redefined therapeutic targets and research priorities accordingly. Reflecting on these medical and commercial pressures, the firm's pharmacologists adapted their work practices and changed the meaning and uses of laboratory models. This was the case when in the first half of the 1960s, clinicians' focus on secondary symptoms of agitation and inhibition was an approach adopted by Geigy's pharmacologists in order to organize preclinical work. In my interpretation, the resulting combination of models traditionally associated with different drug classes, respectively, contributed to the emergence of a 'cross-class', symptom-oriented screening logic.

At the experimental level, this focus on symptomatic targets reached its culminating point at the end of the 1960s, when the standard screening battery was formalized. This screening system enabled the selection of candidate compounds presenting a pharmacological spectrum of activity diverging slightly from that of prototype drugs. The drug selection system could thereby operate at the level of the flexible boundaries between the three psychotropic drug classes. As documented above, pharmacologists could correlate the drug profiles of candidate drugs with commercial products of their indication range and with isolated pharmacological effects associated with the other classes of products. From an internal perspective, this screening logic enabled the alignment of laboratory work with marketing strategies and the issue of sales volumes. At the end of the 1960s, when market studies had a growing impact on the organization of industrial research, the company sought to increase its market shares and moved from the professional psychiatric market to the general practice segment. In this context, the firm's management strengthened its focus on the overlapping action of the three psychotropic drug classes, formulating innovation goals centred on symptomatic targets cutting across different psychiatric conditions. At Geigy, this growing focus on the 'behaviour symptom' unit constituted the bedrock to articulate the firm's shifting marketing orientations and strategies with drug assessment and selection practices. In my opinion, however, this process also contributed to produce a disjunction between the definition of therapeutic targets and their association with distinct psychiatric diagnoses.

NOTES

Gaudillière and Thoms, Introduction

1. The Institute for Medical Statistics was a US company but in 1959 it opened a German branch. Its panel of surveyed pharmacies and physicians was stabilized by the mid-1960s, providing data on global sales as well as on individual products and classes of drugs.

2. 'Der Werbeaufwand marktstarker Arzneimittelhersteller im Zeitraum Januar bis Dezember 1973 und ihr Jahresumsatz', *Arznei-Telegramm*, 5 (1974), pp. 1–34.

3. A short note in the same issue of the journal referred to an article in the *Medical Tribune*, 10 (1974) to prove its ineffectiveness. See *Arznei-Telegramm*, 1 (1974), p. 36.

4. 'Nattermann will auf die Berichterstattung des arznei-telegramm Einfluss nehmen', *Arznei-Telegramm*, 5 (1974), p. 74.

5. 'Werbung bei Ärzten kritisch betrachtet', *Emnid-Informationen*, 27 (July 1958), pp. 4–5.

6. See, for instance, M. Angell, *The Truth about the Drug Companies: How They Deceive Us and What to Do about It* (New York: Random House, 2004); M. Goozner, *The $800 Million Pill: The Truth Behind the Cost of New Drugs* (Berkeley, CA, and Los Angeles, CA: University of California Press, 2004); J. Robinson, *Prescription Games: Life, Death and Money Inside the Global Pharmaceutical Industry* (London: Simon & Schuster, 2001); K. Langbein, H. Weiss, H.-P. Martin and R. Werner, *Gesunde Geschäfte. Die Praktiken der Pharma-Industrie* (Cologne: Kiepenheuer und Witsch, 1981); C. Walter and A. Kobylinski, *Patient im Visier: Die neue Strategie der Pharmakonzerne* (Hamburg: Hoffman und Campe, 2011); M. Keller, 'Geben und einnehmen', Dossier, *Die Zeit*, 19 May 2005, at http://www.zeit.de/2005/21/Pharmafirmen_neu [accessed 11 December 2014].

7. W. Bartmann, *Zwischen Tradition und Fortschritt: aus der Geschichte der Pharmabereiche von Bayer, Hoechst und Schering von 1935–1975* (Stuttgart: Franz Steiner Verlag, 2003); M. Bürgi, *Pharmaforschung im 20. Jahrhundert – Arbeit an der Grenze zwischen Hochschule und Industrie* (Zurich: Chronos Verlag, 2011); A. D. Chandler Jr, *Shaping the Industrial Century: The Remarkable Story of the Evolution of the Modern Chemical and Pharmaceutical Industry* (Cambridge, MA: Harvard University Press, 2009).

8. S. Chauveau, *L'invention pharmaceutique. La pharmacie française entre l'État et la société au XXe siècle* (Paris: Les empêcheurs de penser en rond, 1999); V. Quirke, *Collaboration in the Pharmaceutical Industry: Changing Relationships in Britain and France,*

1935–1965 (New York: Routledge, 2008); D. Tobell, *Pills, Power and Policy: The Struggle for Drug Reform in Cold War America and its Consequences* (Berkeley, CA: University of California Press, 2011); D. Carpenter, *Reputation and Power: Organizational Image and Pharmaceutical Regulation at the FDA* (Princeton, NJ: Princeton University Press, 2010); J.-P. Gaudillière and V. Hess (eds), *Ways of Regulating Drugs in the 19th and 20th Centuries* (Basingstoke and New York: Palgrave Macmillan, 2012); W. Wimmer, 'Wir haben fast immer was Neues': Gesundheitswesen und Innovationen der Pharma-Industrie in Deutschland, 1880–1935* (Berlin: Duncker & Humblot, 1994).

9.   G. Huhle-Kreutzer, *Die Entwicklung arzneilicher Produktionsstätten aus Apothekenlaboratorien, dargestellt an ausgewählten Beispielen* (Stuttgart: Deutscher Apotheker Verlag, 1989).

10.   E. Hickel, *Arzneimittel-Standardisierung im 19. Jahrhundert in den Pharmakopöen Deutschlands, Frankreichs, Großbritanniens und der Vereinigten Staaten von Amerika* (Stuttgart: Wissenschaftliche Verlagsgesellschaft, 1973).

11.   U. Thoms, 'Arzneimittelaufsicht im frühen 19. Jahrhundert. Konflikte und Konvergenzen zwischen Wissen, Expertise und regulativer Politik', in E. J. Engstrom, V. Hess and U. Thoms (eds), *Figurationen des Experten. Ambivalenzen der wissenschaftlichen Expertise im ausgehenden 18. und frühen 19. Jahrhundert* (Frankfurt et al.: Peter Lang Verlag, 2005), pp. 123–46.

12.   On Germany, see Wimmer, 'Wir haben fast immer was Neues'. On France, see Chauveau, *L'invention pharmaceutique*. On ways of regulating, see Gaudillière and Hess (eds), *Ways of Regulating Drugs in the 19th and 20th Centuries*.

13.   For a review, see J.-P. Gaudillière, 'L'industrialisation du médicament: une histoire de pratique entre sciences, techniques, droit et médecine', *Gesnerus*, 64 (2007), pp. 93–108. J.-P. Gaudillière, 'Une manière industrielle de savoir: sciences, innovations et capitalisme au XXème siècle. Le cas de la pharmacie', in C. Bonneuil and D. Pestre (eds), *Les Sciences au XXème siècle* (Paris: Éditions du Seuil, forthcoming).

14.   H. Berghoff (ed.), *Marketinggeschichte: Die Genese einer modernen Sozialtechnik* (Frankfurt and New York: Campus Verlag GmbH., 2007); H. Berghoff, P. Scranton and U. Spiekermann (eds), *The Rise of Marketing and Market Research* (New York: Palgrave Macmillan, 2012); R. Tedlow, *New and Improved: The Story of Mass Marketing in America* (New York: Basic Books, 1990); R. Tedlow, G. Jones (eds), *The Rise and Fall of Mass Marketing* (London: Routledge, 1993).

15.   J. Greene, *Prescribing by Numbers: Drugs and the Definition of Disease* (Baltimore, MD: Johns Hopkins University Press, 2007); E. Siegel Watkins, *The Estrogen Elixir: A History of Hormone Replacement Therapy in America* (Baltimore, MD: Johns Hopkins University Press, 2007); J. A. Greene and E. Siegel Watkins (eds), *Prescribed: Writing, Filling, Using, and Abusing the Prescription in Modern America* (Baltimore, MD: John Hopkins University Press, 2012).

16.   J.-P. Gaudillière (ed.), *How Pharmaceuticals Became Patentable in the Twentieth Century*, special issue, *History and Technology*, 24:2 (June 2008), pp. 99–106.

17.   For doctors' early twentieth century perception of advertising for drugs, see Wimmer, *Wir haben fast immer was Neues*; Thoms, 'Arzneimittelaufsicht'.

18.   J. P. Swann, *Academic Scientists and the Pharmaceutical Industry: Cooperative Research in Twentieth-Century America* (Baltimore, MD: Johns Hopkins University Press, 1988); V. Quirke, *Collaboration in the Pharmaceutical Industry: Changing Relationships in Britain and France, 1935–1965* (New York: Routledge, 2008); N. Rasmussen, 'The Moral Economy of the Drug Company–Medical Scientist Collaboration in Interwar

America', *Social Studies of Science*, 34:2 (2004), pp. 161–85; J.-P. Gaudillière, 'Better Prepared than Synthesized: Adolf Butenandt, Schering AG and the Transformation of Sex Steroids into Drugs', *Studies in History and Philosophy of Science*, 36:4 (2005), pp. 612–44; Wimmer, '*Wir haben fast immer was Neues*'.

19. A. Hüntelmann, 'A *Different* Mode of Marketing? The Importance of Scientific Articles in the Marketing Process of Salvarsan', *History and Technology*, 29 (2013), pp. 116–34; C. Bonah, '"The Strophanthin Question": Early Scientific Marketing of Cardiac Drugs in Two National Markets (France and Germany 1900–1930)', *History and Technology*, 29 (2013), pp. 135–52; Wimmer, '*Wir haben fast immer was Neues*'.

20. See U. Thoms, 'Standardising Selling: Pharmaceutical Marketing, the Enterprise and the Marketing Expert (1900–1990)', in J.-P. Gaudillière and U. Thoms (eds), *Standardizing and Marketing Drugs in the Twentieth Century*, special issue, *History and Technology* 29 (2013), pp. 169–87.

21. According to the FDA, '[e]xpanded access, sometimes called 'compassionate use', is the use of an investigational drug outside of a clinical trial to treat a patient with a serious or immediately life-threatening disease or condition who has no comparable or satisfactory alternative treatment options'. FDA, 'Access to Investigational Drugs outside of a Clinical Trial' (Expanded Access), at http://www.fda.gov/ForConsumers/ByAudience/ForPatientAdvocates/AccesstoInvestigationalDrugs/ucm176098.htm [accessed 30 September 2013].

22. See, amongst others, W. R. Leach, *Land of Desire: Merchants, Power, and the Rise of a New American Culture* (New York: Pantheon Books, 1993); L. Cohen, *A Consumers' Republic: The Politics of Mass Consumption in Postwar America* (New York: Alfred A. Knopf, 2003); V. de Grazia, *Irresistible Empire: America's Advance through Twentieth-Century Europe* (Cambridge, MA: Belknap Press of the Harvard University Press, 2005); A. Chatriot, M.-E. Chessel and M. Hilton (eds), *The Expert Consumer: Associations and Professionals in Consumer Society* (Hants, England: Ashgate Publishing Limited, 2006); C. Kleinschmidt, *Konsumgesellschaft* (Göttingen: Vandenhoeck & Ruprecht, 2008), pp. 13–28; F. Trentmann, *The Making of the Consumer: Knowledge, Power and Identity in the Modern World* (Oxford: Berg Publishers, 2006); P. N. Stearns, *Consumerism in World History: The Global Transformation of Desire* (New York and London: Routledge, 2001); H.-G. Haupt and C. Torp, *Die Konsumgesellschaft in Deutschland 1890–1990* (Frankfurt: Campus Verlag, 2009); N. Gasteiger, *Der Konsument: Verbraucherbilder in Werbung, Konsumkritik und Verbraucherschutz 1945–1989* (Frankfurt: Campus Verlag, 2010).

1 Kessel , Beyond Innovation: Pharmaceutical Marketing, Market Structure and the Importance of the 'Old' in West Germany, 1950–70

1. B. Godin, 'Innovation: The History of a Category', Project on the Intellectual History of Innovation, Working Paper No. 1 (2008), p. 4, at http://www.csiic.ca/PDF/IntellectualNo1.pdf [accessed 2 August 2013].

2. For example: J. Liebenau, 'Innovation in Pharmaceuticals: Industrial R&D in the Early Twentieth Century', *Research Policy*, 14 (1985), pp. 179–87; J. Liebenau, *Medical Science and Medical Industry: The Formation of the American Pharmaceutical Industry* (Baltimore, MD: Johns Hopkins University Press, 1987).

3. Drugs are considered as technologies in Edgerton's sense: D. E. H. Edgerton, *The Shock of the Old: Technology and Global History since 1900* (Oxford: Oxford University Press, 2007).

4. Certainly, Edgerton's remarks essentially refer to consumer and military technologies. But whilst referencing Malaria therapy and contraception he also integrates examples from the history of pharmaceuticals. Edgerton, *The Shock of the Old*, pp. 22–6.

5. D. Dunlop, 'Use and Abuse of Drugs', *British Medical Journal*, 2:5459 (1965), pp. 437–41, on p. 438.

6. Dunlop, 'Use and Abuse of Drugs', p. 438.

7. J. Abraham, 'Pharmaceuticalization of Society in Context: Theoretical, Empirical and Health Dimensions', *Sociology*, 44 (2010), pp. 603–22, on p. 613.

8. NCE is the older term used between the 1960s and the 1990s, while NME has been in use since the 1990s. R. Vos, *Drugs Looking for Diseases: Innovative Drug Research and the Development of the Beta Blockers and the Calcium Antagonists* (Dordrecht, Boston, MA, and London: Kluwer, 1991).

9. Hereafter, I will use the term 'technological innovation' to denote this restrictive understanding of drug innovation and 'commercial innovation' for its understanding in a broader sense. Economic literature differentiates between 'radical' and 'incremental' innovation. See L. A. Stewart, 'The Impact of Regulation on Innovation in the United States: A Cross-Industry Literature Review', in Institute of Medicine of the National Academies (ed.), *Health IT and Patient Safety: Building Safer Systems for Better Care* (National Academies Press: Washington DC, 2012), at http://www.iom.edu//media/ Files/Report%20Files/2011/Health-IT/Commissioned-paper-Impact-of-Regulation-on-Innovation.pdf [accessed 2 August 2013].

10. Anne Rasmussen shows how galenics became an essential tool to obtain patients' acceptance of drugs. See A. Rasmussen, 'Les enjeux d'une histoire des formes pharmaceutiques: La galénique, l'officine et l'industrie (XIXe–début XXe siècle)', *Entreprises et Histoire*, 2:36 (2004), pp. 12–28.

11. See U. Thoms's contribution to this volume.

12. 'Presentation' of the ESF DRUGS programme at http://drughistory.eu/ [accessed 29 August 2013].

13. Yet in contrast to master narratives of a problem-free, successful, inevitable introduction of new therapeutics, many recent studies have shown that drug innovation was less upright, disinterested and driven by humanistic values than claimed by the legends told by some physicians and manufacturers. New studies have shown that not so much the genius of great drug inventors, but more complex configurations of different actors such as manufacturers, scientific personnel both in companies and in universities, subsidiaries and public authorities, have driven forward the introduction of new drugs. See B. Bächi, *Vitamin C für alle! Pharmazeutische Produktion, Vermarktung und Gesundheitspolitik (1933–1953)* (Zurich: Chronos Verlag, 2009); M. Bürgi, *Pharmaforschung im 20. Jahrhundert – Arbeit an der Grenze zwischen Hochschule und Industrie* (Zurich: Chronos Verlag, 2011); J. A. Greene, *Prescribing by Numbers: Drugs and the Definition of Disease* (Baltimore, MD: Johns Hopkins University Press, 2007); T. Pieters, *Interferon: The Science and Selling of a Miracle Drug* (London and New York: Routledge, 2005); C. Ratmoko, *Damit die Chemie stimmt. Die Anfänge der industriellen Herstellung von weiblichen und männlichen Sexualhormonen 1914–1938* (Zurich: Chronos Verlag, 2010).

14. Other uses, for example for diagnosis, are not discussed here.

15. U. Thoms's paper in this volume cites Bayer records using 18,000. Other accounts mention 50,000 or even 70,000 products on the market according to different ways of counting.
16. See, for example, E. Bay, 'Der Arzneimittelmissbrauch des "modernen Menschen"', *Deutsche Medizinische Wochenschrift*, 85:38 (1960), pp. 1676–80; P. Kielholz, 'Tablettensucht. Eine der "Sieben Todsünden des Menschen von heute". Bericht über den Eröffnungsvortrag der Internationalen Fortbildungskongresse der Bundesärztekammer 1967 in Davos und Badgastein', *Deutsches Ärzteblatt – Ärztliche Mitteilungen*, 64:14 (1967), pp. 740–3. Physicians had been complaining about uncontrolled consumption of certain kinds of drugs since the late nineteenth century.
17. Kielholz, 'Tablettensucht', p. 740.
18. See for example the advertisements for Ring-Tablette, *Bunte Münchner Illustrierte*, 12 (1961), p. 20.
19. See for example the painkiller advertisements in the West German tabloid magazine *Bunte Münchner Illustrierte*, particularly the advertisement for Spalt in *Bunte Münchner Illustrierte*, 17 (1961), p. 20.
20. H. U. Zollinger, 'Chronische interstitielle Nephritis bei Abusus von phenacetinhaltigen Analgetika (Saridon usw.)', *Schweizerische Medizinische Wochenschrift*, 85:31 (1955), p. 746.
21. IMS Health GmbH, Company Archives, Der pharmazeutische Markt 1966–1974, 2 vols, vol. 1: *Einheiten* (hereafter DPM 1966–74).
22. The figures are pharmacy purchases and wholesalers' figures. They do not indicate consumption figures, as pharmacy orders do not say how many packages were sold and then consumed. The fact that many drug packages are thrown away without being consumed makes it impossible to quantify consumption reliably.
23. The 1950s number is either five or six because for one product, two different years of introduction are given: 1947 and 1952.
24. It should be kept in mind that neither dosage differences nor package sizes are taken into account in this sales-oriented way of counting drugs. Nevertheless, for this specific therapeutic class of analgesics, package size did not differ much amongst the products. Most were sold in small units of ten or twenty tablets. Bigger package size of 100, 500 or 1,000 pills did not account for much in sales figures. Dosage differences are strongly relevant for therapeutic effects but do not affect the general trend discussed above.
25. Kielholz, 'Tablettensucht', pp. 740–3.
26. 'Die Tablettomanen', *Der Spiegel*, 11:27 (1958), pp. 56–7.
27. The commercial classification used here is that of IMS Health of the 1970s. It is basically one of the first Anatomic Therapeutic Chemical (ATC) classifications.
28. Glutethimide is also a barbiturate derivative.
29. This is mainly due to the fact that commercially pure products are more interesting for clinical practice and therapeutic novelty.
30. IMS Health GmbH, Company Archives, Der pharmazeutische Markt 1974, pp. 609–30 (hereafter DPM 1974).
31. B. Kirk, *Der Contergan-Fall: Eine unvermeidbare Arzneimittelkatastrophe? Zur Geschichte des Arzneistoffs Thalidomid* (Stuttgart: Wissenschaftliche Verlagsgesellschaft, 1999).
32. W. Abelshauser, *Deutsche Wirtschaftsgeschichte. Von 1945 bis zur Gegenwart* (Munich: C. H. Beck, 2011), p. 427 refers to numbers given in R. G. Stokes, 'Assessing the Damages: Forced Technology Transfer and the Chemical Industry', in M. Judt and B. Ciesla

(eds), *Technology Transfer out of Germany after 1945* (Amsterdam: Harwood Academic Publishers, 1996), p. 87. Given that Abelshauser refers to the chemical industry as a whole, his argument should also be valid for the pharmaceutical sector.

33. DPM 1966–74, vol. 1, pp. 271–8.

34. 'Pillen vom Opa', *Der Spiegel*, 29:4 (1975), pp. 100–1.

35. For example, capsules were considered to be genuinely 'modern' galenic forms in contrast to tablets by Swiss manufacturer Ciba. See Minutes of the Pharma-Verkaufskonferenz Meeting, 11 January 1961, Novartis AG Company Archives, Ciba, Vf Ph1: Pharma-Verkaufskonferenz, p.3.

36. The concept of '*icône culturelle*' is developed in D. C. Meyer, 'Icônes culturelles: lecture textuelle et contextuelle', in *Synergies Chine*, 6 (2011), pp. 223–33.

37. See the advertisements in *Bunte Illustrierte*, 1 (1955), no pagination.

38. See the advertisement in *Bunte Illustrierte*, 3 (1955), no pagination.

39. See the advertisements in *Bunte Illustrierte*, 1 (1955), no pagination.

40. I use the term marketing here to encompass all commercial activities intended to increase sales while the term advertising is used restrictively as the print, radio or film products used to encourage sales.

41. 'Kaiserliche Verordnung betreffend den Verkehr mit Arzneimitteln vom 22. Oktober 1901', *Reichsgesetzblatt*, I (1901), p. 380.

42. 'Polizeiverordnung über die Werbung auf dem Gebiete des Heilwesens vom 29 September 1941', *Reichsgesetzblatt*, I (1941), pp. 587–90.

43. *Bunte Illustrierte*, 1 (1955), p. 26.

44. See for example advertisements for the tonics Regipan and Buerlecithin in *Bunte Illustrierte*, 29 (1957), p. 22 and in *Bunte Münchner Illustrierte*, 13 (1961), p. 44.

45. On nervousness at the turn of the twentieth century see W. Eckart, 'Die wachsende Nervosität unserer Zeit. Medizin und Kultur um 1900 am Beispiel einer Modekrankheit', in G. Hübinger, R. vom Bruch and F. W. Graf (eds), *Kultur und Kulturwissenschaften um 1900 II: Idealismus und Positivismus* (Stuttgart: Franz Steiner Verlag, 1997), pp. 207–26.

46. Diagnose 'Neurasthenie', IMS Verschreibungsindex für Pharmazeutika 1968, IMS Health Company Archives, VIP Volumes, p. D183.

47. See advertisement for Regipan and Buerlecithin in *Bunte Illustrierte*, 29 (1957), p. 22.

48. A Frauengold advertisement in *Bunte Illustrierte*, 12 (1955), p. 34, stated: 'Frauengold mobilizes the female organism and brings about natural youthful vigour, a flourishing appearance, inner balance and refreshing beauty sleep'. ('Frauengold mobilisiert den weiblichen Organismus und schenkt auf diesem natürlichen Wege jugendliche Frische, blühendes Aussehen und innere Ausgeglichenheit und einen erquickenden Schönheitsschlaf'.)

49. Diagnose 'Vegetative Dystonie', IMS Verschreibungsindex für Pharmazeutika 1968, IMS Health Company Archives, VIP Volumes, p. D181.

50. Contemporary drug abuse research has confirmed that general practitioners tend to prefer pharmaceuticals with a wide range of indications rather than those with a narrower one. See G. Glaeske, 'Pharmakologische Versorgung und präventive Drogenpolitik: Arzneimittel – legale Alltagsdrogen vom Dealer in weiß?', in B. Schmidt and K. Hurrelmann (eds), *Präventive Sucht- und Drogenpolitik. Ein Handbuch* (Opladen: Leske and Budrich, 2000), pp. 112–28, on p. 114.

51. Specialists were nevertheless seen more often for somatic diseases.

52. The history of the *DSM* is summarized in S. Demazeux, *Qu'est-ce que le DSM? Genèse et*

transformations de la bible américaine de la psychiatrie (Paris: Éditions d'Ithaque, 2013), pp. 25–95.

53. See Jean-Paul Gaudillière's article in this volume.
54. E. Greiser and E. Westermann, *Verordnungen niedergelassener Ärzte in Niedersachsen 1974 und 1976: Untersuchungen zu Verordnungen niedergelassener Kassenärzte für Patienten von RVO-Kassen im ersten Halbjahr 1974 und 1976* (Bonn: Bundesministerium für Arbeit und Sozialordnung, 1979).
55. D. E. H. Edgerton, *The Shock of the Old: Technology and Global History since 1900* (Oxford: Oxford University Press, 2007).
56. See the narrative of a therapeutic revolution in L. Lasagna, 'Recent Trends in Drug Development', in G. Higby and E. C. Stroud (eds), *The Inside Story of Medicines: A Symposium* (Madison, WI: American Institute of the History of Pharmacy, 1997), pp. 217–22, on p. 217. Although critical in account, many studies do comfort the vision of the pharmaceutical industry's capacity to perfectly transform markets in their favour. See, for example, D. Healy, *Let Them Eat Prozac: The Unhealthy Relationship between the Pharmaceutical Industry and Depression* (New York and London: New York University Press, 2004); N. Rasmussen, *On Speed: The Many Lives of Amphetamines* (New York: New York University Press, 2008).
57. B. Bächi, 'Vitamin C für alle! Pharmazeutische Produktion, Vermarktung und Gesundheitspolitik 1933–1953' (Zurich: Chronos-Verlag 2009).
58. J. Abraham, 'Pharmaceuticalization of Society in Context: Theoretical, Empirical and Health Dimensions', in *Sociology*, 44 (2010), pp. 603–22.
59. N. Rose, 'Beyond Medicalisation', *Lancet*, 369 (2007), pp. 700–2, on p. 702.
60. A critical study of pharmaceutical marketing practices that revealed the systematic collection of information on individual physicians' attitudes that was provided by medical representatives is K. Langbein, H. Weiss, H.-P. Martin and R. Werner, *Gesunde Geschäfte. Die Praktiken der Pharma-Industrie* (Cologne: Kiepenheuer und Witsch, 1981).

2 Thoms, Innovation, Life Cycles and Cybernetics in Marketing: Theoretical Concepts in the Scientific Marketing of Drugs and their Consequences

1. Maier, Protokoll der 2. Sitzung der Fachkommission Marktforschung, 4 June 1973, Bayer Archive, 326/23, p. 7, my translation.
2. The situation in the US was similar: out of 500 newly introduced prescription drugs, 400 failed. See C. Winick, 'The Diffusion of an Innovation among Physicians in a Large City', *Sociometry*, 24 (1961), pp. 384–96, on p. 384.
3. The term 'product life cycle' is so self-explanatory that even the special issue of the *Journal of Historical Research in Marketing* on the key terms in marketing did not at all discuss it. Instead the journal published an article on the life course, i.e., the age groups or the different stages of life in marketing research. See M. Bauer and K. J. Auer-Srnka, 'The Life Cycle Concept in Marketing Research', *Journal of Historical Research in Marketing*, 4 (2012), pp. 68–96. For recent work on the topic see, amongst others, H. Siegwart and R. Senti, *Product Life Cycle Management. Die Gestaltung eines integrierten Produktlebenszyklus* (Stuttgart: Schäffer-Poeschel Verlag, 1995); A.-C. Raasch, *Der Patentauslauf von Pharmazeutika als Herausforderung beim Management des*

Produktlebenszyklus (Wiesbaden: Gabler Verlag, 2006).

4. B. Lohff, 'Fortschritt mit der Wissenschaft: Wissenschaft ist Fortschritt. Der Wandel der Fortschrittsidee in der deutschen Medizin im 19. Jahrhundert', in W. Deppert, H. Kliemt, B. Lohff and J. Schaefer (eds), *Wissenschaftstheorien in der Medizin. Ein Symposium* (Berlin and New York: Walter de Gruyter, 1992), pp. 328–54.

5. For a recent understanding of the function of innovation for the development of new drugs, see 'Innovation im Arzneimittelmarkt', at http://wido.de/arz_innovation.html [accessed 6 September 2013].

6. N. Gasteiger, *Der Konsument. Verbraucherbilder in Werbung, Konsumkritik und Verbraucherschutz 1945–1989* (Frankfurt: Campus Verlag, 2010), pp. 64ff.; 'Heilmittelwerbung. Selbstverantwortung statt Vorzensur', *Verbraucherkorrespondenz*, 15:7 (1968), pp. 7–8.

7. J. Liebenau, 'Innovation in Pharmaceuticals: Industrial R&D in the Early Twentieth Century', *Research Policy*, 14 (1985), pp. 179–87.

8. 'Minutes', Pharmaceutische Conferenz, 6–7 November 1900, Bayer Archive 169/3, p. 11ff.

9. As stated by Carl Duisberg in 1899 at a conference at Bayer. See 'Minutes', Pharmaceutische Conferenz, 16–17 November 1899, Bayer Archive 169/3, p. 28.

10. 'Minutes', Pharmaceutische Conferenz, 21 November 1901, Bayer Archive 169/3, p. 35.

11. J. A. Schumpeter, *Business Cycles: A Theoretical, Historical, and Statistical Analysis of the Capitalist Process*, 2 vols (New York: McGraw-Hill, 1939). On Schumpeter, see T. K. McCraw, *Joseph A. Schumpeter: Eine Biografie* (Hamburg: Murmann-Verlag GmbH, 2008); A. Schäfer, *Die Kraft der schöpferischen Zerstörung: Joseph A. Schumpeter. Die Biografie* (Frankfurt: Campus Verlag, 2008).

12. Schumpeter, *Business Cycles*, vol. 1, p. 20.

13. G. Bergler, *Der chemisch-pharmazeutische Markenartikel, PhD. Handelshochschule Nürnberg* (Stuttgart: J. B. Metzlersche Buchdruckerei Stuttgart, 1931), p. 19.

14. For the figures, see R. Landry, N. Amara and N. Becheickh, 'Exploring Innovation Failures in Manufacturing Industries', paper presented at the conference, Entrepreneurship and Innovation: Organizations, Institutions, Systems and Regions, 17–20 June 2008, Copenhagen, CBS, Denmark, p. 2, at http://www2.druid.dk/conferences/viewpaper. php?id=3378&cf=29 [accessed 6 September 2013]; B. Munoz, 'Lessons from 60 years of Pharmaceutical Innovation', *Nature Reviews in Drug Discovery*, 8 (2009), pp. 959–68.

15. P. Ormerod, *Why Most Things Fail: Evolution, Extinction and Economics* (New York: Wiley, 2005); R. Bauer, *Gescheiterte Innovationen. Fehlschläge und technologischer Wandel* (Frankfurt: Campus Verlag, 2006); I. Koehler and R. Rossfeld (eds), *Pleitiers und Bankrotteure: Geschichte des ökonomischen Scheiterns vom 18. bis 20. Jahrhundert* (Frankfurt: Campus Verlag, 2012). For the sales of new and old drugs, see Nils Kessel's paper in this volume.

16. Some of these histories have been written by authors who have otherwise massively criticized pharmaceutical markets. See N. Rasmussen, *On Speed: The Many Lives of Amphetamine* (New York: New York University Press, 2008); D. Healy, *Let Them Eat Prozac: The Unhealthy Relationship between the Pharmaceutical Industry and Depression* (New York: New York University Press, 2004).

17. 'Schering forciert die Forschung. Neue Produkte brachten Umsatzsteigerung', *Die Zeit*, 24 (6 November 1965), p. 36; G. Benz, R. Hahn and C. Reinhardt, *100 Jahre*

chemisch-wissenschaftliches Laboratorium der Bayer AG in Wuppertal-Elberfeld 1896–1996 (Leverkusen: Bayer AG, 1996).

18. Figures taken from Schering Aktiengesellschaft: Bericht über das Geschäftsjahr 1960, Berlin und Bergkamen, Berlin 1969, p. 38; Geschäftsbericht Schering Aktiengesellschaft (Berlin: Schering, 1984), p. 39.

19. Member surveys were conducted yearly starting in 1971/2, but until 1978 research expenses were only given together with license fees. See Bundesverband der Pharmazeutischen Industrie e.V.: Pharma-Daten 1978 (Berlin: BPI, 1978), p. 13.

20. Geschäftsbericht Bayer 1954, p. 3, Bayer Archive, 166/15.

21. K. Steinmüller, 'Zukunftsforschung: Hundert Jahre Geschichte', *Swissfuture – das Magazin für Zukunftsmonitoring*, 3 (2010), at http://www.z-punkt.de/fileadmin/be_user/D_Publikationen/D_Fachartikel/2010_Swissfuture_Geschichte_der_ZF.pdf [accessed 6 September 2013]; A. Schmidt-Gernig, 'Die gesellschaftliche Konstruktion der Zukunft. Westeuropäische Zukunftsforschung und Gesellschaftsplanung zwischen 1950 und 1980', *WeltTrends. Zeitschrift für internationale Politik und vergleichende Studien*, 18 (1998), pp. 63–84.

22. N. Wiener, *Cybernetics or Control and Communication in the Animal and the Machine* (Cambridge, MA: Massachusetts Institute of Technology Press, 1948). These conferences were organized by the Macy Foundation and began in 1946. See the publication of transactions and other documents in C. Pias (ed.), *Cybernetics – Kybernetik: The Macy-Conferences 1946–1953*, 2 vols (Zürich and Berlin: Diaphanes, 2003 and 2004), and a historical account in S. J. Heims, *The Cybernetics Group* (Cambridge, MA: Massachusetts Institute of Technology Press, 1991); I. Clerc, *Am Quellcode des Verhaltens. Die Macy-Konferenzen und die Kybernetisierung verhaltenswissenschaftlicher Theorien* (Heidelberg: Carl-Auer Verlag, 2009).

23. In the past years, systems research and futurology have found considerable interest. From the huge body of literature, see only A. Brinckmann, 'The Studiengruppe für Systemforschung: Systems Research and Policy Advice in the Federal Republic of Germany 1958–1975', *Minerva*, 24 (2006), pp. 149–66; K. F. Hünemörder, 'Die Heidelberger Studiengruppe für Systemforschung und der Aufstieg der Zukunftsforschung in den 1960er Jahren', *Technikfolgenabschätzung. Theorie und Praxis*, 13 (2004), pp. 8–15; R. Kreibich, 'Wissenschaftsverständnis und Methodik der Zukunftsforschung', *Zeitschrift für Semiotik*, 29 (2007), pp. 177–98; A. Schmidt-Gernig, 'Die Geburt der Zukunftsforschung aus dem Geist der Kybernetik', *Zeitschrift für Semiotik*, 29 (2007), pp. 199–210; M. Hagner and E. Hörl (eds), *Die Transformation des Humanen: Beiträge zur Kulturgeschichte der Kybernetik* (Frankfurt: Suhrkamp Verlag, 2008). With a focus on research planning, see A. Malycha and U. Thoms, 'Aufbruch in eine neue Zukunft? Biowissenschaftliche Prognosen in der DDR und der Bundesrepublik in den 1960er und 1970er Jahren', in H. Hartmann and J. Vogel (eds), *Zukunftswissen. Prognosen in Wirtschaft, Politik und Gesellschaft seit 1900* (Frankfurt: Campus Verlag, 2010), pp. 107–34. The very first institute for opinion research had been founded in 1935 by George Gallup, the vice president of the advertising agency Young & Rubicam in New York City. On the history of opinion research in Germany, see A. Kruke, *Demokopie in der Bundesrepublik Deutschland. Meinungsforschung, Parteien und Medien 1949–1990* (Berlin: Droste Verlag, 2007).

24. 'The Ciba Foundation', in A. de Reuck, M. Goldsmith and J. Knight (eds), *Decision Making in National Science Policy: A Ciba Foundation and Science of Science Foundation Symposium* (Boston, MA: Little, Brown and Company, 1968), p. ix, at http://onlineli-

brary.wiley.com/doi/10.1002/9780470719619.fmatter/pdf [accessed 7 September 2013].

25. 'The Ciba Foundation', p. ix.

26. G. E. W. Wolstenholme (ed.), *Man and his Future: A Ciba Foundation Volume* (Boston, MA, and Toronto: Little, Brown and Company, 1963).

27. Between 1954 and 1970 seventeen volumes with the proceedings from the symposia were published.

28. G. E. W. Wolstenholme, C. M. O'Connor and M. O'Connor (eds), for the Ciba Foundation, *Significant Trends in Medical Research* (London: J. & A. Churchill Ltd, 1959).

29. C. H. Waddington, 'Introduction', *The Future as an Academic Discipline*, in Ciba Foundation Symposium, new series, 36 (Amsterdam and New York: Elsevier, 1975), p. 2.

30. For the links between opinion research and the economy see A. Nützenadel, 'Die Vermessung der Zukunft. Empirische Wirtschaftsforschung und ökonomische Prognostik nach 1945', in Hartmann and Vogel (eds), *Zukunftswissen*, pp. 55–75, on pp. 56–8.

31. For a history of mass communication research see M. Schenk, *Medienwirkungsforschung, 2. vollständig überarb. Aufl.* (Tübingen: Mohr Siebeck, 2002); M. Jäckel, *Medienwirkungen. Ein Studienbuch zur Einführung*, 4th rev. edn (Wiesbaden: VS Verlag für Sozialwissenschaften, 2008).

32. Schering had had extremely unfavourable experiences in the 1930s and therefore limited its advertising. Though the firm had spent 127 per cent of the Veramon sales on advertising, there was almost no change in the sales figures. See the report 'Beratung und Revision der Abteilung Dr. Schüssler durch H. F .J. Kropff', Schering Archives, Bayer AG, B02/244, p. 6ff.

33. G. Albus, 'Pharma-Werbung – Probleme und Folgerungen', *Pharmazeutische Industrie*, 28 (1966), pp. 5–7; H. Friesewinkel, 'Der Arzt und die Werbung', *Pharmazeutische Industrie*, 28 (1966), pp. 122–36, 200–5, 287–91, 372–9, 448–54, 535–7.

34. The new ideas and methods were brought to Germany by young German researchers who travelled to the USA, and who then founded their own institutes or began to work in the existing ones. See U. Thoms, 'Standardising Selling: Pharmaceutical Marketing, the Enterprise and the Marketing Expert (1900–1990)', in J.-P. Gaudillière and U. Thoms (eds), *Standardizing and Marketing Drugs in the 20th Century*, special Issue of *History and Technology*, 29 (2013), pp. 169–87.

35. P. F. Lazarsfeld, B. Berelson and H. Gaudet, *The People's Choice: How the Voter Makes up his Mind in a Presidential Campaign* (New York: Duell, Sloane and Pearce, 1944).

36. U. Hansen and M. Bode, *Marketing & Konsum. Theorie und Praxis von der Industrialisierung bis ins 21. Jahrhundert* (Munich: Franz Vahlen, 1999), pp. 109–11.

37. E. Katz, 'The Two-Step-Flow of Communication: An Up-To-Date Report on an Hypothesis', Annenberg School for Communication (ASC) Departmental Papers (Philadelphia, PA: University of Pennsylvania, 1957), at http://repository.upenn.edu/cgi/viewcontent.cgi?article=1279&context=asc_papers [accessed 30 May 2013].

38. E. Katz and H. Menzel, *On the Flow of Scientific Information in the Medical Profession*, unpublished (Columbia University Bureau of Applied Social Research, New York, 1954); H. Menzel, 'Social Determinants of Physicians' Reactions to Innovations in Medical Practice' (PhD dissertation, University of Wisconsin, 1959); H. Menzel and E. Katz, 'Social Relations and Innovation in the Medical Profession: The Epidemiology of a New Drug', *Public Opinion Quarterly*, 27 (1955–6), pp. 337–52. Following publications: H. Menzel, 'Public and Private Conformity under Different Conditions of Acceptance in the Group', *Journal of Abnormal and Social Psychology*, 55 (1957),

pp. 398–402; H. Menzel, J. Coleman and E. Katz, 'Dimensions of Being Modern in Medical Practice', *Journal of Chronic Diseases*, 9 (1959), pp. 20–40; H. Menzel, 'Innovation, Integration, and Marginality: A Survey of Physicians', *American Sociological Review*, 25:5 (1960), pp. 704–13. Several subsequent publications of the trials followed, and in 1966 the detailed full report was published as a book under the title *Medical Innovation: A Diffusion Study*. J. Coleman, H. Menzel and E. Katz, 'Social Processes in Physicians' Adoption of a New Drug', *Journal of Chronic Diseases*, 9:1 (1959), pp. 1–19; J. Coleman, 'The Diffusion of an Innovation among Physicians', *Sociometry*, 20:4 (1957), pp. 253–70; J. Coleman, E. Katz and H. Menzel, *Medical Innovation: A Diffusion Study* (New York: Bobbs-Merrill Co., 1966).

39. T. Caplow, 'Market Attitude: A Research Report from the Medical Field', *Harvard Business Review*, 30 (1952), pp. 105–12; T. Caplow and J. Raymond, 'Factors Influencing the Selection of Pharmaceutical Products', *Journal of Marketing*, 19:1 (1954), pp. 18–23.

40. See R. Ferber and H. G. Wales, 'The Effectiveness of Pharmaceutical Advertising: A Case Study', *Journal of Marketing*, 22:4 (1958), pp. 398–407; R. Ferber and H. G. Wales, *The Effectiveness of Pharmaceutical Promotion* (Urbana, IL: University of Illinois Press, 1958).

41. See R. A. Bauer, 'Information as Source for Risk Reduction', in R. Hancock (ed.), *Proceedings of the American Marketing Association* (Chicago, IL: American Marketing Association, 1960), pp. 389–98; R. A. Bauer, 'Predicting the Future', in J. D. Chalupnik (ed.), *Transportation Noises: Symposium on Acceptability Criteria* (Seattle, WA: University of Washington Press, 1971).

42. R. A. Bauer, 'Risk Handling in Drug Adoption: The Role of Company Preference', *Public Opinion Quarterly*, 25:4 (1961), pp. 546–59; R. A. Bauer and L. H. Wortzel, 'Doctor's Choice: The Physician and his Sources of Information about Drugs', *Journal of Marketing Research*, 3:1 (1966), pp. 40–7.

43. C. van den Bulte and L. L. Gary, 'Medical Innovation Revisited: Social Contagion versus Marketing Effort', *American Journal of Sociology*, 106:5 (2001), pp. 1409–35. This article questions the sufficiency of Katz and Menzel's proof, in their inquiry, of the superior value of the personal contact of 'detail men', as pharmaceutical sales representatives were known then, over advertising. This remains to be checked, but we are following the actor's view here, especially as taken up in general thought.

44. Katz, 'The Two-Step-Flow of Communication', p. 70.

45. E. M. Rogers, *Diffusion of Innovations* (New York: Free Press, 1962, 1971, 1983, 1995 and 2003). The second edition (1971) was published together with F. F. Shoemaker under the title *Communication of Innovations: A Cross-Cultural Approach*. For the German innovation research of those years, see R. Coenen and B. Wingert, 'Konzepte und Ziele der Innovationsforschung', in *Studiengruppe für Systemforschung, Mitteilungen* 1973, pp. 8–9; L. Uhlmann, 'Innovation in Industry: A Discussion of the State-of-Art and the Results of Innovation Research in German-Speaking Countries', *Research Policy*, 4:3 (1975), pp. 312–27.

46. C. F. von Weizsäcker, 'Die Kunst der Prognose', *Bayer-Berichte*, 22 (1969), pp. 12–15.

47. K. Steinbuch, 'Futurologie auf dem Weg zur Systemtheorie', *Bayer-Berichte*, 29 (1972), pp. 22–7; H. Maier-Leibnitz, 'Utopie und Wirklichkeit. Der Forscher in der heutigen Gesellschaft', *Bayer-Berichte*, 38 (1977), pp. 19–23.

48. See for example H. Friesewinkel, 'Der Arzt und die Werbung', *Pharmazeutische Industrie*, 28 (1966), pp. 133–6, 200–5, 286–91, 372–9, 448–54 and 535–41, especially his

comment on p. 372.

49. P. W. Meyer, 'Prognosen – Vorgriff auf die 70er Jahre', *Jahrbuch der Absatz- und Ver-brauchsforschung*, 16 (1970), pp. 193–5.

50. For its history see D. R. Rink and J. E. Swan, 'Product Life Cycle Research: A Litera-ture Review', *Journal of Business Research*, 32 (1979), pp. 219–42.

51. The idea as such is not helpful in analysing the emergence of modern marketing, as it is not able to explain the emergence of modern marketing. See T. Pieters and S. Snelder, 'From King Kong Pills to Mother's Little Helpers – Career Cycles of Two Families of Psychotropic Drugs: The Barbiturates and Benzodiazepines', *Canadian Bulletin of Medical History*, 24 (2007), pp. 93–112; S. Snelders, C. Kaplan and T. Pieters, 'On Cannabis, Chloral Hydrate and Career Cycles of Psychotropic Drugs in Medicine', *Bulletin of the History of Medicine*, 80:1 (2006), pp. 95–114.

52. T. Levitt, 'Exploit the Product Life Cycle', *Harvard Business Review*, 43 (1965), pp. 81–94; C. K. May, 'Planning the Marketing Program throughout the Life Cycle' (PhD dissertation, Columbia University, University Microfilms, Ann Arbor MI, 1961); K. Hoffman, *Der Produktlebensyzklus: eine kritische Analyse* (Freiburg: Rombach, 1972); P. Bischof, *Produktlebensyzklen im Investitionsgüterbereich: Produktplanung unter Berücksichtigung von Wiederständen bei der Markteinführung* (Göttingen: Vanden-hoeck & Ruprecht, 1976).

53. Web of Science, at http://thomsonreuters.com/web-of-science [accessed 30 May 2012]. A search on Google Ngram produces a similar graph, at http://books.google.com/ngrams/graph?content=life+cycle&year_start=1900&year_end=2008&corpus=15&smoothing=1&share= [accessed 7 September 2013].

54. See his famous article, T. Levitt, 'Marketing Myopia', *Harvard Business Review*, 38 (1960), pp. 45–56, on p. 47.

55. May, 'Planning the Marketing Program'.

56. W. E. Cox, 'Product Life Cycles and Promotional Strategy in the Ethical Drug Industry' (PhD dissertation, University of Michigan, 1963). The data was taken from the drug records of Paul De Haen, who had had published regular overviews of newly introduced products since 1949.

57. W. E. Cox, 'Product Life Cycles as Marketing Models', *Journal of Business*, 40:4 (1967), pp. 375–84. The descriptions here are taken from p. 382. Needless to say, there were many variations of this curve.

58. R. Abt, *Der Lebenszyklus ethischer pharmazeutischer Präparate und die Möglichkeiten seiner Beeinflussung* (Basel: Ciba-Geigy, 1971).

59. Abt cited, for example, the work of H. Kahn and A. J. Wiener, *The Year 2000: A Frame-work for Speculation on the Next Thirty-Three Years* (New York: Collier Macmillan Ltd., 1968).

60. Abt, *Der Lebenszyklus*, discusses F. Rosenkranz's model on p. 269.

61. Abt, *Der Lebenszyklus*, p. 284.

62. Abt, *Der Lebenszyklus*, p. 285.

63. G. Dittmar, 'Technische und Kaufmännische Besprechung Nord, Krefeld', 21 April 1970, Bayer Archives 369/586.

64. R. Abt and H. Friesewinkel, *Das Pharmazeutische Marketing* (Wiesbaden: Pharma Team Verlag, 1976).

65. W. Gehrig, *Pharma-Marketing. Instrumente, Organisation und Methoden national und international*, 2nd rev. edn (1987; Landsberg/Lech: Verlag Moderne Industrie, 1992).

66. W. Gehrig, *Zentrales Product-Management im Stammhaus einer Unternehmung der*

pharmazeutischen Industrie (Zurich: Juris Verlag, 1972).

67. H. Weinhold-Stünzi, 'Bedeutung und Stellung des Marketing in der Wirtschaft', *Jahrbuch der Absatz- und Verbrauchsforschung*, 6 (1961), pp. 339–52.
68. 'Sitzt der Marketing-Direktor auf dem richtigen Stuhl?', *Absatzwirtschaft*, 2 (1959), p. 322; 'Sitzt der Marketing-Direktor auf dem richtigen Stuhl?', *Absatzwirtschaft*, 3 (1960), pp. 7, 60–2, 117; 'Marketing Organisation in Deutschland. Heute: Dr. August Oetker, Bielefeld', *Absatzwirtschaft*, 12 (1969), p. 30.
69. See Bayer Archive 168/13; E. Verg, G. Plumpe and H. Schultheis, *Meilensteine – 125 Jahre Bayer* (Leverkusen: Bayer AG, 1988), p. 71.
70. Neuorganisation der Farbenfabriken Bayer, AG, 25 February 1970, Bayer Archives, 369/586.
71. H. A. Baum, 'Ländergeschichte der Pharma nach dem Zweiten Weltkrieg (1945–1984), Teil I, Deutschland', unpublished (Leverkusen, Bayer AG, 1989), Bayer Archives, p. 28.
72. Baum, 'Ländergeschichte der Pharma', p. 170.
73. Baum, 'Ländergeschichte der Pharma', p. 171.
74. See the minutes of this panel, the 'Protokoll über die Sitzung des medizinischen Beraterkreises am Mittwoch, dem 2. Juli 1969 in Elberfeld, Pharmazeutisches Forschungszentraum, 14. Juli 1969', Bayer Archive, 323/136 and 323/137.
75. Baum, 'Ländergeschichte der Pharma', p. 225.
76. 'Report on the Visit to Prof. Fliedner from the Institute for Scientific Cooperation at the University of Regensburg', Bayer Archives, 323/153.
77. 'Neu-Organisation im Pharma-Vertriebsbereich', 2 February 1970, Bayer Archives, 323/153.
78. For the organizational changes, see Baum, 'Ländergeschichte der Pharma', pp. 217–27.
79. See the discussion proposal for the meeting at Hoechst, 12 January 1970, Bayer Archives, 323/153.
80. H. A. Braun, *Geschichte der Pharma nach dem Zweiten Weltkrieg* (Leverkusen: Bayer AG, 1983), pp. 167–70.
81. 'Sitzung der Fachkommission Marktforschung', 28 February 1973, Bayer Archives 323/156.
82. See the contribution of Maier at the second meeting, 'Minutes', '2. Sitzung der Fachkommission Marktforschung', 4 June 1973, Bayer Archives 323/156, p. 7.
83. This topic dominated the fifth meeting, '5. Sitzung der Fachkommission Marktforschung', 11 February 1974, Bayer Archives, 326/23.
84. See the talk by Schütt on the life cycle concept, 'Protocol', 'Referat 'Produktlebenszyklus – Gültigkeit eines Konzepts', Ergebnisprotokoll Fachkommission Marktforschung, 32. Sitzung, 12 November 1980, Bayer Archives 326/23, p. 8.
85. P. Aumann, *Mode und Methode. Die Kybernetik in der Bundesrepublik Deutschland* (Göttingen: Wallstein Verlag, 2009).
86. See, for example, the critiques in R. Polli and V. Cook, 'Validity of the Product Life Cycle', *Journal of Business*, 42:4 (1969), pp. 385–400; G. S. Day, 'The Product Life Cycle: Analysis and Applications Issues', *Journal of Marketing*, 45:4 (1981), pp. 60–7.
87. N. K. Dhalla and S. Yuspeh, 'Forget the Product Life Cycle Concept!', *Harvard Business Review*, 54 (1976), pp. 102–12.
88. N. Elias, *Über den Prozess der Zivilisation. Soziogenetische und psychogenetische Untersuchungen*, 2 vols, 19th edn (Frankfurt: Suhrkamp, 1995).
89. R. Abt, M. Borja, M. M. Menke and J. P. Pezier, 'The Dangerous Quest for Certainty in

Market Forecasting', *Long Range Planning*, 12:2 (1979), pp. 52–62, on p. 52.

90.   P. Herder-Dorneich, *Soziale Kybernetik: die Theorie der Scheine* (Cologne: Kohlhammer, 1965).

91.   P. Herder-Dorneich, *Gesundheitsökonomik. Systemsteuerung und Ordnungspolitik im Gesundheitswesen* (Stuttgart: Ferdinand Enke Verlag, 1980); F. Beske and H. J. Wilhelmy, 'Ziele und Aufgaben der Gesundheits-System-Forschung', *Deutsches Ärzteblatt*, 73:43 (1976), pp. 2729–34; H. Clade, 'Gesundheitsökonomie. Entscheidungshilfen für die Medizin', *Deutsches Ärzteblatt*, 77 (1980), pp. 1127–8.

3 Ravelli, Marketing Epidemics: When Antibiotic Promotion Stimulates Resistant Bacteria

1.   European Center for Disease Prevention and Control and European Medicine Agency, Joint Technical Report, 'The Bacterial Challenge: Time to React', EMEA/576176/2009, 2009, at http://www.ema.europa.eu/docs/en_GB [accessed 20 May 2012].

2.   Infectious Disease Society of America, 'Bad Bugs, No Drugs: As Antibiotic Discovery Stagnates, a Public Health Crisis Brews', July 2004, at http://www.fda.gov/ohrms/dockets/DOCKETS/04s0233/04s-0233-c000005–03-IDSA-vol1.pdf [accessed 16 August 2012], pp. 4, 15–17.

3.   Alliance for the Prudent Use of Antibiotics, 'The Cost of Antibiotic Resistance to US Families and the Health Care System', September 2010, at http://www.tufts.edu/med/apua/consumers/personal_home_5_1451036133.pdf [accessed 20 May 2012].

4.   L. Fleck, *Genesis and Development of a Scientific Fact* (Chicago, IL: University of Chicago Press, 2010).

5.   U. Buchholz et al., 'German Outbreak of Escherichia Coli 0104:H4 Associated with Sprouts', *New England Journal of Medicine,* 365 (2001), pp.1763–70.

6.   M. Finland, 'The Present Status of Antibiotics in Bacterial Infections', *Bulletin of the New York Academy of Medicine*, 27 (1951), pp. 199–220, on p. 217.

7.   L. Hicks, Y.-W. Chien, T. Taylor, M. Haber and K. Klugman, 'Outpatient Antibiotic Prescribing and Nonsusceptible Streptococcus Pneumoniae in the United States, 1996–2003', *Clinical Infectious Disease*, 53 (2011), pp. 632–40; J. J. Granizo, L. Aguilar, J. Casal, C. Garcia-Rey, R. Dal-Re and F. Baquero, 'Streptococcus Pneumoniae Resistance to Erythromycin and Penicillin in Relation to Macrolide and Beta-lactam Consumption in Spain (1979–1997)', *Journal of Antimicrobial Chemotherapy*, 46 (2000), pp. 767–73.

8.   G. A. Jacoby, 'History of Drug-Resistant Microbes', in D. L. Mayers (ed.), *Antimicrobial Drug Resistance*, 2 vols (New York: Humana Press, 2009), vol. 1, pp. 3–7.

9.   B. Cookson, 'Five Decades of MRSA: Controversy and Uncertainty Continues', *Lancet*, 378:9799 (2011), pp.1291–2.

10.   World Health Organization, 'Clinical Pharmacological Evaluation in Drug Control', EUR/ICP/DSE 173 (Copenhagen, 1993).

11.   B. Spellberg, J. Powers, E. Brass, L. Miller and J. Edwards, 'Trends in Antimicrobial Drug Development: Implications for the Future', *Clinical Infectious Diseases*, 38:9 (2004), pp. 1279–86, on p. 1280.

12.   S. Projan, 'Why is Big Pharma Getting out of Antibacterial Drug Discovery?', *Current Opinion in Microbiology*, 6:5 (2003), pp. 427–30; R. Finch and P. Hunter, 'Antibiotic

Resistance: Action to Promote New Technologies. Report on a EU Intergovernemental Conference Held in Birmingham, UK, 12–13 December 2005', *Journal of Antimicrobial Chemotherapy*, 58 (2006), pp. 3–22.

13. S. B. Levy, L. Star and E. D. Kupferberg, 'The Misuse of Antibiotics: The Medical Ethics Forum from Harvard Medical School', *Lahey Clinic Medical Ethics* (2003), pp. 5–8.

14. Adwatch, '"Take a Closer look": Augmentin (amoxicillin with potassium clavulanate) from GlaxoSmithKline', at http://healthyskepticism.org/adwatch/au/2004/augmentin.php [accessed 15 April 2013].

15. B. Lahire, *Portraits sociologiques* (Paris: Nathan, 2002).

16. Les Entreprises du Médicament (Leem), the employers' association gathering most pharmaceutical corporations in France: http://www.leem.org/article/statistiques-de-visite-medicale [accessed 17 December 2014]; *Atlas de la démocratie médicale française 2013*, p. 12: http://www.conseil-national.medecin.fr/sites/default/files/atlas_national_2013.pdf [accessed 17 December 2014].

17. Sanofi-Aventis' internal documentation and listings.

18. Apart from classical factors like market structure or sales force size, inequally distributed among competitors, pharmaceutical markets are frequently transformed by two distinct mechanisms: when a drug loses its patent, because it entails a strong concurrence and a drop in price which puts an end to costly promotional campaigns; and when a drug is withdrawn from the market or loses a part of its indications, which implies that other marketers try to conquer its vacant therapeutic use value.

19. A. Smith, *An Inquiry into the Nature and Causes of the Wealth of Nations*, ed. T. Nelsons and sons (Edinburgh and New York: Paternoster Row, 1901), p. 12.

20. P. Conrad, 'The Shifting Engines of Medicalization', *Journal of Health and Social Behavior*, 46 (2005), pp. 3–14, on p. 3.

21. M. Finland, 'The Present Status of Antibiotics in Bacterial Infections', *Bulletin of the New York Academy of Medicine*, 27 (1951), pp. 210–12.

22. H. J. van Duijn, M. M. Kuyvenhoven, F. G. Schellevis and T. J. M. Verheij, 'Determinants of Prescribing of Second-Choice Antibiotics for Upper and Lower Respiratory Tract Episodes in Dutch General Practice', *Journal of Antimicrobial Chemotherapy*, 56 (2005), pp. 420–2.

23. Q. Ravelli, 'Medico-marketing between Use Value and Exchange Value: How Political Economy Sheds Light on the Biography of Medicines', *Medische antropologie*, 23:2 (2011), pp. 243–54.

24. S. H. Podolsky, 'Pharmacological Restraints: Antibiotic Prescribing and the Limits of Physician Autonomy', in J. A. Greene, *Prescribed: Writing, Filling, Using, and Abusing the Prescription* (Baltimore, MD: John Hopkins University Press, 2012), pp. 46–67.

25. French Code of Public Health, art. L. 5122.

26. The Agence Française de Sécurité Sanitaire et des Produits de Santé is the French equivalent of the Food and Drug Administration.

27. French Code of Public Health, art. L. 5122.

28. E. Sabuncu et al., 'Significant Reduction of Antibiotic Use in the Community after a Nationwide Campaign in France 2002–2007', *PLoS Med* (2009), 6:e1000084, at http://www.plosmedicine.org [accessed 31 January 2013].

29. Agence Française de Sécurité Sanitaire des Produits de Santé, 'Dix ans d'évolution des consommations d'antibiotiques en France', Expert Report (2011), at http://www.afssaps.fr [accessed 31 January 2013].

30. C. Michèle, 'Note de synthèse assurance maladie', *Les assises du médicament*

(March 2011), at http://www.sante.gouv.fr/IMG/pdf/Michele_Carzon [accessed 15 April 2013].

31. C. Michèle, 'Note de synthèse assurance maladie', p. 3.

32. Commission des Comptes de la Sécurité Sociale, 'Les Comptes de la Sécurité Sociale', September 2011, at http://www.securite-sociale.fr/IMG/pdf/ccss2011-9-versiondefinitive.pdf [accessed 17 December 2014].

33. Q. Ravelli, *La stratégie de la bactérie* (Paris: Le Seuil, 2015), p. 80.

34. P. Rubin, 'The FDA's Antibiotic Resistance', *Regulation*, 27:4 (2004), pp. 34–7.

35. European Medicine Agency, Innovative Drug Development Approaches, London, 22 March 2007, doc. ref. EMEA/127318/2007, at http://www.emea.europa.eu/docs/en_GB/document_library/Other/2009/10/WC500004913.pdf [accessed 17 December 2014].

36. H. L. Leavis, 'Epidemic and Nonepidemic Multidrug-Resistant *Enteroccocus Faecium*', *Emerging Infectious Diseases*, 9:9 (2003), pp. 1108–15, on p. 1109.

37. 'Expanded access, also called "compassionate use", is a regulation that makes promising drugs and devices available to patients with serious or immediately life-threatening diseases': Food and Drug Administration, 'Understanding Expanded Access / Compassionate Use', at http://www.fda.gov/ForPatients/Other/expandedAccess/ucm20041768.htm [accessed 17 December 2014]. In the FDA anti-infective committee, experts talked about 'compassionate use' clinical trials: http://www.fda.gov/ohrms/dockets/ac/98/transcpt/3383t1.pdf [accessed 17 December 2014], pp. 75, 287, and 288.

38. Food and Drug Administration, Public Health Service, Department of Health and Human Services, 'Anti-infective Drugs Advisory Committee, 63rd meeting', open session, 19 February 1998, at http://www.fda.gov/ohrms/dockets/ac/98/transcpt/3383t1.pdf [accessed 17 December 2014], p. 24.

39. C. Rosenthal, *Les capitalistes de la science. Enquête sur les démonstrateurs de la Silicon Valley et de la NASA* (Paris: CNRS Editions, 2007).

40. Food and Drug Administration, 'Anti-infective Drugs Advisory Committee, 63rd meeting', pp. 284–5.

41. D. Carpenter, *Organizational Image and Pharmaceutical Regulation at the FDA* (Princeton, NJ: Princeton University Press, 2010).

4 Felder, Gaudillière and Thoms, Ads, Ads, Ads: The GEPHAMA Database and its Uses

1. See W. Wimmer, 'Die Pharmazeutische Industrie als "ernsthafte" Industrie: Die Auseinandersetzungen um die Laienwerbung im Kaiserreich', *Medizin in Gesellschaft und Geschichte*, 11 (1992), pp. 73–86; for the role of the moral economy of science, see U. Thoms, 'Arzneimittelaufsicht im frühen 19. Jahrhundert. Konflikte und Konvergenzen zwischen Wissen, Expertise und regulativer Politik', in E. Engstrom, V. Hess and U. Thoms (eds), *Figurationen des Experten* (Frankfurt: Peter Lang, 2005), pp. 123–46; H. Zimmermann, *Arzneimittelwerbung in Deutschland vom Beginn des 16. bis Ende des 18. Jahrhunderts: Dargestellt vorzugsweise an Hand von Archivalien der Freien Reichs-, Handels- und Messe-Stadt Frankfurt am Main: mit einer Einführung in das Wesen der Werbung unter besonderer Berücksichtigung ihrer Frühformen in antiker und mittelalterlicher Heilmittelwirtschaft* (Marburg: E. Mauersberger, 1968); S. Bernschneider-Reif,

Laboranten, Destillatores, Balsamträger: das laienpharmazeutische Olitätenwesen im Thüringer Wald vom 17. bis zum 19. Jahrhundert (Frankfurt and New York: Peter Lang, 2001); E. Ernst, *Das 'industrielle' Geheimmittel und seine Werbung. Arzneifertigwaren in der zweiten Hälfte des 19. Jahrhunderts in Deutschland* (Würzburg: Jal Verlag, 1975); W. H. Helfand, *Quack, Quack, Quack: The Sellers of Nostrums in Prints, Posters, Ephemera and Books: An Exhibition on the Frequently Excessive and Flamboyant Seller of Nostrums as Shown in Prints, Posters, Caricatures, Books, Pamphlets, Advertisements and Other Graphic Arts over the Last Five Centuries*, catalogue to an exhibition of the same title at the Grolier Club, 18 September–23 November 2002, and the Philadelphia Museum of Art, 2005 (New York: Grolier Club, 2002); E. S. Juhnke, *Quacks and Crusaders: The Fabulous Careers of John Brinkley, Norman Baker, and Harry Hoxsey* (Lawrence, KS: University Press of Kansas, 2002).

2. F. Mildenberger, *Medikale Subkulturen in der Bundesrepublik Deutschland und ihre Gegner (1950–1990). Die Zentrale zur Bekämpfung der Unlauterkeit im Heilgewerbe* (Stuttgart: Steiner, 2011). In France, post-war debates on pharmaceutical publicity led to the enactment of a series of decrees after World War II. On this subject see Anne-Sophie Mazas in this volume.

3. See A. Hüntelmann, 'A *Different* Mode of Marketing? The Importance of Scientific Articles in the Marketing Process of Salvarsan', *History and Technology* (forthcoming); W. Wimmer, *'Wir haben fast immer was Neues': Gesundheitswesen und Innovationen der Pharma-Industrie in Deutschland, 1880–1935* (Berlin: Duncker & Humblot, 1994).

4. One famous German example is Rudolf Mosse's Advertising Expedition, which bought advertising space from newspapers and magazines and sold it to those who were willing to place ads. See D. Reinhardt, *Von der Reklame zum Marketing. Geschichte der Wirtschaftswerbung in Deutschland* (Berlin: Akademie Verlag GmbH, 1993), pp. 110–14.

5. For the history of the *Deutsche Medizinische Wochenschrift* see especially C. Staehr, *Spurensuche. Ein Wissenschaftsverlag im Spiegel seiner Zeitschriften 1886–1986* (Stuttgart and New York: Thieme Verlag, 1986) and for the history of medical bulletins in general, S. Stöckel, G. Rüve, W. Lisner and T. Möller (eds), *Das Medium Wissenschaftszeitschrift seit dem 19. Jahrhundert. Verwissenschaftlichung der Gesellschaft – Vergesellschaftung von Wissenschaft* (Stuttgart: Franz Steiner Verlag, 2009).

6. While many works have been written on journals of the eighteenth and early nineteenth century, when the scientific public developed, the modern scientific medical journal has so far been given little attention in the history of science, and recent studies have not focused on advertisements at all even though they played a significant role in the economic existence of the journals. See U. Thoms, 'Medizinische Zeitschriften und Pharma-Marketing, 1920–1980', *Medizinhistorisches Journal*, forthcoming.

7. H. H. Eulner, *Die Entwicklung der medizinischen Spezialfächer an den Universitäten des deutschen Sprachgebietes* (Stuttgart: Ferdinand Enke Verlag, 1970).

8. 'Bericht der Bundesregierung über die Lage von Presse und Rundfunk in der Bundesrepublik Deutschland (1978)', Deutscher Bundestag, 8. Wahlperiode, Drucksache 8/2264, p. 45.

9. Today, the practice has changed. After the printing houses themselves founded special departments to market the ads, they were once again scattered throughout the issues. See for instance today's *Deutsches Ärzteblatt*.

10. On these methods, see G. H. Stempel and B. H. Westley, *Research Methods in Mass Communication*, 2nd edn (1989; Englewood Cliffs, NJ: Prentice-Hall Inc., 1991); and

V. Gehrau, B. Fretwurst, B. Krause and G. Daschmann (eds), *Auswahlverfahren in der Kommunikationswissenschaft* (Cologne: Halem, 2005). See also the unpublished manuscript, U. Thoms, 'Sampling Methods' (Berlin, 2009).

11. In the case of Germany, the ads were collected for the period 1910–80, but due to organisational problems the French ads were collected only for 1910–70.

12. R. W. Pollay, 'The Subsiding Sizzle: A Descriptive History of Print Advertising, 1900–1980', *Journal of Marketing*, 49:3 (July 1985), pp. 24–37, on p. 25.

13. The idea that marketing can shape markets has in particular been pursued by scholars such as David Healy and Jeremy Greene, although in the former case with little investigation of marketing activities. See for example J. Greene, *Prescribing by Numbers: Drugs and the Definition of Disease* (Baltimore, MD: Johns Hopkins University Press, 2007); D. Healy, *Let Them Eat Prozac: The Unhealthy Relationship between the Pharmaceutical Industry and Depression* (New York: New York University Press, 2004).

14. The collection of ads, their photographing and indexing was performed by Stephan Felder and Fabien Moll-François. S. Felder, 'Werbegesetzgebung und ihr Einfluss auf die visuellen Werbestrategien der pharmazeutischen Industrie im 20. Jahrhundert' (Advertising legislation and its impact on the visual advertising strategies of the pharmaceutical industry in the twentieth century) (unpublished manuscript, Charité Universitätsmedizin Berlin, 2010), which he wrote as a student qualification work, provided the first results of the study, demonstrating the usefulness of the German part of the database for a social history of drug marketing.

15. The group of painkillers covers the treatment of many ailments and today has become a group of everyday drugs available over the counter. As such, their marketing follows different schemes than those of the other groups, which are mainly made up of prescription drugs.

16. For reasons of differentiated access to the sources, the time period taken into account for both journals is slightly different. For the *Concours Médical* the most recent years could not be included while for the *Deutsche Medizinische Wochenschrift* the gaps are more evenly distributed. The following table has therefore been restricted to the period for which a comparison is possible.

17. For these difficulties and the reactions of pharmaceutical companies, see for example S. H. Linder, *Hoechst. Ein I.G. Farben Werk im Dritten Reich* (Munich: C. H. Beck, 2005), pp. 56–61. In France, the rising investments in advertising, including pharmaceutical advertising, are well reflected in *Vendre*, a journal entirely devoted to the discussion of publicity practices, which was started in 1921.

18. On these aspects see U. Thoms, 'Standardizing Selling: Pharmaceutical Marketing, the Enterprise and the Marketing Expert (1900–1990)', in J.-P. Gaudillière and U. Thoms (eds), *Standardizing and Marketing Drugs in the 20th Century*, special issue, *History and Technology* 29 (2013), 29 (2013), pp. 169–87.

19. See more specifically in this volume the chapters by Ulrike Thoms, Jean-Paul Gaudillière, Christian Bonah and Lucie Gerber.

20. For the new theoretical models see, for instance, R. Abt and H. Friesewinkel, *Das Pharmazeutische Marketing* (Wiesbaden: Pharma Team Verlag, 1976); P. Herbin, *La publicité pharmaceutique* (Lagny: Éditions de la Gourdine, 1970). New journals included *Medizin und Werbung* and *Pharmazeutische Industrie* in Germany, and *La Pharmacie Industrielle* in France.

21. On both points, see Anne-Sophie Mazas in this volume on the French situation.

22. For this aspect see Tricia Close-Koenig and Ulrike Thoms in this volume and U. Thoms 'The German Pharmaceutical Industry and the Standardization of Insulin before the Second World War', in A. von Schwerin, H. Stoff and B. Wahrig (eds), *Biologics: A History of Agents Made from Living Organisms in the Twentieth Century* (London: Pickering & Chatto, 2013), pp. 151–72.

23. D. Reinhardt, *Von der Reklame zum Marketing. Geschichte der Wirtschaftswerbung in Deutschland* (Berlin: Akademie Verlag GmbH, 1993), pp. 202–30; R. W. Pollay, 'The Subsiding Sizzle: A Descriptive History of Print Advertising, 1900–1980', *Journal of Marketing*, 49:3 (July 1985), pp. 24–37.

24. 'Pictures' as defined here may be drawn, painted or photographed.

25. On the growing impact of aesthetics on advertising see Reinhardt, *Von der Reklame zum Marketing*, pp. 49–87.

26. See indications of this in this volume in the chapters by Anne-Sophie Mazas and Jean-Paul Gaudillière; see Lucie Gerber's contribution for Ciba-Geigy's policy, and see Thoms's remarks on the targeted choice of pink as a colour attached to Schering's new pill, Femovan, in U. Thoms, 'The Contraceptive Pill, the Pharmaceutical Industry and Changes in the Patient–Doctor Relationship in Germany', in T. Ortiz et al. (eds), *Gendered Drug Standards from Historical and Socio-anthropological Perspectives* (Farnham: Ashgate, forthcoming). See also J. Greene, 'The Same but Not the Same: Pharmaceutical Trademarks and the Limits of Equivalence', in J.-P. Gaudillière and U. Thoms (eds), *Standardizing and Marketing Drugs in the 20th Century, History and Technology*, special issue 29 (2013), pp. 210–26.

27. B. Schmitt and A. Simonson, *Marketing Aesthetics* (New York: Free Press, 1997), p. 223 ff.

28. Pollay, 'The Subsiding Sizzle', p. 28.

29. See G. Bergler, 'Der chemisch-pharmazeutische Markenartikel. Darstellung des Wesens, des Absatzformen und des Kampfes um den Markt' (Dissertation, Tübingen University, 1931).

30. This was also the case for anti-diabetics. See Tricia Close-Koenig and Ulrike Thoms in this volume.

31. According to S. Felder, 'Werbegesetzgebung und ihr Einfluss auf die visuellen Werbestrategien der pharmazeutischen Industrie im 20. Jahrhundert' (Advertising legislation and its impact on the visual advertising strategies of the pharmaceutical industry in the twentieth century), (unpublished manuscript, Charité Universitätsmedizin Berlin, 2010), p. 30, in the entire sample of German ads the percentage of drugs that pointed to drug effects was 1 per cent in 1930, 9.6 per cent in 1960, 19.4 per cent in 1965, 19.3 per cent in 1970 and 33 per cent in 1975.

32. See 'Gesetz über die Werbung auf dem Gebiete des Heilwesens', Bundesgesetzblatt 1965, part I, pp. 604–9, see section 11, para. 4, and the discussion in Felder, 'Werbegesetzgebung und ihr Einfluss', p. 28.

33. Reichsgesetzblatt 1941, I, pp. 587–9.

34. Felder, 'Werbegesetzgebung und ihr Einfluss', pp. 29–30.

35. It is important to note that in several of the years there were not enough ads to calculate meaningful percentages.

36. There is a vast bulk of literature on the construction of diseases beginning with M. Foucault, *History of Madness* (Banbury: Routledge, 2007), first published in French as *Folie et déraison: Histoire de la folie à l'âge classique* (Paris: Plon, 1961). For a general perspective see C. E. Rosenberg and J. Golden, *Framing Disease: Studies in Cultural*

History, Health and Medicine in American Society (Piscataway, NJ: Rutgers University Press, 1992), where this perspective is especially developed. For the case of mental disorders, see E. Shorter, *A History of Psychiatry: From the Era of the Asylum to the Age of Prozac* (New York: John Wiley & Sons, 1997); A. Tone, *The Age of Anxiety: A History of America's Turbulent Affair with Tranquilizers* (New York: Basic Books, 2009); K. Ingenkamp, *Depression und Gesellschaft. Zur Erfindung einer Volkskrankheit* (Bielefeld: Transcript Verlag, 2012); D. Healy, *The Antidepressant Era* (Cambridge, MA: Harvard University Press, 1997); D. Healy, *Let Them Eat Prozac: The Unhealthy Relationship between the Pharmaceutical Industry and Depression* (New York: New York University Press, 2004); L. D. Hirschbein, *American Melancholy: Constructions of Depression in the Twentieth Century* (Piscataway, NJ: Rutgers University Press, 2009); A. Haggett, *Desperate Housewives, Neuroses and the Domestic Environment, 1945–1970* (London: Pickering & Chatto, 2012); D. Herzberg, *Happy Pills in America: From Miltown to Prozac* (Baltimore, MD: Johns Hopkins University Press, 2009); M. C. Smith, *A Social History of the Minor Tranquilizers: The Quest for Small Comfort in the Age of Anxiety* (New York: Pharmaceutical Products Press, 1985); N. Rasmussen, *On Speed: The Many Lives of Amphetamine* (2008; New York: New York University Press, 2009); A. Ehrenberg, *La Fatigue d'être soi. Dépression et société* (Paris: Odile Jacob, 1998); V. Hess and H.-P. Schmiedebach (eds), *Am Rande des Wahnsinns: Schwellenräume einer urbanen Moderne* (Vienna: Böhlau, 2012).

37. Lucie Gerber and Jean-Paul Gaudillière in this volume show the potential of a closer investigation for a specific group of psychotropic drugs.

38. N. Henckes, 'Reshaping Chronicity: Neuroleptics and the Changing Meanings of Therapy in French Psychiatry, 1950–1975', *Studies in History and Philosophy of Biological and Medical Sciences*, 42:4 (2011), pp. 434–42.

39. From the vast amount of literature see for instance A. Götz, *Totgeschwiegen 1933–1945. Die Geschichte der Karl-Bonhoeffer-Nervenklinik* (Berlin: Hentrich, 1988); W. Süß, *Der 'Volkskörper' im Krieg. Gesundheitspolitik, Gesundheitsverhältnisse und Krankenmord im nationalsozialistischen Deutschland 1939–1945* (Munich: Oldenbourg Wissenschaftsverlag, 2003).

40. For the propaganda against addiction to tranquilizers and sedatives see, for instance, Herzberg, *Happy Pills in America* and N. Rasmussen, 'Goofball Panic: Barbiturates, "Dangerous" and Addictive Drugs and the Regulation of Medicine in Postwar America', in J. Greene and E. Siegel Watkins (eds), *Prescribed: Writing, Filling, Using and Abusing the Prescription in Modern America* (Baltimore, MD: John Hopkins University Press, 2012), pp. 23–45; D. Herzberg, 'Busted for Blockbusters: "Scrip Mills", Quaalude and Prescribing Power in the 1970s', in Greene and Siegel Watkins (eds), *Prescribed*, pp. 207–31. These papers document a development that was not only to be found in America, but had a similar shape in Germany and France.

41. 'Anxiolytic' is well documented in our sample. As a concept it had been adopted from the USA. In Germany the anxiolytic agent is not present, but the concept 'Anxiolyse' is mentioned in adverts for antidepressants (i.e., SSRIs) during the later period, and this is what produces the increase.

42. L. Haller, *Cortison. Geschichte eines Hormons* (Zurich: Chronos Verlag, 2012). 43. From the emerging literature on 'stress' see, for example, M. Jackson, *The Age of Stress: Science and the Search for Stability* (Oxford: Oxford University Press, 2013); P. Kury, *Der überforderte Mensch. Eine Wissensgeschichte vom Stress zum Burnout* (Frankfurt: Campus Verlag, 2012).

5 Bonah, Marketing Film: Audio-Visuals for Scientific Marketing and Medical Training in Psychiatry: The Sandoz Example in the 1960s

1. For a development of this argument see S. Hilger, *'Amerikanisierung' deutscher Unternehmen: Wettbewerbsstrategien und Unternehmenspolitik bei Henkel, Siemens und Daimler-Benz (1945/49–1975)* (Stuttgart: Franz Steiner Verlag, 2004); W. Feldenkirchen and S. Hilger, *Menschen und Marken. 125 Jahre Henkel 1876–2001* (Düsseldorf: Henkel KGaA, 2001); and C. Kleinschmidt, *Der produktive Blick. Wahrnehmung amerikanischer und japanischer Management- und Produktionsmethoden durch deutsche Unternehmer 1950–1985* (Berlin: Akademie Verlag GmbH., 2002). For a more critical appreciation of the American influence see H. Berghoff (ed.), *Marketinggeschichte: Die Genese einer modernen Sozialtechnik* (Frankfurt and New York: Campus Verlag GmbH., 2007). For a critical appraisal of marketers' self-promotion see R. Bubik, *Geschichte der Marketing-Theorie. Historische Einführung in die Marketing-Lehre* (Frankfurt: Lang, 1996), p. 108, and especially the contributions of Ulrike Thomas, Jean-Paul Gaudillière and Lucie Gerber in this volume.

2. Postgraduate professional training became mandatory by law in France in 1973 (Law on postgraduate training, 1973). The role of medical films and the link with financing from the pharmaceutical industry are discussed extensively in the journal *Médecine/Cinéma*. See, for, P. Chantelou, 'Médecine/cinéma ou les difficultés de l'information indépendante sur le film médical', *Médecine/Cinéma*, 17 (1973), pp. 2–3.

3. For drug testing and evaluation, see C. Gradmann and J. Simon (eds.), *Evaluating and Standardizing Therapeutic Agents 1890–1950* (London: Palgrave, 2010). For the history of clinical trials see H. M. Marks, *The Progress of Experiment: Science and Therapeutic Reform in the United States, 1900–1990* (New York: Cambridge University Press, 1997); H. M. Marks, '"Until Science, the True Apollo of Medicine, Has Risen": Collective Investigation in Britain and the United States', *Medical History*, 50 (2006), pp. 147–66. J.-P. Gaudillière, 'The Singular Fate of Industrial Screening in Twentieth-Century Pharmacy: Some Thoughts about Drug Standardisation and Drug Regulation', in C. Bonah, C. Masutti, A. Rasmussen and J. Simon, (eds.), *Harmonizing Drugs: Standards in 20th Century Pharmaceutical History* (Paris: Glyphe, 2009), pp. 153–80. H. M. Marks, 'Histories of Therapeutic Research', in C. Bonah et al. (eds), *Harmonizing Drugs*, pp. 81–100. I. Löwy, 'Producing Pharmaceutical Standards at the Margins: Chemical Contraceptives between the Laboratory and the Field', in Bonah et al. (eds), *Harmonizing Drugs*, pp. 297–322. O. Keel, *La medicine des preuves. Une histoire de l'expérimentation thérapeutique par essais cliniques contrôlés* (Montréal: Presses de l'Université de Montréal, 2011). The phrase used in French for 'promotional information' is *information promotionnelle*. See P. Chantelou, 'Information "promotionnelle" par le film: Armour Montagu / La folie de Copp et la calcitonine', *Médecine/Cinéma*, 13 (1972), p. 17; P. Chantelou, 'Information "promotionnelle" par le film: Choay / La série "Coagulation" et les anticoagulants et thrombolytiques', *Médecine/Cinéma*, 15 (1972), p. 7.

4. For Germany after World War I, see U. Thoms, 'Standardizing Selling: Pharmaceutical Marketing, the Pharmaceutical Company and the Marketing Expert (1900–1980)', *History & Technology*, 29:2 (2013), pp. 169–87. For France, see T. Cramer, *Die Rückkehr ins Pharmageschäft. Marktstrategien der Farbenfabriken vormals Friedrich Bayer*

& Co. in Lateinamerika nach dem Ersten Weltkrieg (Berlin: Wissenschaftlicher Verlag, 2010). For marketing theories and practices in France in the pharmaceutical sector, see S. Chauveau, 'De la transfusion à l'industrie. Une histoire des produits sanguins en France (1950 – fin des années 1970)', in S. Chauveau (ed.), *Entreprises et Histoire*, 36, special issue: 'Industries du médicament et du vivant' (2005), pp. 103–19; S. Chauveau, 'Malades ou consommateurs? La consommation de médicaments en France dans le second XXe siècle', in A. Chatriot, M.-E. Chessel and M. Hilton (eds.), *Au nom du consommateur: Consommation et politique en Europe et aux États-Unis au XXe siècle* (Paris: Éditions La Découverte, 2004), pp. 182–98; S. Chauveau, *L'invention pharmaceutique. La pharmacie française entre l'État et la société au XXe siècle* (Paris: Les empêcheurs de penser en rond, 1999); S. Chauveau, 'Marché et publicité des médicaments', in C. Bonah and A. Rasmussen (eds.), *Histoire et médicament aux XIXe et XXe siècles* (Paris: Glyphe Éditions, 2005), pp. 189–213; M. A. Beale, *Advertising and the Politics of Public Persuasion in France, 1900–1939* (PhD dissertation, University of California Berkeley, university microfilms, 1991); M.-E. Chessel, *La Publicité: Naissance d'une profession 1900–1940* (Paris: CNRS Éditions, 1998).

5. P. Chantelou, 'Comment des cinémathèques scientifiques favorisent un cinéma de création et comment un réalisateur-créateur leur apporte une conception réaliste du film médical', *Médecine/Cinéma*, 14 (1972), pp. 9–11, on p. 9.

6. For recent interest in medical film in general, see L. J. Reagan, N. Tomes and P. A. Treichler, *Medicine's Moving Pictures: Medicine, Health, and Bodies in American Film and Television* (Rochester: University of Rochester Press, 2007); G. Harper and A. Moor (eds), *Signs of Life: Cinema and Medicine* (London: Wallflower Press, 2005); C. Bonah and A. Laukötter, 'Moving Pictures and Medicine in the First Half of the 20th Century: Some Notes on International Historical Developments and the Potential of Medical Film Research', *Gesnerus*, 66:1 (2009), pp. 121–45; K. Ostherr, *Cinematic Prophylaxis: Globalization and Contagion in the Discourse of World Health* (Durham: Duke University Press, 2005); L. D. Friedman (ed.), *Cultural Sutures: Medicine, Media and Morals* (Durham: Duke University Press, 2004); D. Cantor, 'Uncertain Enthusiasm: The American Cancer Society, Public Education, and the Problems of the Movie, 1921–1960', *Bulletin of the History of Medicine*, 81:1, 2007, pp. 39–69.

7. P. Chantelou, 'Le cinéma médical: essai de situation', *Médecine/Cinéma*, 7 (1969), pp. 7–13, on p. 7. The same volume supposes, in the context of the presentation of a new concept, the 'Cine-books' (*Ciné-livres*) by the Theraplix laboratories, that 'everybody knows that pharmaceutical companies pay ever increasing attention to audio-visuals and it is unnecessary to publish a journal devoted to medical film to recognize their growing influence in medical teaching and postgraduate professional training'. Anon., 'Entendre, voir, lire: Ciné-livres', *Médecine/Cinéma*, 7 (1969), pp. 20–1.

8. For a concrete example in Switzerland, Geigy, see the contribution by Lucie Gerber in this volume.

9. V. Hediger and P. Vonderau (eds.), *Films that Work: Industrial Film and the Productivity of Media* (Amsterdam: Amsterdam University Press, 2009); G. Leblanc, *Quand l'entreprise fait son cinéma: la médiathèque de Rhône-Poulenc (1972–1981)* (Vincennes: Cinéthique Presses Universitaires de Vincennes, 1983).

10. T. Elsaesser, 'Archives and Archaeologies: The Place of Non-fiction Film in Contemporary Media', in Hediger and Vonderau (eds.), *Films that Work*, pp. 19–34, on p. 22.

11. P. Chantelou, 'Comment des cinémathèques scientifiques favorisent un cinéma de

création et comment un réalisateur-créateur leur apporte une conception réaliste du film médical', *Médecine/Cinéma*, 14 (1972), pp. 9–11.

12. T. Elsaesser, 'Archives and Archaeologies: The Place of Non-fiction Film in Contemporary Media', in V. Hediger and P. Vonderau (eds), *Films that Work: Industrial Film and the Productivity of Media* (Amsterdam: Amsterdam University Press, 2009), pp. 19–34. For exemplary studies see, T. Lefebvre, *Cinéma et discours hygiéniste (1890–1930)* (Paris: Université Paris III, Thèse UFR Cinéma et audiovisuel, 1996); M. S. Pernick, *The Black Stork: Eugenics and the Death of 'Defective' Babies in American Medicine and Motion Pictures since 1915* (New York: Oxford University Press, 1996); T. Boon, 'Films and the Contestation of Public Health in Interwar Britain' (PhD dissertation, London University, 1999); J. Parascandola, 'VD at the Movies: PHS Films of the 1930s and 1940s', *Public Health Reports*, 111:2 (1996), pp. 173–5. For an unpublished overview: A. Nichtenhauser, *A History of Medical Film*, unpublished manuscript (National Library of Medicine, Nichtenhauser papers, Washington, DC, 1954).

13. Hediger and Vonderau (eds), *Films that Work*; V. Hediger and P. Vonderau (eds), *Filmische Mittel, industrielle Zwecke. Das Werk des Industriefilms* (Berlin: Vorwerk 8 Verlag, 2007); C. R. Acland and H. Wasson (eds), *Useful Cinema* (Durham: Duke University Press, 2011); Y. Zimmermann (ed.), *Schaufester Schweiz: Dokumentarische Gebrauchsfilme 1896–1964* (Zurich: Limmat Verlag, 2011); U. Jung and M. Loiperdinger (eds), *Geschichte des dokumentarischen Films in Deutschland. Band 1: Kaiserreich 1895–1918* (Stuttgart: Reclam Philipp Jun, 2005); K. Kreimeier, A. Ehmann and J. Goergen (eds), *Geschichte des dokumentarischen Films in Deutschland. Band 2: Weimarer Republik 1918–1933* (Stuttgart: Reclam Philipp Jun, 2005).

14. For 'utility' see V. Hediger, '"Dann sind Bilder also *nichts*!" Vorüberlegungen zur Konstitution des Forschungsfelds "Gebrauchsfilm"', *Montage/AV*, 14:2 (2005), pp. 11–22; Y. Zimmermann, '"What Hollywood Is to America, the Corporate Film Is to Switzerland": Remarks on Industrial Film as Utility Film', in Hediger and Vonderau (eds), *Films that Work*, pp. 101–17. For 'ephemeral' see P. Vonderau, 'Vernacular Archiving: An Interview with Rick Prelinger', in Hediger and Vonderau (eds.), *Films that Work*, pp. 51–61; R. Prelinger, *The Field Guide to Sponsored Films* (San Francisco: National Film Preservation Foundation, 2006); Elsaesser, 'Archives and Archaeologies', p. 23. These films are sometimes designated as well as non-theatrical or non-fiction films. See also R. M. Barsam, *Nonfiction Film: A Critical History* (New York: E. P. Dutton, 1973).

15. Many sponsored, or ephemeral, films are also orphan works, since they lack copyright owners and active custodians to guarantee their long-term preservation. See Hediger and Vonderau (eds), *Films that Work* and the earlier differing German version, V. Hediger and P. Vonderau (eds), *Filmische Mittel, industrielle Zwecke. Das Werk des Industriefilms* (Berlin: Vorwerk 8 Verlag, 2007); Kreimeier, Ehmann and Goergen (eds), *Geschichte des dokumentarischen Films*.

16. Hediger, 'Introduction', in *Films that Work*, pp. 9–16. For the figure of 400,000 films for the US see Vonderau, 'Vernacular Archiving', p. 53; J. Goergen, 'Industrie und Werbefilme', in Kreimeier, Ehmann and Goergen (eds), *Geschichte des dokumentarischen Films*, pp. 33–8; J. Goergen, 'In filmo veritas! Inhaltlich vollkommen wahr. Werbefilme und ihre Produzenten', in Kreimeier, Ehmann and Goergen (eds), *Geschichte des dokumentarischen Films*, pp. 348–63. It is estimated as well that one-third to one-half of the films have been lost due to neglect.

17. C. Bonah and A. Laukötter, 'Moving Pictures and Medicine in the First Half of the 20th Century: Some Notes on International Historical Developments and the

Potential of Medical Film Research', *Gesnerus*, 66:1 (2009), pp. 121–46. More generally: A. Nichtenhauser, *A History of Motion Pictures in Medicine* (unpublished book manuscript, *c.*1950), Adolf Nichtenhauser History of Motion Pictures in Medicine Collection, MS C 380, Archives and Modern Manuscripts Program, History of Medicine Division, National Library of Medicine, Bethesda MD. For Shell, see C. Bonah, 'Health Crusades: Environmental Approaches as Public Health Strategies against Infections in Sanitary Propaganda Films, 1930–1960', in V. Berridge and M. Gorsky (eds), *Environment, Health and History* (London: Palgrave Macmillan, 2011), pp. 152–75.

18. For a history of UFA documentary films see H. M. Bock and M. Töteberg (eds), *Das Ufa-Buch. Kunst und Krisen, Stars und Regisseure, Wirtschaft und Politik* (Frankfurt: Zweitausendeins, 1994); K. Kreimeier, *The UFA Story: A History of Germany's Greatest Film Company 1918–1945* (New York: Hill & Wang Publishers, 1996) [K. Kreimeier, *Die UFA-Story. Geschichte eines Filmkonzerns* (Munich-Vienna: Hanser, 1992)]; K. Kreimeier, 'Die Gründung der Ufa-Kulturabteilung', in Kreimeier, Ehmann and Goergen, *Geschichte des dokumentarischen Films*, pp. 70–4. More generally: Bonah and Laukötter, 'Moving Pictures and Medicine'.

19. O. Wagner 'The Cinematograph in the Service of Medical and Biological Research in Medicine in its Chemical Aspects', Reports from the Medico-Chemical Research Laboratories of the IG-Farbenindustrie Aktiengesellschaft (1934), pp. 391–404; Dr Weintraud, Chronologische Darstellung der Entwicklung der Bayer-Filmstelle, unpublished typescript, 46 pp., Bayer Archives Box 92/1/1.

20. M. Loiperdinger, *Julius Pinschewer. Klassiker des Werbefilms* (Berlin: Absolut Medien GmbH, 2010); A. Amsler, *Wer dem Werbefilm verfällt ist verloren für die Welt. Das Werk von Julius Pinschewer 1883–1961* (Zurich: Chronos Verlag, 1997). For further indications see the bibliography in Amsler.

21. For research and educational film elements see U. von Keitz, 'Wissen als Film. Zur Entwicklung des Lehr- und Unterrichtsfilms', in Kreimeier, Ehmann and Goergen (eds), *Geschichte des dokumentarischen Films in Deutschland*, pp. 120–50; T. Boon, *Films of Fact: A History of Science in Documentary Films and Television* (London: Wallflower Press, 2008); D. Orgeron, M. Orgeron and D. Streible (eds), *Learning with the Lights off: Educational Film in the United States* (New York: Oxford University Press, 2012). For product-specific advertising, see Goergen, 'Industrie und Werbefilme', pp. 33–8; Goergen, 'In filmo veritas', pp. 348–63. For a detailed analysis: C. Bonah, 'In the Service of Industry and Human Health: The Bayer Corporation, Industrial Film and Promotional Propaganda, 1934 to 1943', in C. Bonah, D. Cantor and A. Laukötter (eds), *Communicating Good Health* (Rochester: Rochester University Press, forthcoming).

22. S. Legg, 'Shell Film Unit: Twenty-One Years', *Sight and Sound*, 23 (1954), pp. 209–11.

23. M. Fedunkiw, 'Malaria Films: Motion Pictures as Public Health Tool', *American Journal of Public Health*, 93:7 (2003), pp. 1046–57. In her historical analysis of malaria films Fedunkiw draws exclusively from US and British productions. The first Bayer *Malaria* film, coproduced in black and white with sound by the UFA and Bayer, directed by Ulrich Kayser, dates back to 1934 and lasts twenty-four minutes. A second film, *Malaria. Experimentelle Forschung und klinische Ergebnisse*, was presented as produced by Bayer's Scientific-Pharmaceutical Department, by Leverkusen (*c.*1934). It seems to have been the chemical compound–oriented complement to *Malaria* (UFA/Bayer) and a disease and public health–oriented version of the film. See also Bonah, 'Health Crusades', pp. 152–75.

24. For Pinschewer, see Goergen, 'Industrie und Werbefilme', pp. 33–8; Goergen, 'In filmo

veritas', pp. 348–63. For Ruttmann, see J. Goergen, *Walter Ruttmann. Eine Dokumentation. Mit Beiträgen von Paul Falkenberg, William Uricchio, Barry A. Fulks* (Berlin: Freunde der Deutschen Kinemathek, 1989). For Ruttmann's role during the Nazi period see P. Zimmermann and K. Hoffmann (eds), *Geschichte des dokumentarischen Films in Deutschland. Band 3: Drittes Reich 1933–1945* (Stuttgart: Reclam Philipp Jun, 2005).

25. V. Vignaux, *Jean Benoit-Lévy ou le corps comme utopie* (Paris: Association française de recherche sur le cinéma, 2007). D. Cantor, 'Uncertain Enthusiasm: The American Cancer Society, Public Education, and the Problems of the Movie, 1921–1960', *Bulletin of the History of Medicine*, 81:1 (2007), pp. 39–69; D. Cantor, 'Between Movies, Markets, and Medicine: The Eastern Film Corporation, Frank A Tichenor, and Medical and Health Films in the 1920s', in Bonah, Cantor and Laukötter (eds), *Communicating Good Health*.

26. G. Pessis, *Entreprise et Cinéma. Cent ans d'images* (Paris: La Documentation Française, 1997); V. Hediger and P. Vonderau (eds), *Films that Work: Industrial Film and the Productivity of Media* (Amsterdam: Amsterdam University Press, 2009); V. Hediger and P. Vonderau (eds), *Filmische Mittel, industrielle Zwecke. Das Werk des Industriefilms* (Berlin: Vorwerk 8 Verlag, 2007).

27. G. Leblanc, 'L'âge d'or du cinéma médical et l'aventure de *Médecine/Cinéma*. Entretien avec Gérard Leblanc', *Sociétés & Représentations*, 28:2 (2009), pp. 107–18; G. Leblanc, *Quand l'entreprise fait son cinéma: la médiathèque de Rhône-Poulenc (1972–1981)* (Vincennes: Cinéthique Presses Universitaires de Vincennes, 1983).

28. R. Odin (ed.), *L'âge d'or du documentaire. Europe: Années cinquante. France, Allemagne, Espagne, Italie. Tome 1* (Paris: L'Harmattan, 1998).

29. For the film corpus approach, see C. Bonah, D. Cantor and A. Laukötter (eds), *Communicating Good Health* (Rochester: Rochester University Press, forthcoming).

30. For the corporate history of Sandoz, see H. Fritz, *Industrielle Arzneimittelherstellung. Die pharmazeutische Industrie in Basel am Beispiel der Sandoz AG* (Stuttgart: Wissenschaftliche Verlagsgesellschaft 1992); L. Straumann and D. Wildmann, *Schweizer Chemieunternehmen im "Dritten Reich"*, Independent Expert Commission Switzerland – World War 2 (Zurich: Chronos Verlag, 2001), vol. 7; C. Zeller, *Globalisierungsstrategien – Der Weg von Novartis* (Berlin and Heidelberg: Springer Verlag, 2001);T. Studer, 'Die Geschichte der Sandoz im Lichte ihrer Diversifikationen', *Sandoz Bulletin*, 22 (1986), pp. 16–45.

31. Julien Duvivier's major films included, between 1930 and 1960, *La Bandera, Pépé le Moko, Panique, Voici le temps des assassins* and *Marianne de ma jeunesse*. During World War II, unlike most notably Marcel Carné, Duvivier left to work in the United States. He made five films in those years: *Lydia*; two anthology films; *Tales of Manhattan* with stars including Charles Boyer and Rita Hayworth; *Flesh and Fantasy* with Edward G. Robinson, Charles Boyer and Barbara Stanwyck; *The Impostor*, a remake of *Pépé le Moko* with Jean Gabin again; and *Destiny* (1944), a Reginald Le Borg film to which Duvivier contributed without taking any credit. See http://www.imdb.com/name/nm0245213/bio [accessed 2 May 2013].

32. This and the following account are based on an interview with Eric Duvivier by C. Bonah and E. Simon, 29 January 2012, Paris.

33. *Syndrome hébéphréno-catatonique was* produced in 1971 for the Laboratories Lagrange: '*Stéréotypies gestuelles, maniérisme, discordance psychomotrice, désorganisation idéo-verbale, évoluant depuis 2 ans chez un adolescent ayant suivi une scolarité normale jusqu'à la quatrième. 10 minutes*' (Stereotyped gestures, mannerisms, psychomotor discordance,

ideo-verbal disorganization, developing for two years in a teenager who had normal school development until eighth grade. Ten minutes). *État démentiel* was produced for Delagrange in 1971 with the description, 'Femme de 62 ans sans antécédent neuro-psychiatrique. Début de la maladie il y a un an, par des troubles mnésiques et une déso-rientation spatiale. Pas de signes neurologiques en foyer EEG globalement perturbé, gamma-encéphalogramme normal. Maladie d'Alzheimer probable' (Sixty-two-year-old woman with no neuropsychiatric history. Onset of the disease a year ago, with memory and disorientation problems. No neurological signs, EEG disrupted overall, normal gamma brainwave. Probable Alzheimer's disease).

34. Interview with Eric Duvivier by C. Bonah and E. Simon, 29 January 2012, Paris.

35. T. Lefebvre, *La Chair et le Celluloïd. Le cinéma chirurgical du docteur Doyen* (Brionne: Jean Doyen éditeur, 2004). Note that this very first example already held ambiguities and led to disputes over who was the 'author' of a film: the 'directing' physician, Doyen, or Parnaland, the film 'operator', to use the term used during the first decade of moving pictures for the artist/photographer directing the camera. Lefebvre, *Cinéma et discours hygiéniste*.

36. The reference to the theory of a two-step flow of communication propounded by Paul Lazarsfeld and Elihu Katz is anachronistic here but reveals practices existing before they were theorized and turned into a strategic target by the 1960s–70s. Since the 1930s and the 1940s the pharmaceutical industry, in its move to scientific marketing, has targeted 'leading clinicians' as 'opinion leaders' in order to enhance corporate interests indirectly through them. Scientific film marketing has amply employed this method and films have served as an amplifier for leading clinicians' voices and images. No direct reference to the Lazarsfeld–Katz model has been made by film authors, even in the 1960s and 1970s. For the two-step model in the pharmaceutical industry see Ulrike Thoms's paper in this volume.

37. P. Chantelou, 'Comment des cinémathèques scientifiques favorisent un cinéma de créa-tion et comment un réalisateur-créateur leur apporte une conception réaliste du film médical', *Médecine/Cinéma*, 14 (1972), pp. 9–11, on p. 9.

38. The following is based on the ScienceFilm production records deposited at the Centre Régional de l'Image (CRI) Nancy, Fonds Duvivier. For further references to physician gatherings, see P. Chantelou, 'Information "promotionnelle" par le film: Armour Mon-tagu / La folie de Copp et la calcitonine', *Médecine/Cinéma*, 13 (1972), p. 17. For a very critical appraisal of such events see P. Chantelou, 'Le cinéma médical: essai de situation', *Médecine/Cinéma*, 7 (1969), pp. 7–13.

39. Archives CRI Nancy, Fonds Duvivier, Box 176; J. P. Martin, *Henri Michaux* (Paris: Gallimard, 2003); R. Bellour, *Henri Michaux ou une mesure de l'être* (Paris: Gallimard, 1965). For the English title of the film, the translation used here is that of the English-language copy in Archives CRI Nancy, Fonds Duvivier, Box 176.

40. The official and identified version of the film accessible on the online MEDFILM platform or website corresponding to the original version of the film deposited at CRI Nancy is thirty-four minutes long. See http://medfilm.unistra.fr [accessed 5 September 2013].

41. Film script, Archives CRI Nancy, Fonds Duvivier, Box 176, Filmscript, p. 1.

42. Archives CRI Nancy, Fonds Duvivier, Box 176.

43. *Images du monde visionnaire* (dir. E. Duvivier), at 00:08.

44. *Images du monde visionnaire*, at 00:19.

45. See for example the film *L'Ordre* produced for Sandoz and directed by Jean-Daniel

Pollet in 1974, at http://www.youtube.com/watch?v=RIPGsbAUFvM [accessed 5 September 2013]. For patient views in the work of Duvivier, see for example *Le monde du Schizophrène* (1961) at http://medfilm.unistra.fr/wiki/Le_monde_du_schizophr%C3%A8ne_%281961%29 [accessed 5 September 2013]; *Autoportrait d'un schizophrène* (1977), Fonds Eric Duvivier code no. 464, at http://medfilm.unistra.fr/wiki/Autoportrait_d%27un_schizophr%C3%A8ne_%281977%29 [accessed 5 September 2013]; *Phobie d'impulsion* (1967), Fonds Eric Duvivier code no. 172, at http://medfilm.unistra.fr/wiki/Phobie_d%27impulsion_%281967%29 [accessed 5 September 2013]; *Re-née ou le rendez-vous avec le temps* (1993), Fonds Eric Duvivier code no. 536, at http://medfilm.unistra.fr/wiki/Re-n%C3%A9e_ou_le_rendez-vous_avec_le_temps [accessed 5 September 2013]. For details and descriptions of these films see the medical film database MEDFILM at http://medfilm.unistra.fr [accessed 5 September 2013].

46. For a list of films screened in medical professionals' meetings in 1972, for example, see Anon., 'Programmes cinématographiques dans les congrès', *Médecine/Cinéma*, 14 (1972), pp. 12–13.

6 Mazas, Images, Visualization and the Practices of Scientific Marketing in Post-War France

1. P. Herbin, *La publicité pharmaceutique* (Lagny: Éditions de la Gourdine, 1970), p. 63.
2. A. Janser and B. Junod (eds), *Corporate Diversity, Swiss Graphic Design and Advertising by Geigy, 1940–1970* (Zurich: Zürcher Hochschule der Künste, Zürcher Fachhochschule and Lars Müller Publishers, 2009), p. 36.
3. J. Greene, *Prescribing by Numbers: Drugs and the Definition of Disease* (Baltimore, MD: Johns Hopkins University Press, 2007).
4. R. Barthes, *Mythologies* (Paris: Éditions du Seuil, 1957); J. Baudrillard, *Le Système des objets* (Paris: Éditions Gallimard, 1968); J. Baudrillard, *La Société de consommation, ses mythes, ses structures* (Paris: Éditions Denoël, 1970).
5. R. Beasley and M. Danesi, *Persuasive Signs: The Semiotics of Advertising* (Berlin: Walter de Gruyter, 2002), p. 73.
6. M.-E. Chessel, *La publicité en France. Naissance d'une profession (1900–1940)* (Paris: CNRS Éditions, 1998), ch. 1.
7. Chessel, *La publicité en France*, p. 40.
8. Chessel, *La publicité en France*, p. 64.
9. Chessel, *La publicité en France*, p. 214, author's translation.
10. For an example of such reorganization, see the paper by Jean-Paul Gaudillière in this volume.
11. R. Bartels, *The History of Marketing Thought*, 2nd edn (Columbus, OH: Grid Inc., 1976); G. Jones and R. S. Tedlow (eds), *The Rise and Fall of Mass Marketing* (London: Routledge, 1993); R. S. Tedlow, *News and Improved: The Story of Mass Marketing in America* (New York: Basic Books, 1990).
12. J. Greene, *Prescribing by Numbers: Drugs and the Definition of Disease* (Baltimore, MD: Johns Hopkins University Press, 2007).
13. For the use of films in drug advertising see Christian Bonah's contribution in this volume.
14. This corpus is a limited sample of the database established in the framework of the

GEPHAMA research project based on the collection and systematic indexing of all the advertisements published in *Concours Médical* from 1910 to 1970 with a five-year periodicity. On the establishment and general use of this data see the paper by Stefan Felder, Jean-Paul Gaudillière and Ulrike Thoms in this volume.

15. On the general trajectory of marketing at Geigy, see A. Janser and B. Junod (eds), *Corporate Diversity, Swiss Graphic Design and Advertising by Geigy, 1940–1970* (Zurich: Zürcher Hochschule der Künste, Zürcher Fachhochschule and Lars Müller Publishers, 2009); on the differentiation of national markets and publicity material, see the example of Geigy's antidepressants in J.-P. Gaudillière and L. Gerber, 'Marketing Larved Depression: Physicians, Pharmaceutical Firms and the Redefinition of Mood Disorders in the 1960s–1970s' (forthcoming).

16. See Jean-Paul Gaudillière's contribution in this volume.

17. P. Herbin, *La publicité pharmaceutique* (Lagny: Éditions de la Gourdine, 1970), p. 147.

18. J.-P. Gaudillière and V. Hess (eds), *Ways of Regulating Drugs in the 19th and 20th Centuries* (Basingstoke and New York: Palgrave Macmillan, 2012), p. 14.

19. Gaudillière and Hess (eds), *Ways of Regulating Drugs*, p. 14.

20. S. Chauveau, *L'invention pharmaceutique. La pharmacie française entre l'État et la société au XXe siècle* (Paris: Les empêcheurs de penser en rond, 1999), ch. 5.

21. J. Lallement, 'L'industrie pharmaceutique devant la loi' (PhD dissertation, Faculté de Droit de l'Université de Paris, 1944).

22. C. Bonah and J.-P. Gaudillière, 'Faute, accident ou risque iatrogène? La régulation des événements indésirables du médicament à l'aune des affaires Stalinon et Distilbène', *Revue française des affaires sociales*, 3–4 (2007), pp. 123–51.

23. S. Chauveau, 'Le statut légal du médicament en France, XIXe–XXe siècles', in C. Bonah and A. Rasmussen (eds), *Histoire et médicament au XIXe et XXe siècles* (Paris: Éditions Glyphe, 2005), pp. 87–113, on p. 104.

24. O. Diamant-Berger and G. Sabat, G., *Information médicale et publicité pharmaceutique, Réglementation et revue de jurisprudence* (Paris: Masson et Cie, 1974), p. 25.

25. Decree-Law No. 63–253, 14 March 1963.

26. See Stephen Felder, Jean-Paul Gaudillière and Ulrike Thoms in this volume.

27. The first two instances of such manuals were P. Herbin, *Comment concevoir et rédiger votre publicité* (Paris: La Publicité, 1938) and P. Lafont, *La publicité pharmaceutique* (Paris: Librairie des Études de Vente, 1936).

28. See, for instance, R. Labasque, *Introduction à l'étude des cas concrets de publicité, vente, propagande* (Paris: Chez L'auteur, 1959); C.-R. Hass, *La Publicité: théorie, technique et pratique* (Paris: Dunod, 1965).

29. See A. Fourcade, 'Méthode sémiologique appliquée au pré-testing des messages publicitaires', in *Les apports de la sémiotique au marketing et à la publicité: séminaire IREP, 15–16 juin 1976* (Paris: IREP, 1976), pp. 67–83, on p. 78.

30. J.-M. Floch, *Sémiotique, Marketing et communication: Sous les signes, les stratégies* (Paris: Presses Universitaires de France, 1990), p. 106.

31. Floch, *Sémiotique, Marketing et communication*, p. 105.

32. Floch, *Sémiotique, Marketing et communication*, p. 85.

33. Fourcade, 'Méthode sémiologique', p. 80.

34. Floch, *Sémiotique, Marketing et communication*, pp. 84–5.

35. R. Beasley and M. Danesi, *Persuasive Signs: The Semiotics of Advertising* (Berlin: Walter de Gruyter, 2002), p. 50.

36. Floch, *Sémiotique, Marketing et communication*, p. 81.

37. A. Janser and B. Junod (eds), *Corporate Diversity, Swiss Graphic Design and Advertising by Geigy, 1940–1970* (Zurich: Zürcher Hochschule der Künste, Zürcher Fachhochschule and Lars Müller Publishers, 2009), p. 104.

38. J.-P. Gaudillière and L. Gerber, 'Marketing Larved Depression: Physicians, Pharmaceutical Firms and the Redefinition of Mood Disorders in the 1960s–1970s' (forthcoming).

39. Felder, Gaudillière and Thoms in this volume.

40. For a chronology on the use of colours and photographs in *Concours Medical* see Felder, Gaudillière and Thoms in this volume.

41. Regarding the use of cultural codes related to the female body in medical images, see L. Jordanova, *Sexual Visions: Image of Gender in Science and Medicine between the Eighteenth and the Twentieth Centuries* (Madison, WI: University of Wisconsin Press, 1993), ch. 7.

42. Beasley and Danesi, *Persuasive Signs*, p. 39.

43. J. Williamson, *Decoding Advertisements (Ideas in Progress)* (London: Marion Boyars Publishers Ltd, 1994), p. 22.

44. Beasley and Danesi, *Persuasive Signs*, p. 46.

45. About the general use of colours as a mood set, see Hass, *La Publicité*, pp. 110–11.

46. Slogans were widely used for drug advertising throughout the entire century. The difference here is their new relation to laboratory science and clinical research.

47. Organométril visa file, 25 May 1979, Archives of the Commission de contrôle de la publicité.

48. Session report, 24 March 1977, Archives of the Commission de contrôle de la publicité.

49. Herbin, *La publicité*, p. 140.

50. Geigy Archives Basel, Produktwerbung Pharma: Anafranil, Schweiz und Deutschland 1978–1984.

51. Floch, *Sémiotique, Marketing et communication*, p. 83, author's translation.

52. Gaudillière and Gerber, 'Marketing Larved Depression'.

7 Close-Koenig and Thoms, A Balancing Act: Antidiabetic Products and Diabetes Markets in Germany and France

1. In this paper, we use Insulin (uppercase) when it refers to a product commercialized under a trademark, and insulin (lowercase) when referring to the generic substance. On the early history of insulin see amongst others, M. Bliss, *The Discovery of Insulin* (Chicago, IL: Chicago University Press, 1982); P. Dilg, 'Zur Frühgeschichte der industriellen Insulin-Herstellung in Deutschland', *Pharmazie in unserer Zeit*, 30 (2001), pp. 10–15; K. Federlin, *75 Jahre Insulin Hoechst. Vom Naturstoff zum Designerprotein* (Frankfurt: Hoechst, 1999); C. Feudtner, *Bittersweet: Diabetes, Insulin, and the Transformation of Illness* (Chapel Hill, NC: University of North Carolina Press, 2003); C. Sinding, 'L'invention de l'insuline. Entre physiologie, clinique et industrie pharmaceutique', *Médecine/sciences*, 17:11 (2001), pp. 1176–81; C. Sinding, 'Making the Unit of Insulin: Standards, Clinical Work, and Industry, 1920–1925', *Bulletin of the History of Medicine*, 76 (2002), pp. 231–70; C. Sinding, 'The Specificity of Medical Facts: The Case of Diabetology', *Studies in the History and Philosophy of Science, Part C*, 35 (2004), pp. 545–59; U. Thoms, 'The German Pharmaceutical Industry and the Standardization of Insulin before WWII', in A. von Schwerin, H. Stoff and B. Wahrig (eds), *Biologics: A History of Agents Made from Living Organisms in the Twentieth Century* (London:

Pickering & Chatto, 2013).

2. 'Inquiries for supplies', University of Toronto Archives (hereafter UTA), Collection: University of Toronto, Board of Governors, Insulin Committee, A1982–0001/001(01).

3. This is testified by the many newspaper clippings in 'Produkte A-Z: Insulin', Bayer Archive 186/8.

4. M. Mareck, 'Global, Local or Glocal? The Debate Continues', *Research World*, 45 (2014), pp. 26–9.

5. Although in France Albert Calmette initially offered the Institut Pasteur's services for the control of insulin, there are no traces of any activity related to insulin in the Institut Pasteur archives. 'Letter from A. Calmette to the Insulin Committee', 22 October 1923, UTA, Collection: University of Toronto, Board of Governors, Insulin Committee, A1982–2001/062(01); 'Report to the Insulin Committee on F. Lorne Hutchison's Mission to Europe in the Summer of 1924', 14 January 1925, UTA, Collection: University of Toronto, Board of Governors, Insulin Committee, A1982 – 0001/006(01), p.27. For the early history of the German committee, see Thoms, 'The German Pharmaceutical Industry'; F. Umber, 'Werden und Wirken des Deutschen Insulinkomitees', *Deutsche Medizinische Wochenschrift*, 58 (1932), pp. 1150–60. That firms had to pay 5 per cent of sales is mostly forgotten in the discussion on the altruism of the Toronto group. See in contrast the negotiations of Hoffman La Roche with the Toronto Insulin Committee, 'F. Hoffmann-La-Roche & Co, lt. Comp., Chemical Works, Basel, to M. F. Lorne Hutchison, c/o Messrs Thomas Cook & Son, Ludgate Circus, London', 2 September 1924, UTA, Collection: University of Toronto, Board of Governors, Insulin Committee, A1982 – 0001/006(01), A1982–0001/005(11).

6. Thoms, 'The German Pharmaceutical Industry'. For the Canadian and the international perspective, see M. Cassier and C. Sinding, '"Patenting in the Public Interest": Administration of Insulin Patents by the University of Toronto', *History and Technology*, 24 (2008), pp. 153–71; and Sinding, 'Making the Unit of Insulin'.

7. See the introduction of this volume and the paper by Stephan Felder, Jean-Paul Gaudillière and Ulrike Thoms.

8. Antidiabetics are medication and products that help the body to resorb blood sugar and make it available to the body. These numbers are a result of sampling in every seventh issue of the journals of every fifth year (1920, 1925, 1930, etc.).

9. This accounts for all products that were advertised as antidiabetics, including such products as oral insulin. There were a total of 1,042 ads that had diabetes as an indication for the product, including instruments, water and food products marketed for diabetics. These numbers are a result of sampling in every issue of the journals of every fifth year.

10. J.-P. Gaudillière, 'Une marchandise pas comme les autres. Historiographie du médicament et de l'industrie pharmaceutique en France au XXe siècle', in C. Bonah and A. Rasmussen (eds), *Histoire et médicament au XIXe et XXe siècle* (Paris: Glythe, 2005), pp. 115–48.

11. For recent critiques of the cooperation of the pharmaceutical industry and the German Diabetes Association (DDB), see *Transparenzmängel, Korruption und Betrug im deutschen Gesundheitswesen. Kontrolle und Prävention als gesellschaftliche Aufgabe. Grundsatzpapier von Transparency Deutschland. 5. Auflage* (Berlin: Transparency Deutschland, 2008); E. Feyerabend and K. Görlitzer, *Ungleiche Partner. Patientenselbsthilfe und Wirtschaftsunternehmen im Gesundheitssektor* (Ersatzkassen und ihre

Verbände: Siegburg, 2008); M. Zerahn, 'Im Dienst von Schering & Co', *taz*, 15 June 2006, at http://www.taz.de/1/archiv/archiv/?dig=2006/06/15/a0180 [accessed 25 June 2013]; M. Bunjes, 'Pharmaindustrie unterwandert Patienten-Blogs', *Der Blinde Fleck. Initiative Nachrichtenaufklärung*, 23 February 2008, at http://www.derblindefleck.de/index.php/2009/02/23/pharmaindustrie-unterwandert-patienten-blogs/ [accessed 12 July 2012]; M. Mennessier, 'Des associations de malades financées par les labos', *Le Figaro*, 12 October 2012, at http://sante.lefigaro.fr/actualite/2012/10/12/19281-associations-malades-financees-par-labos [accessed 24 June 2013]; A. Bazot, J.-P. Davant and B. Toussaint, 'Patients et firmes pharmaceutiques: halte aux liaisons dangereuses', *Le Monde*, 28 May 2009, at http://www.lemonde.fr/idees/article/2009/05/28/patients-et-firmes-pharmaceutiques-halte-aux-liaisons-dangereuses-par-alain-bazot-jean-pierre-davant-et-bruno-toussaint_1199165_3232.html [accessed 24 June 2013].

12. For a comparison, see P. Herbin, *La publicité pharmaceutique* (Lagny: De la Gourdine, 1970); J. Lallement, 'L'industrie pharmaceutique devant la loi' (PhD dissertation, Faculté de Droit de l'Université de Paris, 1944); H. U. A. Kleist and H. G. Hoffmann, *Heilmittelwerbegesetz, Kommentar zum Gesetz über die Werbung* (Frankfurt: pmi Verlag, 1979).

13. For an analysis see M. Keller, 'Geben und einnehmen', *Die Zeit*, 21, 19 May 2005, at www.zeit.de/2005/21/Pharmafirmen_neu [accessed 10 May 2013]; B. Lerner, 'Ill Patient, Public Activist: Rose Kushner's Attack on Breast Cancer Chemotherapy', *Bulletin of the History of Medicine*, 81 (2007), pp. 224–40.

14. There are remarkable parallels in the history of the German diabetes association and the consumer association, the most obvious of which is their development during the Weimar period. Cornelius Torp has underscored the central significance of the 1930s for the development of the consumer movement: C. Torp, *Konsum und Politik in der Weimarer Republik* (Göttingen: Vandenhoeck & Ruprecht, 2011).

15. For an alternative view of drugs and drug prescriptions, see J. Greene and E. Watkins, *Prescribed: Writing, Filling, Using and Abusing the Prescription in Modern America* (Baltimore, MD: John Hopkins University Press, 2012); U. Thoms, 'The Contraceptive Pill, the Pharmaceutical Industry and Changes in the Patient–Doctor Relationship in Germany', in T. Ortiz et al. (eds), *Gendered Drug Standards from Historical and Socio-Anthropological Perspectives* (Farnham: Ashgate 2013) pp. 153–76; Nils Kessel's contribution to this volume.

16. The Afssaps is the French equivalent of the US Food and Drug Administration (FDA).

17. Although we refer to a semiotic approach to advertising, the limited space here does not allow us to produce an in-depth semiotic analysis of the ads. From the massive body of relevant research, see D. J. Umiker-Sebeok (ed.), *Marketing and Semiotics: New Directions in the Study of Signs for Sale* (Berlin: Mouton de Gruyter, 1987), especially pp. 41 ff.; J. M. Floch, *Semiotics, Marketing and Communication: Beneath the Signs, the Strategies* (Basingstoke: Palgrave Macmillan, 2001); J. Williamson, *Decoding Advertisements: Ideology and Meaning in Advertising* (London: Boyars, 1978); R. Beasley and M. Danesi, *Persuasive Signs: the Semiotics of Advertising* (Berlin: Mouton de Gruyter, 2002).

18. This ad was run a second time, while the third print advertisement for Insulin was published much later, in 1975, in the *Deutsches Medizinisches Wochenblatt*. It was for Insulin by Hoechst, the largest German insulin producer.

19. Advertisement for insulin A. B. Brand with the text 'Proven in diabetes by greatest purity and highest efficiency: "Englisch Insulin A.B. Brand". Cheap prices!' *Deutsches*

Ärzteblatt, 59:23 (1930).

20. It was not common to use the superlative in pharmaceutical advertising at that time; it was rather more typical of quackery. Here its use may be explained by the fact that this was a foreign product.

21. This was due to a change made in America in the standardization methods, which had not been communicated: U. Thoms, 'The German Pharmaceutical Industry and the Standardization of Insulin before WWII', in A. von Schwerin, H. Stoff and B. Wahrig (eds.), *Biologics: A History of Agents Made from Living Organisms in the Twentieth Century* (London: Pickering & Chatto, 2013), pp. 151–72.

22. Other insulin ads, such as one for Insulyl by Dr Roussel, provided the address of a pharmacy that carried it: *Concours Médical* (*CM*), 29 November 1925, p. 2770; *CM*, 28 June 1925, p. 1562.

23. In fact only Hoechst (Frankfurt), Bayer (Elberfeld), C. A. F. Kahlbaum (Berlin), Merck (Darmstadt) and Schering (Berlin) were granted the 'Tested by the German Insulin Committee' label.

24. See 'Hoffmann la Roche's Letter to M. F. Lorne Hutchison', 2 September 1929, UTA, Collection: University of Toronto, Board of Governors, Insulin Committee, A1982–0001/005(11), pp. 68–70.

25. M. Cassier, 'Patents and Public Health in France: Pharmaceutical Patent Law in-the-Making at the Patent Office between the Two World Wars', *History and Technology*, 24 (2008), pp. 135–51.

26. In 1924, the Toronto Insulin Committee was informed that the Société N. V. Organon held the trademark for 'Insulin, Neerlandicum' in France. 'Patents and Trademarks', *c.*1924, 'Patents and Trademarks – List of Countries', UTA, Collection: University of Toronto, Board of Governors, Insulin Committee, A1982–0001/024(05), p. 12; 'Countries in Which the Name "Insulin" Has Already Been Registered so as to Not Infringe on the Insulin Trademark. A Trademark', 1 June 1927, 'Patents and Trademarks – List of Countries', UTA, Collection: University of Toronto, Board of Governors, Insulin Committee, A1982–0001/024(05).

27. See the ad for Insulin Bayer, undated (*c.*1920s), Bayer Archives, 166/08: Insulin. In the case of Hoechst, Insulin occupies most of the space of a 1924 advertisement but is placed amongst four other of the firm's drugs, shown at the corners of the ad. The other drugs were to benefit from the glory of Insulin. See the advertisement for Insulin Hoechst (18 June 1929), and the advertisement for Insulin Hoechst intended for publication in *Therapeutische Berichte* (18 December 1926), Bayer Archives, 166/08: Insulin.

28. See the files Insulin, Nativ-Insulin and Depot Insulin at Bayer Archives, 166/08: Insulin.

29. See Thoms, 'The German Pharmaceutical Industry' and the correspondence of Schering-Kahlbaum in Landesarchiv Berlin A Rep 229, Nr. 263.

30. The production cost of 100 units of insulin thus dropped from 22 Pfennig in 1939 to 17.4 Pfennig in 1941, or by 20 per cent, which did not result in retail price reductions. See 'Bericht der Insulinabteilung über den Monat Januar', 18 February 1942, Landesarchiv Berlin, Rep. B, Nr. 161.

31. *CM*, 12 May 1940, p. 790.

32. On some of the Bayer Archives inserts there are notes stating that 97,000 copies were printed of single inserts. See for example the advertisement for Insulin Hoechst, 21 May 1930, Bayer Archives, 166/08, Insulin.

33. Insert for *Ärztliche Mitteilungen* and *Wirtschaftliche Ärzteblätter*, 21 May 1930, Bayer

Archives, 166/08, Insulin. There are more like this that we will not discuss in depth here as that would go beyond the framework of this contribution.

34. This was the first insert found to be distributed beyond medical doctors. Advertisement 'Bei Diabetes Insulin Hoechst–Sionon', 31 January 1934, Bayer Archives, 166/08: Insulin.

35. See the ad for Insulin Hoechst, 'Garantiert rein und haltbar, genau eingestellt nach der internationalen Einheit, zuverlässig wirksam, unter ständiger klinischer Kontrolle. Neues Indikationsgebiet: Mastkuren bei Tuberkulose' (Guaranteed pure and durable, adjusted exactly to the international standard, reliably effective, under constant clinical monitoring. New indication: fattening cures for tuberculosis). According to a note it was published in *Zeitschrift für Tuberkulose*, a journal specializing in tuberculosis. Bayer Archives, 166/08: Produkte A-Z, Insulin (Werbung). See 'Auszug aus der Niederschrift über die Wissenschaftliche Besprechung vom 15.8.1938', Bayer Archives, 166/08: Insulin; B. Felder, 'Menschenversuche mit Insulin. Die Insulin-Koma-Therapie im Kontext von Eugenik, Euthanasie und wissenschaftlicher Profilierung am Beispiel der klinischen Psychiatrie in den baltischen Staaten der Zwischenkriegszeit 1920–1930', *Gesundheitswesen*, 73 (2011), p. A13; H. Leinfelder, 'Die Geschichte der Insulin- und Cardiazol-Schocktherapie in der Psychiatrie von 1922 bis 1945' (PhD dissertation, Ulm, 2003); T. Walther, *Die Insulin-Koma-Behandlung. Erfindung und Einführung des ersten modernen psychiatrischen Schockverfahrens* (Berlin: Antipsychiatrieverlag, 2000); J. L. Crammer, 'Insulin Coma Therapy for Schizophrenia', *Journal of the Royal Society for Medicine*, 93:6 (2000), pp. 332–3; K. Jones, 'Insulin Coma Therapy in Schizophrenia', *Journal of the Royal Society for Medicine*, 93:6 (2000), pp. 147–9.

36. For example, advertisements for Endopancrine, *CM*, 3, March 1935, p. 644. They, as well as those for Insulyl, further included a long list of indications, which included fattening cures, liver failure, cirrhosis, heart failure, arrhythmia, asystole, menorrhagia, dysmenorrhea, asthma, hives, hyperemesis gravidarum, malnutrition, chronic ulcers, in addition to schizophrenia, in L. Vidal, *Dictionnaire de spécialités pharmaceutiques* (Paris: Office de Vulgarisation Pharmaceutique): (1940), p. 960; (1943), p. 562; (1950), p. 662.

37. A blotting paper advertisement for Insulanol was found in the Archives Roussel (no reference number). See also entries for Insulanol in Vidal, *Dictionnaire de spécialités pharmaceutiques* (1925), p. 213; Vidal, *Dictionnaire de spécialités pharmaceutiques* (1940), p. 956.

38. Glykorator, *Der Diabetiker*, 1, 1951, back cover; Clinitest, *CM*, 14 May 1955, p. 2108, for example is one of the ten ads that year; IniematicStar, *Journal des diabétiques*, ads in all issues in 1960, 1965, 1970.

39. Though German researchers and clinicians had been at the forefront of diabetes research, the standardization of diabetes treatment, and especially of the diabetes diet, took quite a while in Germany. See D. Oyen, E. A. Chantelau and M. Berger, *Zur Geschichte der Diabetesdiät* (Berlin: Springer-Verlag 1985).

40. These were advertised in the French general medical journals *CM* and *PM* and accounted for a surge in advertisements with diabetes as in indication in the 1960s and 1970s.

41. On these problems, see C.-R. Prüll, 'Auf der Suche nach dem "Zucker-Mädchen". Sexualität und Partnerschaft im Journal "Der Diabetiker" (1951–1970)', *Medizinhistorisches Journal*, 47 (2012), pp. 31–60.

42. *Journal des diabétiques*, 39 (1956), p. 12.

43. Ad for Bols Liqueurs, *Der Diabetiker*, 6 (1955), p. 61. In these liqueurs the sugar was replaced by artificial sweeteners, albeit the drinks contained the full amount of alcohol, which would charge the blood glucose balance.

44. M. Hauff, *Neue Selbsthilfebewegung und staatliche Sozialpolitik. Eine analytische Gegenüberstellung* (Wiesbaden: Deutscher Unversitätsverlag 1989); R. Geene et al., 'Entwicklung, Situation und Perspektiven der Selbsthilfeunterstützung in Deutschland', *Bundesgesundheitsblatt*, 52 (2009), pp. 11–20; A. Trojahn, 'Selbsthilfebewegung und Public Health', in T. Schott and C. Hornberg (eds), *Die Gesellschaft und ihre Gesundheit* (Wiesbaden: VS Verlag für Sozialwissenschaften, 2011), pp. 87–104. See also T. Oka and T. Borkaman, 'The History, Concepts and Theories of Self-Help Groups: From an International Perspective', *The Japanese Journal of Occupational Therapy*, 34 (2000), pp. 718–22; A. Mold, 'Patient Groups and the Construction of the Patient-Consumer in Britain: An Historical Overview', *Journal for Social Policy*, 39 (2010), pp. 505–21; M. Akrich, C. Méadel and V. Rabeharisoa, *Se mobiliser pour la santé. Des associations de patients témoignent* (Paris: Les Presses Mines ParisTech, 2009).

45. Jeremy Greene refers to this as a 'paternalistic top-down' group. J. Greene, *Prescribing by Numbers: Drugs and the Definition of Disease* (Baltimore, MD: Johns Hopkins University Press, 2007), p. 87.

46. *WEFRA Heilmittelwerbung*, 7th edn (Frankfurt: Werbegesellschaft Frankfurt, G. Toepfer & Co, 1965), p. 117. The 'diabetesgate' website, for example, initiated by the German Diabetic Association, offers advertising options: the price was EUR 400 to place a note or an ad in the patient section of the website, while only EUR 300 was charged for a note in the medical section, at http://www.diabetesgate.de/mediadaten_aktuell_10_07.pdf [accessed 18 February 2013].

47. For the early history of this association in Germany, see W. Stemmer, 'Deutscher Diabetiker-Bund 1931–1943', *Subkutan*, 20 (1981), pp. S13–17; W. Stemmer, '5 bewegte Jahrzehnte. Ein kritischer Rück- und Ausblick', *Subkutan*, 20 (1981), pp. S24–30; S. Roth, 'Entwicklung und Aufgaben des Deutschen Diabetiker-Bundes' (MD dissertation, Düsseldorf, 1993).

48. Stemmer, 'Deutscher Diabetiker-Bund', p. 15.

49. R. S. Frick, 'Zehn Jahre Deutscher Diabetiker-Bund e.V.', *Der Diabetiker*, 11 (1961), pp. 19–23. The bulletin was renamed *Diabetes-Journal* in 1971.

50. 'Neue Satzungen des DDB', *Der Diabetiker*, 1 (1951), pp. 7–8, on p. 7.

51. For up to 1960, see Frick, 'Zehn Jahre Deutscher Diabetiker-Bund e.V.'; for later years there are no exact figures, only estimates. For these, see Stemmer, '5 bewegte Jahrzehnte', p. 29; Roth, 'Entwicklung und Aufgaben des Deutschen Diabetiker-Bundes', p. 38.

52. In 1958 membership fees only covered 30 per cent of the organization's budget, with 20 per cent coming from the federal government and 50 per cent from other welfare institutions. The federal government supported the DDB with DM 3,000 per year starting in 1951 and from 1954 onwards with DM 5,000 per year, along with another DM 5,000 a year in support of summer camps for diabetic children. R. Krapp, 'Die Jahreshauptversammlung des DDB am 21. Juli 1958', *Der Diabetiker*, 8 (1958), pp. 238–40.

53. H. D. Reichhelm, 'Versammlung des Deutschen Diabetiker-Bundes e.V. in Wuppertal am 26. Juli 1953', *Der Diabetiker*, 3 (1953), pp. 151–3. Unfortunately, the financial reports do not specify the income from these payments.

54. H. D. Engelhardt, *Leitbild Menschenwürde. Wie Selbsthilfeinitiativen den Gesundheits- und Sozialbereich demokratisieren* (Frankfurt: Campus, 2011). It might be argued that

the group was professionalized relatively early and quickly, whereas many other patient self-help groups were set up only after 1980. S. Borelli and R. Bauerdorf, *Medizinische Selbsthilfegruppen in Deutschland* (Cologne: Deutscher Ärzteverlag, 1990), p. 34; B. Borgetto, 'Selbsthilfe im Gesundheitswesen. Stand der Forschung und Forschungs-bedarf', *Bundesgesundheitsblatt–Gesundheitforschung–Gesundheitsschutz*, 45 (2002), pp. 26–32; J. Matzat, 'Zum Stand der Selbsthilfe in Deutschland', in A. Weber (ed.), *Gesundheit–Arbeit–Rehabilitation* (Regensburg: S. Roderer Verlag, 2008), pp. 242–50.

55. 'Extrait des statuts', *Journal des Diabétiques*, 1 (1947), p. 2.

56. 'Extrait des statuts', p. 2.

57. These included: *Memento; Nouveau Memento de Diabète, Le Guide du Diabétique et Le Carnet de Santé* and *Feuilles détachables pour le Manuel*.

58. The annual (one-page) financial reports were published in the April issues of the journal. D. Coppeaux, 'Rapport financier', *Journal des Diabétiques*, 14 (1950), p. 13; G. Piquet, 'Compte rendu financier', *Journal des Diabétiques*, 34 (1955), p. 16; G. Piquet, 'AFD Compte rendu financier', *Journal des Diabétiques*, 50 (1960), p. 14; M. Fombar-let, 'Compte rendu financier pour l'exercice 1964', *Journal de l'AFD*, 74 (1965), p. 15.

59. At this time the German journal appeared monthly with around sixty to seventy pages per issue, but this number varied over time. In the 1960s, it was at about forty per issue.

60. For example, L. Justin-Besacon, 'Les cures thermales chez les diabétiques', *Journal des Diabétiques*, 2 (1947), pp. 4–7; M. Rathery, 'La seringue à insuline', *Journal des Diabé-tiques*, 29 (1954), pp. 19–22.

61. This was calculated in terms of the number of pages the ads occupied, where many were half of quarter of a page.

62. 'Ce Bulletin peut reparaître grâce à l'appui fourni par nos annonces. Elles nous aident ... Pensez à elle ...'. This note appeared in a box occupying one-third of a page in every issue from 1947 to the early 1950s.

63. 'Diabetiker beachten den Anzeigenteil. Seine Informationen sind nicht weniger wichtig wie der Anzeigenteil', *Wir Zuckerkranken*, 1 (1931), p. 24.

64. The statement 'Le laboratoire Choay est heureux de pouvoir aider à la publication de ce journal', was published in nearly every *Journal des Diabétiques* issue from 1950 to 1968.

65. For example: Laboratoires Somedix, 32 rue de l'Ardèche, Paris VIIIe; Thérapeutique hormonale et Opothérapie, 48 rue de la Procession, Paris XVe; Insulines Novo, dis-tributeurs pour la France, Laboratoires du Dr. H. Martinet, 16 rue du Petit-Musc, Paris IVe. These ad spaces devoted to insulin producers ceased to appear in 1968.

66. This was done, however, without the body of information that such literature provided.

67. C. Sinding, 'Les multiples usages de la quantification en médecine: le cas du diabète sucré', in G. Jorland, A. Opinel and G. Weisz (eds), *Body Counts: Medical Quantifica-tion in Historical and Sociological Perspectives* (Montreal and Kingston: McGill-Queens University Press, 2005), pp. 127–44.

68. C. Sinding, 'The Specificity of Medical Facts: The Case of Diabetology', *Studies in the History and Philosophy of Science, Part C*, 35 (2004), pp. 545–59.

69. Insulines Zinc NOVO, *Le diabète* (1955), p. 62, 68, 166; (1960), p. 224. Other uses of the term include Somedia's Dolipol advertising slogan, 'équilibre du diabète': for exam-ple, Dolipol, *Concours Médical* (1955), pp. 35, 52, 1244, 1818, 2102, 4649, 4972; A. Hervouet, *Le diabète, maîtrise, soin et équilibre* (Paris: Maison de la pédagogie, 1994). *Balance* is also the name of the Diabetes UK magazine.

70. C. Sinding, 'Une molécule espion pour les diabétologues. L'innovation en médecine entre science et morale', *Sciences Sociales et Santé*, 18 (2000), pp. 95–120.

71. H. Hauner, 'Diabetesepidemie und Dunkelziffer', in G. Nuber, *Deutscher Gesundheits-bericht Diabetes* (Mainz: Kirchheim, 2011), pp. 8–13, on p. 9.

72. They ultimately had to reduce their prices. 'Bericht des Bundeskartellamtes über seine Tätigkeit in den Jahren 1983/1984 sowie über Lage und Entwicklung auf seinem Aufgabengebiet (§ 50 GWB)', *Plenarprotokolle des Deutschen Bundestages*, 10, Wahlperiode, Drucksache 10/3550, pp. 17–18.

8 Malich, Variation in Drugs and Women: Standardization as a Tool for Scientific Marketing of Oral Contraceptives in France and West Germany (1961–2006)

1.   L. V. Marks, *Sexual Chemistry: A History of the Contraceptive Pill* (New Haven, CT: Yale University Press, 2001), p. 2.

2.   United Nations, Department of Economic and Social Affairs, Population Division 'World Contraceptive Use 2011', at http://www.un.org/esa/population/publications/contraceptive2011/wallchart_front.pdf [accessed 10 February 2014].

3.   H. Cook, *The Long Sexual Revolution: English Women, Sex, and Contraception, 1800–1975* (Oxford: Oxford University Press, 2004); Marks, *Sexual Chemistry*; E. Siegel Watkins, *On the Pill: A Social History of Oral Contraceptives, 1950–1970* (Baltimore, MD: Johns Hopkins University Press, 1998).

4.   R. Dose, *Die Durchsetzung der chemisch-hormonellen Kontrazeption in der Bundesrepublik Deutschland* (Berlin: Wissenschaftszentrum Berlin, 1989); E. M. Silies, *Liebe, Lust und Last: Die Pille als weibliche Generationserfahrung in der Bundesrepublik 1960–1980* (Göttingen: Wallstein Verlag, 2010).

5.   S. Chauveau, 'Les espoirs déçus de la loi Neuwirth', *Clio: Histoire, femmes et sociétés*, 18 (2003), pp. 223–39; X. Gauthier, *Naissance d'une liberté. Contraception, avortement: le grand combat des femmes au XXe siècle* (Paris: Robert Laffont, 2002); L. Toulemon and H. Leridon, 'Vingt années de contraception en France: 1968–1988', *Population*, 4 (1991), pp. 777–812.

6.   C. A. Bayly et al., 'AHR Conversation: On Transnational History', *American Historical Review*, 111:5 (2006), pp. 1441–64.

7.   Marks, *Sexual Chemistry*, pp. 126–37, 216–36; Silies, *Liebe, Lust und Last*, pp. 425–35.

8.   Siegel Watkins, *On the Pill*; Silies, *Liebe, Lust und Last*; K. Theweleit, '"What Did We Do to Our Song, Girl ... (Boy)": Zu Pillen, zur Pille und zu einigen Schicksalen des Sexuellen in Deutschland von 1960 bis heute', in G. Staupe and L. Vieth (eds), *Die Pille: Von der Lust und von der Liebe* (Berlin: Rowohlt, 1998), pp. 21–49.

9.   N. Gane, 'When We Have Never Been Human, What Is to Be Done? Interview with Donna Haraway', *Theory, Culture & Society*, 23:7–8 (2006), pp. 135–58.

10. French: *Comptes Rendus de la Société Française de Gynécologie (CR)*, *Gynécologie pratique (GP)*, *Gynécologie et Ontologie (GO)*, *Gynécologie (G)*, *Journal de gynécologie obstétrique et biologie de la reproduction (JG)* and *Gynécologie obstétrique pratique (GOP)*. German: *Der Gynäkologe (DG)*, published since 1968 and *Geburtshilfe und Frauenheilkunde (GF)*, published since as far back as 1939.

11. Schering AG is designated as the manufacturer of the first European pill in S. Sieg 'Anovlar - die erste europäische Pille, zur Geschichte eines Medikaments', in G. Staupe and L. Vieth (eds), *Die Pille: Von der Lust und von der Liebe* (Berlin: Rowohlt, 1998),

pp 131–44, on p. 131.

12. G. Rose, *Visual Methodologies: An Introduction to Interpreting Visual Materials* (London: Sage, 2012), pp. 1–32.

13. K. Theweleit, '"What Did We Do to Our Song, Girl … (Boy)": Zu Pillen, zur Pille und zu einigen Schickalen des Sexuellen in Deutschland von 1960 bis heute', in G. Staupe and L. Vieth (eds), *Die Pille: Von der Lust und von der Liebe* (Berlin: Rowohlt, 1998), pp. 21–49, on p. 28.

14. E. M. Silies, *Liebe, Lust und Last: Die Pille als weibliche Generationserfahrung in der Bundesrepublik 1960–1980* (Göttingen: Wallstein Verlag, 2010), p. 102.

15. J.-P. Gaudillière and V. Hess (eds), *Ways of Regulating: Therapeutic Agents between Plants, Shops, and Consulting Rooms* (Berlin: Max Planck Institut für Wissenschaftsgeschichte, 2008), pp. 1–15; B. Kirk, *Der Contergan-Fall: Eine unvermeidbare Arzneimittelkatastrophe? Zur Geschichte des Arzneistoffs Thalidomid* (Stuttgart: Wissenschaftliche Verlagsgesellschaft, 1999).

16. Silies, *Liebe, Lust und Last*, p. 8.

17. Silies, *Liebe, Lust und Last*, pp. 156–8.

18. '*Beratung junger Ehepaare*' and '*Beratung junger Mütter*' (Schering's Anovlar, 1964), '*Familienplanung*' (Organon's Lyndiol, 1969) and '*verantwortungsvolle Elternschaft*' (Boehringer's Ovulen, 1968).

19. '*Antikonzeption*' (Eli Lilly's Estirona 21, 1969) or '*Konzeptionsverhütung*' (Schering's Microlut, 1972).

20. S. Chauveau, 'Les espoirs déçus de la loi Neuwirth', *Clio: Histoire, femmes et sociétés*, 18 (2003), pp. 223–39; A. F. Khanine, '1967–1997: les 30 ans de la pilule. Quelles libérations pour les femmes? Interview de Lucien Neuwirth', *Lunes*, 2 (1998), pp. 20–5.

21. Chauveau, 'Les espoirs déçus', p. 237.

22. Gynaecology and obstetrics were fused at the beginning of the nineteenth century in many countries such as Germany, Britain and the USA. In France, however, the field was divided into four different groups in 1949: (1) a combination of obstetrics and gynaecology (OBGYN); (2) surgical gynaecology; (3) obstetrics; and (4) medical gynaecology. The first and fourth group played the leading roles in the debate on contraception. See I. Löwy and G. Weisz, 'French Hormones: Progestins and Therapeutic Variation in France', *Social Science and Medicine*, 60 (2005), pp. 2609–22.

23. X. Gauthier, *Naissance d'une liberté. Contraception, avortement: le grand combat des femmes au XXe siècle* (Paris: Robert Laffont, 2002), pp. 68–88.

24. Löwy and Weisz, 'French Hormones', p. 2615.

25. Chauveau, 'Les espoirs déçus'; L. Toulemon and H. Leridon, 'Vingt années de contraception en France : 1968–1988', *Population*, 4 (1991), pp. 777–812, on p. 785.

26. D. Serfaty, *Contraception* (Issy-les-Moulineaux: Masson, 2007), p. 2; Toulemon and Leridon, 'Vingt années de contraception', p. 785.

27. Similar indications were listed in many countries in the first years after introduction of the pill, for instance in the USA. Watkins, *On the Pill*, p. 37. Nevertheless, French marketing was forced to use this strategy for a longer time and more intensely.

28. *Comptes Rendus de la Societé Française de Gynécologie* (*CR*), 33 (1963), p. 55.

29. The advertisement for Enidrel is for example very similar to the design of other hormonal drugs with related indications but without contraceptive properties, e.g., Progestérone Retard by SEPP.

30. The statue shown in the German ad is the work of the Danish painter and sculptor Kai Nielsen (1882–1925).

31. *Gynécologie pratique* (*GP*), 16 (1965), p. xii.
32. Schering Archives, Bayer AG, 1967.
33. To distinguish them from the very similar appearance of advertising for oral contraception, marketing for hormonal medication without contraceptive effects also used this characteristic sentence by stating explicitly that these products would not stop the ovarian function, e.g., Colpormon, *CR*, 33 (1963), p. 130.
34. According to Gaudillière and Hess, *Ways of Regulating*, pp. 1–15, there are four different ways of regulating drugs: administrative, industrial, public and professional. In the case I am discussing, those that are relevant are the first two.
35. A. Daemmrich, *Pharmacopolitics: Drug Regulation in the United States and Germany* (Chapel Hill, NC: University of North Carolina Press, 2004), pp. 3–5.
36. Watkins, *On the Pill*, pp. 135–6; Silies, *Liebe, Lust und Last*, pp. 105–12.
37. *Journal de gynécologie obstétrique et biologie de la reproduction* (*JG*), 3 (1974), p. xii.
38. C. Gradmann and J. Simon, 'Introduction: Evaluating and Standardizing Therapeutic Agents, 1890–1950', in C. Gradmann and J. Simon (eds), Evaluating and Standardizing Therapeutic Agents, 1890–1950 (Basingstoke and New York: Palgrave Macmillan, 2010), pp. 1–12.
39. Most advertising and marketing theories differentiate two strategies: the 'USP' (unique selling proposition), which identifies the specific and unique qualities of a product, and the 'UAP' (unique advertising proposition). In marketing, the latter is the more important and frequent strategy, since it is brought into play when products are interchangeable. A. Janoschka defines it as follows: 'UAPs are artificially created arguments which are often emotionally loaded'. A. Janoschka, *Web Advertising: New Forms of Communication on the Internet* (Philadelphia, PA: John Benjamins Publishing Company, 2004), p. 16. In the analysed advertising material for hormonal contraceptives, UAP-based argumentation prevails.
40. J.-P. Gaudillière, 'The Visible Industrialist: Standards and the Manufacture of Sex Hormones', in C. Gradmann and J. Simon (eds), *Evaluating and Standardizing Therapeutic Agents, 1890–1950* (Basingstoke and New York: Palgrave Macmillan, 2010), pp. 174–201.
41. L. V. Marks, *Sexual Chemistry: A History of the Contraceptive Pill* (New Haven, CT: Yale University Press, 2001), p. 138; E. Siegel Watkins, *On the Pill: A Social History of Oral Contraceptives, 1950–1970* (Baltimore, MD: Johns Hopkins University Press, 1998), p. 1.
42. J.-P. Gaudillière, 'Introduction: Drug Trajectories', *Studies in History and Philosophy of Biological and Biomedical Sciences*, 36 (2005), pp. 603–11.
43. Gradmann and Simon, 'Introduction: Evaluating and Standardizing'.
44. *Gynécologie et Ontologie* (*GO*), 68 (1969), p. xxiii.
45. For example, Lyndiol 2,5, *Der Gynäkologe* (*DG*), 1 (1968), and Anovlar 21, *Gynécologie pratique* (*GP*), 19 (1968), p. xii.
46. Schering Archives, 1967.
47. Planovin, *DG*, 1 (1968); Stédiril, *Geburtshilfe und Frauenheilkunde* (*GF*), 29 (1969); Lovelle, *DG*, 27 (1994).
48. Marks, *Sexual Chemistry*, pp. 138–82; Siegel Watkins, *On the Pill*, pp. 73–102.
49. For example, Sinovula, *DG*, 7 (1974), p. A13.
50. For example, Lyndiol, *GF*, 32 (1972); Oraconal, *DG*, 7 (1974), pp. 21–2.
51. For example, TriStep, *DG*, 17 (1984), p. A43.
52. *GF*, 32 (1972).

53. Neorlest 21, *DG*, 7 (1974), pp. A10–A11.

54. For example, Ovariostat, *GO*, 68 (1969), p. xxiii.

55. N. Rose, *The Politics of Life Itself: Biomedicine, Power, and Subjectivity in the Twenty-First Century* (Princeton, NJ: Princeton University Press, 2007), p. 10.

56. Marks, *Sexual Chemistry*, pp. 76–7.

57. D. Serfaty, *Contraception* (Issy-les-Moulineaux: Masson, 2007), p. 2. L. Toulemon and H. Leridon, 'Vingt années de contraception en France: 1968–1988', *Population*, 4 (1991), pp. 777–812, on pp. 781–3, describe slightly varying numbers for the year 1988 in a different sample. According to them, 32 per cent of all French women between the ages of eighteen and forty-nine years used oral contraception. The pill was especially preferred by young women, with 50 per cent of twenty-year-old women using it.

58. B. J. Oddens et al., 'Contraception in Germany: A Review', *Advances in Contraception*, 9 (1993), pp. 105–16, on p. 106.

59. *GF*, 29 (1969), pp. viii–ix; *DG*, 7 (1974), p. A53.

60. *DG*, 12 (1979), pp. 34–5.

61. *DG*, 12 (1979), p. A53.

62. *DG*, 7 (1974), p. A17; *Journal de gynécologie obstétrique et biologie de la reproduction* (*JG*), 3 (1974), p. xii.

63. See the Ulrike Thoms's article on innovation in this volume and her paper 'The Contraceptive Pill, the Pharmaceutical Industry and Changes in the Patient–Doctor Relationship in Germany', in T. O. Gómez, M. J. Santesmases, A. Ignaciuk and N. Tschudy (eds), *Gendered Drug Standards from Historical and Socio-Anthropological Perspectives* (Farnham: Ashgate, 2014), pp. 153–76.

64. *DG*, 12 (1979), p. A53.

65. 'Mehr als Aknetherapie' and 'Wechselwirkung Selbstbewusstsein'.

66. *DG*, 27 (1994), p. A40.

67. *Gynécologie obstétrique pratique* (*GOP*), 2 (1989), pp. 7, 9.

68. *DG*, 22 (1989), back cover.

69. 'Typus 2: Sie will, was andere wollen' and 'Typus 3: Eigentlich weiß sie alles besser'.

70. See for example Minesse, *JG*, 28 (1999), back cover.

71. Microgynon, *DG*, 27 (1994).

72. Serfaty, *Contraception*, p. 2.

73. United Nations, 'World Contraceptive Use 2009 and 2011', at http://www.un.org/esa/population/publications/contraceptive2011/wallchart_front.pdf [accessed 10 February 2014]. The study includes only women fifteen to forty-nine years old who are married or living with a partner. Single women are excluded.

74. Oddens et al., 'Contraception in Germany', p. 106.

75. Bundeszentrale für gesundheitliche Aufklärung, 'Pille und Kondom: Bevorzugte Verhütungsmittel', 199, at http://publikationen.sexualaufklaerung.de/index.php?docid=611 [accessed 14 August 2013].

76. Bundeszentrale für gesundheitliche Aufklärung, 'Verhütungsverhalten Erwachsener 2011', at http://www.bzga.de/infomaterialien/sexualaufklaerung/studien/verhuetungsverhalten-erwachsener-2011/?uid=ffbb14a4e7d883b3c6ac01b5b6b0ce10 [accessed 11 March 2014].

77. Silies, *Liebe, Lust und Last*, p. 103.

78. *GF*, 62 (2002); *DG*, 36 (2003).

79. *DG*, 36 (2003).

9 Gaudillière, Marketing Loops: Clinical Research, Consumption of Antidepressants and the Reorganization of Promotion at Geigy in the 1960s and 1970s

1. H. Marks, *The Progress of Experiment: Science and Therapeutic Reform in the United States, 1900–1990* (Cambridge: Cambridge University Press, 2000); I. Löwy, *Between Bench and Bedside: Science, Healing and Interleukine-2 in a Cancer Ward* (Cambridge, MA: Harvard University Press, 1996); P. Keating and A. Cambrosio, *Cancer on Trial: Oncology as a New Style of Practice* (Chicago, IL: University of Chicago Press, 2012).

2. S. Chauveau, *L'invention pharmaceutique. La pharmacie française entre l'État et la société au XXe siècle* (Paris: Les empêcheurs de penser en rond, 1999); V. Quirke, *Collaboration in the Pharmaceutical Industry: Changing Relationships in Britain and France, 1935–1965* (New York: Routledge, 2008); J. Greene, *Prescribing by Numbers: Drugs and the Definition of Disease* (Baltimore, MD: Johns Hopkins University Press, 2007); D. Tobell, *Pills, Power and Policy: The Struggle for Drug Reform in Cold War America and its Consequences* (Berkeley, CA: University of California Press, 2011); D. Carpenter, *Reputation and Power: Organizational Image and Pharmaceutical Regulation at the FDA* (Princeton, NJ: Princeton University Press, 2010); J.-P. Gaudillière and V. Hess (eds), *Ways of Regulating Drugs in the 19th and 20th Centuries* (Basingstoke and New York: Palgrave Macmillan, 2012).

3. The notions of 'use value' and 'exchange value' have long been part of Marxist-inspired political economy and linked to the exploitation of labour and the appropriation of surplus value. Here it is understood in a more anthropological sense, with no specific reference to the labour-related theory of value, as a way of pointing to the two dimensions of creating value for economic goods through market operations.

4. On patents see J.-P. Gaudillière (ed.), *How Pharmaceuticals Became Patentable in the Twentieth Century, History and Technology*, special issue, 24:2 (June 2008).

5. V. Balz, *Zwischen Wirkung und Erfahrung – eine Geschichte der Psychopharmaka*, (Bielefeld: Transcript Verlag, 2010); D. Healy, *The Antidepressant Era* (Cambridge, MA: Harvard University Press, 1997); J. P. Swazey, *Chlorpromazine in Psychiatry: A Study of Therapeutic Innovation* (Cambridge, MA: Massachusetts Institute of Technology Press, 1974).

6. N. Rasmussen, *On Speed: The Many Lives of Amphetamine* (2008; New York: New York University Press, 2009); D. Herzberg, *Happy Pills in America: From Miltown to Prozac* (Baltimore, MD: Johns Hopkins University Press, 2009).

7. Healy, *The Antidepressant Era*; D. Healy, *Let Them Eat Prozac: The Unhealthy Relationship between the Pharmaceutical Industry and Depression* (New York: New York University Press, 2004).

8. *Geigy heute: die jüngste Geschichte, der gegenwärtige Aufbau und die heutige Tätigkeit der J.R. Geigy AG., Basel und der ihr nahestehenden Gesellschaften: Jubiläumsschrift zum 200 jährigen Bestehen des Geigy-Unternehmens 1958* (Basel: Birkhäuser, 1958).

9. One issue underlying the emergence of a system of scientific marketing at Geigy is that the merger with Ciba actually triggered a significant reshaping of activities, including clinical research and marketing. The chapter does not however address the status of marketing at Ciba before the merger nor therefore the resources that it brought into the new entity. This remains to be investigated. For an economic history of the merger see P. Erni, *Die Basler Heirat. Die Geschichte der Fusion Ciba-Geigy* (Zürich: Buchverlag der Neuen Zürcher Zeitung, 1979).

10. A. Janser and B. Junod (eds), *Corporate Diversity, Swiss Graphic Design and Advertising by Geigy, 1940–1970* (Zürich: Zürcher Hochschule der Künste, Zürcher Fachhochschule and Lars Müller Publishers, 2009), pp. 8–28.

11. Between 1959 and 1961, the number of medical representatives in France and West Germany grew from 114 to 166, a 40 per cent increase, which parallels that of the sales force in the United States, where Geigy had established a subsidy. Geigy Pharmaka Jahresbericht 1959 and 1961, PP1 A, Produktion Pharma Geigy Pharmaka, Jahresberichte, Geigy Archiv Basel (hereafter GAB).

12. 'Ärzte Besucher Kontakte und Informationen', Werkezeitung Geigy, March 1968, GAB.

13. Geigy Pharmaka Jahresbericht 1964 and 1965, PP1 A, Produktion Pharma Geigy Pharmaka, Jahresberichte, GAB.

14. See D. Healy, *The Antidepressant Era* (Cambridge, MA: Harvard University Press, 1997), ch. 1.

15. This statement is based on our own comparison of the Tofranil promotion material for France and Switzerland kept under specific labelling in Geigy's archives. See PP 22/6 and PP 22/7 Produktion Pharma, Psychopharmaka, Tofranil, GAB.

16. D. Healy, *The Psychompharmacologists*, 3 vols (London: Chapman & Hall, 1996), vol. 2, ch. 5.

17. This is well reflected in both the resulting research papers. See for example P. Kielholz, F. Labahardt, R. Battegay, W. Rümmele and H. Feer, 'Therapie der Depressionen und der depressiven Krankheitszustände', *Deutsche Medizinische Wochenschrift*, 88 (1963), pp. 1617–24 and their presentation in Geigy's promotional material, which juxtaposed short medical histories of individual patients and tables of qualitatively evaluated efficacy for various types of depression (as in 'La sécurité avec le Tofranil – 3: Comment agit le Tofranil?', brochure, PP 22/6 Produktion Pharma, Psychopharmaka, Tofranil, GAB).

18. 'La sécurité avec le Tofranil – 4: Électrochoc ou Tofranil ?', brochure, PP 22/6 Produktion Pharma, Psychopharmaka, Tofranil, GAB.

19. N. Henckes, 'Narratives of Change and Reform Processes: Global and Local Transactions in French Psychiatric Hospital Reform after the Second World War', *Social Science & Medicine*, 68:3 (2009), pp. 511–18; N. Henckes, 'Un tournant dans les régulations de l'institution psychiatrique: la trajectoire de la réforme des hôpitaux psychiatriques en France de l'avant-guerre aux années 1950', *Genèses*, 76:3 (2010), pp. 76–98.

20. L. Gerber and J.-P. Gaudillière, 'Marketing Masked Depression: Physicians, Pharmaceutical Firms and the 1960s–1970s Redefinition of Mood Disorders', forthcoming.

21. Jahresbericht 1965, Medizinische Abteilung, PP 42, Medizinische Abteilung, Jahresberichte, 1964–1967, GAB.

22. 'Richtlinien für Prüfungsprogramme', Klinische Forschung Medizin II, Oktober 1968, PP 52, GAB Produktion Pharma, Medizinische Abteilung, Planung und Organisation 1969–1971, GAB.

23. See V. Balz, *Zwischen Wirkung und Erfahrung*; J. Angst, R. Battegay and W. Pöldinger, 'Zur Methodik der statistischen Bearbeitung des Therapieverlaufs depressiver Krankheitsbilder', 'Verlaufsprotokolle für elektronische Datenverarbeitung Psychiatrischer Pharmakotherapie Antidepressiva', April 1964, PP 52 Produktion Pharma, Medizinische Abteilung. Planung und Organisation 1969–1971, GAB.

24. M. Worboys, 'The Hamilton Rating Scale for Depression: The Making of a "Gold Standard" and the Unmaking of Chronic Illness, 1960–1980', *Chronic Illness*, 21 November 2012, DOI: 10.1177/1742395312467658, at http://chi.sagepub.com/

content/early/2013/07/12/1742395312467658.full.pdf [accessed 27 August 2013]. See also Lucie Gerber in this volume.

25. R. Oberholzer, 'Organisation der Pharmamarktforschung', 31 August 1966, FB 1–0 Leitung Medizinische Abteilung, GAB.

26. Geigy Pharmaceuticals, 'Review of Psychotherapeutic Marketing for Marketing/Research', 9 October 1968, PP 36 Produktion Pharma, Pharmaforschung Quartalberichte, 1965–1970, GAB.

27. A. Fuchs, 'Der Markt für Psychopharmaka', report to the production department, 3 August 1967, PP 36 Produktion Pharma, Pharmaforschung Quartalberichte, 1965–1970, GAB.

28. P. Erni, *Die Basler Heirat. Die Geschichte der Fusion Ciba-Geigy* (Zürich: Buchverlag der Neuen Zürcher Zeitung, 1979).

29. PH 4.02 Division Pharmaforschung Konzern, Research Conference Basel-U.S.A., 1974, CGAB.

30. PH 4.02 Division Pharmaforschung Konzern, Research Conference Basel-U.S.A., 1973, CGAB.

31. PH 4.02 Division Pharmaforschung Konzern, Research Conference Basel-U.S.A., 1975, CGAB.

32. Produktinformation für das Marketing Ludiomil, Bisherige Ergebnisse in der Schweiz – Supplement zur Marketing Information – Product Management, June 1973, Ciba-Geigy Archives Basel (CGAB)

33. P. Kielholz (ed.), *Depressive Zustände. Erkennung, Bewertung, Behandlung* (Bern, Stuttgart and Vienna: Verlag Hans Huber, 1972), pp. 180–268.

34. O. de S. Pinto, S. P. Afeiche, E. Bartholini and P. Loustalot, 'Internationale Erfahrungen mit Ludiomil', in P. Kielholz (ed.), *Depressive Zustände. Erkennung, Bewertung, Behandlung* (Bern, Stuttgart and Vienna: Verlag Hans Huber, 1972), pp. 254–65.

35. PH 7.04 Division Pharma – Präparate und Information – Produktinformation für das Marketing Ludiomil – Supplement zur Marketing Information – Product Management, April 1973, Ciba-Geigy Archives Basel (CGAB).

36. 'Troubles fonctionnels sans support organique – Dépression larvée? Tofranil Thymoleptique Geigy', PP 22/6 Produktion Pharma, Psychopharmaka, Tofranil, GAB.

37. The remaining flyers are collected in PP 22/6 Produktion Pharma, Psychopharmaka, Tofranil, GAB.

38. One can only speculate about the decision not to pursue the use of 'larved depression' in France. One motive might have been the reluctance of local psychiatrists to grant the category any legitimacy (for a discussion on this, see L. Gerber and J.-P. Gaudillière, 'Marketing Masked Depression: Physicians, Pharmaceutical Firms and the 1960s–1970s Redefinition of Mood Disorders', forthcoming).

39. Anafranil 10 mg, Antidépresseur de pratique courante, PP 22/2 Produktion Pharma – Produktwerbung Anafranil, GAB.

40. J. J. López Ibor, 'Larvierte Depressionen und Depressionsäquivalente', in P. Kielholz (ed.), *Depressive Zustände. Erkennung, Bewertung, Behandlung* (Bern, Stuttgart and Vienna: Verlag Hans Huber, 1972), pp. 38–48. Here larved depression was not a depression proper but an alternative mental process resulting in a fundamental camouflage of the mood disorder.

41. PH 7.04 Division Pharma – Präparate und Information – Produktinformation für das Marketing Ludiomil, July 1974, CGAB.

42. The topic of the meeting was not depression, its treatment or the use of antidepressants

in general practice, but larved depression, its status and specificities.

43. Gerber and Gaudillière, 'Marketing Masked Depression'.

44. J. Angst, 'Die larvierte Depression in transkultureller Sicht', in P. Kielholtz (ed.), *Die larvierte Depression* (Bern: Verlag Hans Huber, 1973), pp. 276–81.

45. P. Kielholtz (ed.), *Die larvierte Depression* (Bern: Verlag Hans Huber, 1973), p. 286.

46. This is a minimum figure as it only refers to the successive printings alluded to in the 'Produktinformation für das Marketing' files.

47. W. Pöldinger, 'Zusammenfassende Darstellung der Fragen und Ergebnisse einer Umfrage bei Algemeinpraktiken und nichtpsychiatrischen Fachärzten in der Bundesrepublik Deutschland, in Berlin, Frankreich, Österreich und der Schweiz', in P Kielholtz (ed.), *Die larvierte Depression*, pp. 123–39.

48. Internationale Produkt Werbung Ludiomil – Schweiz – 1973–1979 – CGAB.

49. Internationale Produkt Werbung Ludiomil.

50. Internationale Produkt Werbung Ludiomil.

51. Internationale Produkt Werbung Ludiomil. See for instance, 'Comment survient et comment s'exprime la dépression masquée?' (How does masked depression occur and how is it expressed?), flyer for the Swiss market, April 1975, Internationale Produkt Werbung Ludiomil. The English translation of the titles of the series mentioned in the text are 'Behind the façade', 'What one is thinking of' and 'Larved depression in routine practice'.

52. PH 4.02 Division Pharmaforschung Konzern, Research Conference Basel-U.S.A., 1979, CGAB.

53. PH 4.02 Division Pharmaforschung Konzern, Research Conference Basel-U.S.A., 1979, CGAB.

54. For a discussion of the specificities of the French case, i.e., the role played by the early rise of ambulatory care as an alternative to asylums and by the psychiatrists' local culture in the rapid and widespread use of antidepressants, see Gerber and Gaudillière, 'Marketing Masked Depression'.

55. N. Kessel and C. Bonah, 'What Was It All About? Reframing Drug Innovation, Sales and Consumption Approaches 1960–1980', communication presented at the conference, 'Is This the End? The Eclipse of the Therapeutic Revolution', September 2012, Zurich, at http://www.academia.edu/3666556/Is_this_the_End_The_eclipse_of_the_therapeutic_revolution [accessed 27 August 2013].

56. See the introductory chapter in J.-P. Gaudillière and V. Hess (eds), *Ways of Regulating Drugs in the 19th and 20th Centuries* (Basingstoke and New York: Palgrave Macmillan, 2012), pp. 1–16.

10 Gerber, Marketing Loops: The Development of Psychopharmacological Screening at Geigy in the 1960s and 1970s

1. 'Proceedings of the Conference on Experimental Neuroses and Allied Problems. Under the Auspices of the Inter-divisional Committee on Borderline Problems of the Life Sciences', National Research Council, 17–18 April 1937, Washington DC, p. 5.

2. J. P. Swazey, *Chlorpromazine in Psychiatry: A Study of Therapeutic Innovation* (Cambridge, MA: Massachusetts Institute of Technology Press, 1974); A. Ehrenberg, *La Fatigue d'être soi. Dépression et société* (Paris: Odile Jacob, 1998); D. Healy, *The Antidepressant Era* (Cambridge, MA: Harvard University Press, 1997); A. Tone, *The Age of*

Anxiety: A History of America's Turbulent Affair with Tranquilizers (New York: Basic Books, 2009).

3. C. Bonah and S. Massat-Bourrat, 'Les "agents thérapeutiques". Paradoxes et ambiguïtés d'une histoire des remèdes aux XIXe et XXe siècles', in C. Bonah and A. Rasmussen (eds), *Histoire et Médicament aux XIXe et XXe siècles* (2005; Paris: Éditions Glyphe, 2008, pp. 23–64, on pp. 45–57.

4. D. Healy, *The Antidepressant Era*, p. 65.

5. D. Healy, *The Antidepressant Era*, pp. 59–68.

6. A. Delini-Stula, 'Animal Models in the Research of Depression and their Experimental Validation' (PhD dissertation, University of Basel, 1998), p. 8.

7. P. Pignarre, *Le grand secret de l'industrie pharmaceutique* (Paris: La Découverte, 2003).

8. N. Rasmussen, *On Speed: The Many Lives of Amphetamine* (2008; New York: New York University Press, 2009), p. 151. J.-P. Gaudillière, 'Hormones: régimes d'innovation et stratégies d'entreprise: les exemples de Schering et Bayer', *Entreprises et Histoire*, 36 (2004), pp. 84–102; J. Lesch, 'Chemistry and Biomedicine in an Industrial Setting: The Invention of the Sulfa Drugs', in S. H. Mauskopf (ed.), *Chemical Sciences in the Modern World* (Philadelphia: University of Pennsylvania Press, 1993), pp. 158–215.

9. J. Greene, *Prescribing by Numbers: Drugs and the Definition of Disease* (Baltimore, MD: Johns Hopkins University Press, 2007).

10. This twofold analytical pathway to document the transformations of marketing practices in the pharmaceutical sector was developed by the GEPHAMA project.

11. W. F. Bynum, '"C'est un malade": Animal Models and Concepts of Human Diseases', *Journal of the History of Medicine and Allied Sciences*, 45:3 (1990), pp. 397–413; I. Löwy, 'The Experimental Body', in R. Cooter and J. Pickstone (eds), *Medicine in the Twentieth Century* (London: Harwood Publishers, 2000), pp. 435–49; I. Löwy and J.-P. Gaudillière, 'Disciplining Cancer: Mice and the Practice of Genetic Purity', in J.-P. Gaudillière and I. Löwy (eds), *The Invisible Industrialist: Manufactures and the Production of Scientific Knowledge* (London: Macmillan, 1998), pp. 209–49; K. Rader, *Making Mice: Standardizing Animals for American Biomedical Research, 1900–1955* (Princeton, NJ: Princeton University Press, 2004); Healy, *The Antidepressant Era*; Ehrenberg, *La Fatigue d'être soi*; Rasmussen, *On Speed*; L. D. Hirschbein, *American Melancholy: Constructions of Depression in the Twentieth Century* (Piscataway NJ: Rutgers University Press, 2009).

12. A. Broadhurst, 'The Discovery of Imipramine from a Personal Point of View', in T. A. Ban, D. Healy and E. Shorter (eds), *The Rise of Psychopharmacology and the Story of CINP* (1998; East Kilbride: CINP, 2010), pp. 69–75, on p. 71.

13. Protokoll der Arbeitsgebiet-Besprechung über Mental Drugs, 5 February 1960, Geigy Archives, Basel (hereafter GAB), PP 130/1, Jahresberichte der Pharmazeutischen Abteilung 1960–1966, Spartenbericht Pharmazeutika 1965 (hereafter JAP), p. 2.

14. Jahresbericht 1955, GAB, WI 40/57, Wissenschaftliche Tätigkeit, Forschung, Berichte der Chemiker, Häfliger, F. D., 1940–1956, on p. 25.

15. R. Domenjoz and W. Theobald, 'Zur Pharmakologie des Tofranil r (N-(3-DIMETHYLAMINOPROPYL)-IMINODIBENZYL-HYDROCHLORID)', *Archives Internationales de Pharmacodynamie et de Thérapie*, 120:3–4 (1959), pp. 450–89, on pp. 450–1; A. Delini-Stula, 'From Animal Experiments to Clinical Dosing: Some Aspects of Preclinical Development of Antidepressants', in S. G. Dahl and L. F. Gram (eds), *Clinical Pharmacology in Psychiatry* (Berlin and Heidelberg: Springer Verlag, 1989), pp. 288–95.

16. I. Löwy, 'The Experimental Body', in R. Cooter and J. Pickstone (eds), *Medicine in the Twentieth Century* (London: Harwood Publishers, 2000), pp. 435–49, on p. 436.

17. For early neurophysiologically oriented investigations on the antidepressant action mechanism of imipramine, see E. B. Sigg, 'Pharmacological Studies with Tofranil', *Canadian Psychiatric Association Journal*, 4, supplement (1959), pp. 75–83; J. Axelrod, L. G. Whitby and G. Hertting, 'Effect of Psychotropic Drugs on the Uptake of 3H-Norepinephrine by Tissues', *Science,* 133:3450 (1961), pp. 383–4, quoted in A. Delini-Stula, 'Animal Models in the Research of Depression and their Experimental Validation' (PhD dissertation, University of Basel, 1998), p. 60.

18. A. Delini-Stula, 'Serendipität oder die Faszination von "Zufällen". Entdeckung der trizyklischen Antidepressiva', *Pharmazie in unserer Zeit*, 37:3 (2008), pp. 194–7, on p. 196.

19. On the engineering processes required when using living organisms to construct experimental research devices, see: R. E. Kohler, *Lords of the Fly: Drosophila Genetics and the Experimental Life* (Chicago, IL: University of Chicago Press, 1994).

20. Domenjoz and Theobald, 'Zur Pharmakologie', p. 485–7; Aktennotiz über eine Besprechung das Sachgebiet Psychopharmaka vom 17 August 1967, 17 August 1967, GAB, PP 38 Produktion Pharmaka Pharma Forschung Zielsetzung Forschungprojekte Stellungsnahmen D–7 1967–1970 (hereafter PP 38), pp. 10–13.

21. A. Delini-Stula, 'Serendipität oder die Faszination von "Zufällen"', p. 196.

22. R. Domenjoz and W. Theobald, 'Zur Pharmakologie des Tofranil r (N-(3-DIMETHYLAMINOPROPYL)-IMINODIBENZYL-HYDROCHLORID)', *Archives Internationales de Pharmacodynamie et de Thérapie*, 120:3–4 (1959), pp. 450–89; E. Costa, S. Garattini and L. Valzelli, 'Interactions between Reserpine, Chlorpromazine and Imipramine', *Experientia*, 16:10 (1960), pp. 461–3.

23. Domenjoz and Theobald, 'Zur Pharmakologie'; Costa, Garattini and Valzelli, 'Interactions between Reserpine, Chlorpromazine and Imipramine', p. 463.

24. Domenjoz and Theobald, 'Zur Pharmakologie', pp. 470–1.

25. While pharmacogenic models were dominant, in the 1960s Geigy's pharmacologists followed multiple leads and methodologies to develop new preclinical test methods. For instance, starting in 1962, the pharmacologist Clara Morpurgo devoted considerable time and efforts to adapt, more or less successfully, operant conditioning methods. For a summary see Anhang zu Quartalsbericht 1965, GAB, WI 40/173, Wissenschaftliche Tätigkeit – Forschung Berichte der Chemiker – Dr. W. Theobald, Pharmakologie Labor, 1961–1964, hereafter, WI 40/173 W.T.W.T, pp. 1–5.

26. E. B. Sigg, L. Gyermek and R. T. Hill, 'Antagonism to Reserpine Induced Depression by Imipramine, Related Psychoactive Drugs, and Some Autonomic Agents', *Psychopharmacologia*, 7:2 (1965), pp. 144–9, on p. 144.

27. E. B. Sigg, 'Pharmacological Studies with Tofranil', *Canadian Psychiatric Association Journal*, 4, supplement (1959), pp. 75–83; A. Delini-Stula, 'Serendipität oder die Faszination von "Zufällen". Entdeckung der trizyklischen Antidepressiva', *Pharmazie in unserer Zeit*, 37:3 (2008), pp. 194–7, on p. 195.

28. A. Delini-Stula, 'Animal Models in the Research of Depression and their Experimental Validation' (PhD dissertation, University of Basel, 1998), pp. 96–104.

29. R. Hazard et al., *Manuel de pharmacologie* (Paris: Masson et Cie, 1969), p. 110.

30. E. D. Freis, 'Mental Depression in Hypertensive Patients Treated for Long Periods with Large Doses of Reserpine', *New England Journal of Medicine*, 251:25 (1954), pp. 1006–8; I. Kass and E. C. Brown, 'Treatment of Hypertensive Patients with Rau-

wolfia Compounds and Reserpine: Depressive and Psychotic Changes', *Journal of the American Medical Association*, 159:16 (1955), pp. 1513–16.

31. A. Delini-Stula, 'Animal Models in the Research of Depression and their Experimental Validation' (PhD dissertation, University of Basel, 1998), p. 79.

32. R. Domenjoz and W. Theobald, 'Zur Pharmakologie des Tofranil r (N-(3-DIMETHYLAMINOPROPYL)-IMINODIBENZYL-HYDROCHLORID)', *Archives Internationales de Pharmacodynamie et de Thérapie*, 120:3–4 (1959), pp. 450–89; S. Garattini, A. Giachetti, L. Pieri and R. Re, 'Antagonists of Reserpine Induced Eyelid Ptosis', *Medicina Experimentalis. International Journal of Experimental Medicine*, 3 (1960), pp. 315–31; F. Sulser, J. Watts and B. B. Brodie, 'On the Mechanism of Antidepressant Action of Imipraminelike Drugs', *Annals of the New York Academy of Sciences*, 96 (1962), pp. 279–88; B. M. Askew, 'A Simple Screening Procedure for Imipramine-like Antidepressant Agents, *Life Sciences*, 10 (1963), pp. 725–30; A. Delini-Stula, 'Animal Models', p. 60.

33. Domenjoz and Theobald, 'Zur Pharmakologie', pp. 474–6.

34. The antagonism of imipramine on palpebral ptosis is not specific to tricyclic antidepressants. Chlorpromazine, even at very high doses, does not, however, counteract this functional disturbance of the autonomic nervous system. G. Halliwell, R. M. Quinton and F. E. Williams, 'A Comparison of Imipramine, Chlorpromazine and Related Drugs in Various Tests Involving Autonomic Functions and Antagonism of Reserpine', *British Journal of Pharmacology and Chemotherapy*, 23 (1964), pp. 330–50, on pp. 338–9.

35. Domenjoz and Theobald, 'Zur Pharmakologie', p. 487.

36. B. B. Brodie, P. Dick, P. Kielholz, W. Pöldinger and W. Theobald, 'Preliminary Pharmacological and Clinical Results with Desmethylimipramine (DMI) G 35020, a Metabolite of Imipramine', *Psychopharmacologia*, 2 (1961), pp. 467–74.

37. B. Hermann, W. Schindler and R. Pulver, 'Papierchromatographischer Nachweis von Stoffwechselprodukten des Tofranils', *Medicina Experimentalis: International Journal of Experimental Medicine*, 1 (1959), pp. 381–5.

38. J. R. Gillette et al., 'Isolation from Rat Brain of a Metabolic Product, Desmethylimipramine, that Mediates the Antidepressant Activity of Imipramine (Tofranil)', *Experientia*, 17 (1961), pp. 417–18.

39. A. Delini-Stula, 'Animal Models', p. 80.

40. 'Aktennotiz über Telefongespräch mit Dr. B. Brodie', 6 July 1961, GAB, PP130/1, Jahresberichte der Pharmazeutischen Abteilung 1960–1968, Spartenbericht Pharmazeutika 1965 (hereafter PP130/1 JPA), p. 1.

41. F. Sulser, M. H. Bickel and B. B. Brodie, 'On Mechanism of the Anti-depressant Action of Imipramine', in W. D. M. Paton (ed.), *Proceedings of the First International Pharmacological Meeting*, 10 vols, vol. 8: *Pharmacological Analysis of Central Nervous Action* (New York: Macmillan, 1962), pp. 123–9, on pp. 123–6.

42. Brodie, Dick, Kielholz, Pöldinger and Theobald, 'Preliminary Pharmacological and Clinical Results', p. 469.

43. Brodie, Dick, Kielholz, Pöldinger and Theobald, 'Preliminary Pharmacological and Clinical Results', p. 472.

44. Protokoll einer Besprechung über Mental Drugs, 8 May 1961, GAB, PP 130/1 JPA, p. 5.

45. Quartalsbericht IV / 1961. 1. Oktober – 31 Dezember, GAB, WI 40/173 WT.W.T, p. 2.

46. Protokoll der Arbeitsgebiet-Besprechung über Mental Drugs vom 5. Februar 1960, 10.00–12h im Sitzungzimmer 62.2.23, 5 February 1960, GAB, PP130/1 JAP, on p. 3.

47. Tofranil, Thymoleptique, Dissipe la dépression, GAB, PP 22/7 Produktion Pharma

Tofranil, p. 25.

48. Tofranil, Thymoleptique, Dissipe la dépression, GAB, PP 22/7 Produktion Pharma Tofranil, p. 25.

49. 2. La sécurité avec le Tofranil, GAB, PP 22/7 Produktion Pharma Tofranil, unpaginated.

50. 2. La sécurité avec le Tofranil, GAB, PP 22/7 Produktion Pharma Tofranil, unpaginated.

51. 1. La sécurité avec le Tofranil, GAB, PP 22/7 Produktion Pharma Tofranil, unpaginated.

52. Amongst others, ambulatory treatment of endogenous depressions was complicated because these syndromes often evolve in a periodic manner. The condition waxes and wanes between asymptomatic periods and acute phases. This relapsing character of severe depressions commanded strict monitoring of the patients. Geigy Pharmaka Jahresberichte – 1961, GAB, PP 130/1 JAP, p. 21; P. Kielholz et al., 'Therapie des Depressionen und der depressiven Krankheitszustände', *Deutsche Medizinische Wochenschrift*, 88:34 (1963), pp. 1617–24.

53. Jahresbericht der Pharmazeutische Abteilung, GAB, PP 130 Geigy Pharmaka, Jahresbericht der Pharmazeutische Abteilung, 1947–69, p. 5.

54. Quartalsbericht IV/1963, 1 Oktober–31 Dezember, Mit Übersicht 1963, GAB, WI 40/173 WT.W.T, p. 12.

55. A. Ehrenberg, *La Fatigue d'être soi. Dépression et société,* (Paris: Odile Jacob, 1998), p. 82.

56. 'Minutes of Discussions on Mental Drugs', 15 August 1962, GAB, PP 130/1 JAP, p. 2; P. Kielholz and W. Pöldinger, 'Die ambulante Behandlung von Depressionen', *Schweizerische Medizinische Wochenschrift*, 94:28 (1964), pp. 981–8.

57. P. Kielholz et al., 'Therapie der Depressionen', pp. 1617–24.

58. Aktennotiz über eine Besprechung das Sachgebiet Psychopharmaka vom 17 August 1967, 17 August 1967, GAB, PP 38, p. 11.

59. Aktennotiz über eine Besprechung das Sachgebiet Psychopharmaka vom 17 August 1967, 17 August 1967, GAB, PP 38, pp. 11–12. Save for the search for stronger sedative effects, Geigy's main goals in searching for new antidepressants after the introduction of imipramine were to find more potent drugs with fewer side effects and a faster onset of action.

60. Aktennotiz über eine Besprechung das Sachgebiet Psychopharmaka vom 17 August 1967, 17 August 1967, GAB, PP 38, p. 13.

61. See, for example, Quartalsbericht IV 1962, 1 Oktober – 31 Dezember. Mit Übersicht 1962, GAB, WI 40/173W.T W.T., p. 9. The archives contain figures enabling quantification of the uses of each preclinical test for each quarter. Nevertheless, it must be stressed that these figures do not allow precise measurement of the proportionate use of each procedure to search for the various classes of drugs, and the narcosis potentiation test was also used in searching for a neuroleptic drug.

62. For a historical account of the development of this experimental procedure, see J. P. Swazey, *Chlorpromazine in Psychiatry: A Study of Therapeutic Innovation* (Cambridge, MA: Massachusetts Institute of Technology Press, 1974), pp. 54–6.

63. R. Hazard et al., *Manuel de pharmacologie* (Paris: Masson et Cie, 1969), p. 76.

64. Substanzen I. Besprechung über Zielsetzung vom 16.8.1968–14:15 –17:45 h, 5 November 1968, GAB, PP 38, p. 6; Aktennotiz über eine Besprechung das Sachgebiet Psychopharmaka vom 17 August 1967, 17 August 1967, GAB, PP 38, p. 13.

65. Quartalsbericht, Department Forschung Pharma, 1/68, GAB, Produktion Pharma – Pharma Forschung Quartalsbericht 1965–1970, hereafter PPFQ, p. 6.
66. Ansprache von Herrn Dr. h.c. W. G. Stoll. Anlaesslich der ordentliche Generalversammlung der J. R. Geigy A. G. Basel, 30 March 1967, GAB, p. 7 (emphasis mine).
67. Betrifft Organisationsplan, 15 July 1961, GAB, Organisations Reglemente der J. R. Geigy A. G. 1964–66.
68. Quartalsbericht II, 1967, 15 July 1967, GAB, PPFQ, p. 5.
69. Quartalsbericht, Department Forschung Pharma 1/68, GAB, PPFQ, p. 9.
70. Aktennotiz über eine Besprechung das Sachgebiet Psychopharmaka vom 17 August 1967, 17 August 1967, GAB, PP 38; 'Review of Psychotherapeutic Market for Research/Marketing Liaison Meeting – 14 October 1968, 9 October, 1968', GAB, PP 38.
71. Aktennotiz über eine Besprechung das Sachgebiet Psychopharmaka vom 17 August 1967, 17 August 1967, GAB, PP 38; 'Review of Psychotherapeutic Market for Research/Marketing Liaison Meeting – 14 October 1968, 9 October, 1968', GAB, PP 38, p. 2.
72. Aktennotiz über eine Besprechung das Sachgebiet Psychopharmaka vom 17 August 1967, 17 August 1967, GAB, PP 38; 'Review of Psychotherapeutic Market for Research/Marketing Liaison Meeting – 14 October 1968, 9 October, 1968', GAB, PP 38, p. 1.
73. Aktennotiz über eine Besprechung das Sachgebiet Psychopharmaka vom 17 August 1967, 17 August 1967, GAB, PP 38; 'Review of Psychotherapeutic Market for Research/Marketing Liaison meeting – 14 October 1968, 9 October, 1968', GAB, PP 38, p. 7.
74. Zentralwirksame Substanzen 1, 5 November 1968, GAB, PP 38, p. 1.
75. Quartalsbericht Department Forschung Pharma 1/68, GAB, PPFQ, p. 9.
76. Der Markt für Psychopharmaka, 3 August 1967, GAB, PP 38, p. 2.
77. Zentralwirksame Substanzen 1, 5 November 1968, GAB, PP 38, pp. 6, 8.
78. Betrifft: Wirkungsbild zentral aktiver Substanzen. Pendenz Chemie und Pharmakologie der Besprechung vom 16.8.68 über Zielsetzung, 'Zentralwirksame Substanzen I', 12 March 1969, GAB, PP 38.
79. A. Delini-Stula, private interview, 13 July 2011, Basel.
80. Betrifft: Wirkungsbild zentral aktiver Substanzen, 12 March 1969, GAB, PP 38, pp. 2–3.
81. R. Hazard et al., *Manuel de pharmacologie* (Paris: Masson et Cie, 1969), p. 74.
82. A. Delini-Stula, 'Animal Models in the Research of Depression and their Experimental Validation' (PhD dissertation, University of Basel, 1998), p. 26. For a historical discussion of the pharmacology of tranquilizer drugs, see C. E. Guise-Richardson, 'Protecting Mental Health in the Age of Anxiety: The Context of Valium's Development, Synthesis, and Discovery in the United States, to 1963' (PhD Dissertation, Iowa State University, 2009), pp. 226–53.
83. Betrifft: Wirkungsbild zentral aktiver Substanzen, 12 March 1969, GAB, PP 38, p. 3.
84. Delini-Stula, 'Animal Models', pp. 24–6.
85. H. Steinberg, J. Knight and A. V. S. de Reuck (eds), *Animal Behaviour and Drug Action* (Boston, MA: Little, Brown and Company, 1964), p. 399.
86. Delini-Stula, 'Animal Models', p. 26.
87. Betrifft: Wirkungsbild zentral aktiver Substanzen, 12 March 1969, GAB, PP 38, p. 2.
88. Betrifft: Wirkungsbild zentral aktiver Substanzen, 12 March 1969, GAB, PP 38, p. 1.
89. Division Pharma Forschung Konzern Research Conference Basel-USA, 1971 I, Ciba-

Geigy Archives, Basel (hereafter CBAG), PH 4.02, p. 31 (emphasis mine).

90. Conclusions, Division Pharma Forschung Konzern, Research Conference Basel-USA, 1976 I, CBAG, PH4.02, p. 1; Second Session, Thursday P.M., Division Pharma Forschung Konzern, Research Conference Basel-USA, 1975 I, CGAB, PH 4.02, p. 1.

91. Stellungnahme der Arbeitsgruppen ZNS, der Ressorts Pharma Chemie und Pharmakologie, zur Zielsetzung in der Bearbeitung von Substanzen mit Wirkung auf das Zentralnervensystems (ZNS), GAB, PP 38, p. 11.

INDEX

advertisements, 9–12, 18–19, 24, 63–9, 71, 74, 78, 84, 105, 108–9, 111–17, 119, 123, 130–1, 134, 136–41, 146–50, 152–3, 155–6, 158, 161–4

advertising, 181 *See also* scientific marketing; *See also* promotion; *See also* publicity, 1–2, 5–8, 10–12, 16, 18–19, 22–3, 26, 30–2, 34, 36–7, 39, 44, 46, 49, 54, 63–71, 75, 77, 79–80, 84, 87–92, 96, 101, 103, 105–6, 108–12, 114–17, 119, 121–2, 130–2, 134–42, 146–9, 152–4, 156, 160, 162–4, 170, 179

    strategy, 23 *See also* promotional strategy

amoxicillin, 46

antibiotics, 9, 31, 43–9, 51–6, 58–62, 111, 129

antidepressant, 13, 93, 119, 121, 169–73, 176, 178, 181, 183, 187, 191, 193, 195–205, 207, 210

antidiabetics, 12, 21, 67, 130–1, 143

anxiety, 80–1, 85, 119, 177, 179, 181, 184, 191, 200–3

anxiolytics, 80

artificial sweetener, 136

barbiturate, 21

Bayer, 4, 19, 29–30, 32, 35, 38, 48, 64, 90–2, 101, 131, 135–7, 189

brand, 10, 31, 48, 71–2, 84, 121, 132, 134, 150, 164, 170

branding, 22, 26, 31, 72, 165

brochure, 201 *See also* flyer; *See also* leaflet, 125, 136, 179, 182

bulletin, 177 *See also* journal, 1, 64–5, 135–43

business, 4–5, 9, 19, 29–32, 34–6, 40–1, 45, 64, 105, 110, 113, 129, 134, 143, 205

capitalism, 4, 163, 168

chemotherapy, 3, 168, 172, 177, 191

chlorpromazine, 13, 99, 171, 178, 191, 204, 207

Choay, 134, 141

chronic disease, 130

clinic, 211 *See also* hospital, 13, 137, 141, 193, 195, 199–200

clinical
    practice, 13, 191
    trials, 4, 6–7, 9, 13, 46, 50, 52–4, 57–61, 88, 116, 122, 156, 167, 173, 176–7, 179–80, 186, 189, 193, 199, 205

colour code, 71, 121–2

colour concept *See* colour code

communication, 2, 6, 9, 32–5, 37–8, 66, 69, 87, 89–90, 101, 109, 118, 124, 130, 137, 142, 154, 165

conflict of interests, 2, 189

consumer, 165 *See also* patient, 12–13, 30, 39, 46, 54, 109, 131, 136, 141, 146, 154–5, 159–64

consumption, 3, 8, 10, 14, 20, 26, 44, 47, 54–5, 57, 78, 80, 111, 124, 126, 131, 164, 167, 175, 187

contraception, 145–50, 152–5, 163–5

contraceptive, 165 *See also* pill, the, 12, 146, 149–50, 152, 154–6, 158, 164

cost, 1, 13, 37, 56, 135, 175, 211

cybernetics, 9, 30, 32, 35–6, 38, 40–2, 109

database, 11, 64–7, 72, 76, 78, 83–5